NEUROSCIENCE RESEARCH PROGRESS

SPATIAL, LONG-AND SHORT-TERM MEMORY

FUNCTIONS, DIFFERENCES AND EFFECTS OF INJURY

NEUROSCIENCE RESEARCH PROGRESS

Additional books in this series can be found on Nova's website
under the Series tab.

Additional e-books in this series can be found on Nova's website
under the e-book tab.

NEUROSCIENCE RESEARCH PROGRESS

SPATIAL, LONG-AND SHORT-TERM MEMORY

FUNCTIONS, DIFFERENCES AND EFFECTS OF INJURY

EDWARD A. THAYER
EDITOR

New York

Library of Congress Cataloging-in-Publication Data

Library of Congress Control Number: 2015955203

ISBN: 978-1-63484-148-1

Published by Nova Science Publishers, Inc. † New York

CONTENTS

PREFACE

Memory is one of the earliest cognitive functions to show decline during aging and some neurodegenerative diseases and this decline has a social and economic impact on individuals, families, the health care system, and society as a whole. This book examines spatial, long-and short term memory loss. The aim of the first chapter is to discuss and detail several well-established spacial-memory behavioral tests, focusing specially on the MWM, describing the principal advantages or disadvantages of these memory tasks. Chapter two examines the importance of the AMPAr and its specific subunits in LTP processes as well as the formation and utilization of spatial memory representations. Chapter three studies grizzly bears and examines their spatial and visual memory. Chapter four introduces a study to show that difficulty encoding relational information between spatial locations presented in random positions simultaneously is responsible for impaired visuospatial working memory. Chapter five describes short and long term memory functions in children with idiopathic epilepsy and assesses a novel cognitive behavioral group intervention aiming to improve memory deficits in this population whose deficits are specified and their background capacities are preserved. Chapter six studies the emergence of self-reference effect in episodic memory during early childhood. Chapter seven analyzes an optical memory model of the human brain. Chapter eight studies an fNIRS study on adaptive memory. The final chapter identifies the synaptic and structural mechanisms that drive plasticity, as well as describes the purported processes responsible for short- and long-term memory.

Chapter 1 – Memory is one of the earliest cognitive functions to show decline during aging and some neurodegenerative diseases and this decline has a social and economic impact on individuals, families, the health care system, and society as a whole. Therefore, scientists have been experimenting to find methods to prevent the memory loss associated with neurodegeneration. The main strategy involved in these experiments is the use of animal models to assess hippocampal-based spatial memory. This kind of memory encodes, stores, recognizes and recalls spatial information about the environment and the agent's orientation within it and it is essential for independence, safety and a good quality of life.

In order to understand the pathophysiology of brain aging and to gain insight into the potential mechanisms underlying spatial memory dysfunctions many rodent behavioral tasks have been specifically designed, including Morris water maze (MWM), radial arm water maze (RAWM), Barnes maze or T-maze. Among them, the most widely employed spatial working memory test is MWM. Theoretically, preclinical rodent cognitive testing would assess identical cognitive domains to those examined through neuropsychological testing in human. However, researchers need to be aware of the advantages as well as of the potential weaknesses of the available behavioral models in terms of their ability to model cognitive changes observed in human.

The aim of this chapter is to discuss and detail several well-established spacial-memory behavioral tests, focusing specially on the MWM, describing the principal advantages or disadvantages of these memory tasks. Moreover it will review the most important studies demonstrating its accuracy and sensitivity to detect spatial memory dysfunction in different animal models of neurodegenerative and neuropsychiatric diseases. It is their hope that this review will assist researchers in selecting an appropriate behavioral paradigm to investigate different aspects of neurodegenerative pathology and disease progression.

Chapter 2 – The ability to acquire and utilize spatial memory representations in the brain is key for successful navigation through novel and familiar environments. This ability is critically dependent on cellular, synaptic and systems mechanisms within medial temporal lobe structures of the mammalian brain. One such structure, the hippocampus, appears to play an important role in integrating relationships amongst stimuli in the environment, forming neural representations of those relationships and utilizing that information to navigate seamlessly through a variety of surroundings. For efficient navigation, synaptic responses within the hippocampus should show potentiated responses when presented with either novel or familiar spatial cues. A key feature underlying this ability, and an important cellular mechanism of memory and spatial memory specifically, is long-term potentiation (LTP). LTP describes a process whereby increases in the strength of synapses lead to highly efficient signal transmission between neurons and through neural networks. The induction of LTP nominally requires the interplay between N-methyl-D-aspartate receptors (NMDAr) and α-amino-3-hydroxy-5-methylisoxazole-4-propionic acid receptors (AMPAr) while the expression of LTP appears to be largely dependent on changes in AMPAr composition. The current chapter examines the importance of the AMPAr and its specific subunits (GluR1 – GluR4) in LTP processes as well as the formation and utilization of spatial memory representations. A summary of *in vitro* work will be provided to examine how different subunit compositions of the AMPAr contribute to the induction and expression of LTP. This will be compared and contrasted with work examining *in vivo* hippocampal AMPAr subunit manipulations and outcomes on spatial behavioral processes.

Chapter 3 – The authors wished to determine the efficacy of cues from different modalities in order to better understand the cues that grizzlies may utilize to recall the location of food. In this study, two captive grizzly bears (*Ursus arctos horribillis*; one male juvenile and one adult female) at the Detroit Zoological Society were tested for the use of spatial memory under two testing conditions; spatial and visual. The female completed only the spatial condition whereas the male completed first visual and then spatial cue testing. The bears were presented with three of six baited sites in their outdoor habitat. In the spatial condition, the same sites were always baited. In the visual condition, differently colored containers varied by location but the same colors consistently predicted food. Neither bear utilized spatial or visual cues in order to reduce time spent foraging at unbaited sites, and no learning was demonstrated across the course of 12 to 36 sessions. The authors conclude that the reduced cost of foraging in captive environments mitigates against motivation to use the most efficient foraging strategies for animals with large home ranges.

Chapter 4 – There have been a substantial number of reports indicating the existence of children who have intact verbally based learning but not visuospatially based learning.

Rourke (1995) and Semrud-Clikeman, Walkowiak, Wilkinson, & Christopher (2010) described these children as having nonverbal learning disabilities (NLD). Normally, they show a large discrepancy between high verbal and lower performance scores on IQ testing, and generally have a pattern of cognitive and emotional impairment coupled with postulated right hemisphere brain dysfunction. Cornoldi et al. (2003) indicated that children with NLD who exhibited low visuospatial intelligence but intact verbal intelligence showed deficits in visual and spatial working memory (more specifically a storage component for visuospatial coded materials in the working memory system called the visuospatial sketchpad, or VSSP). It could be argued that because children with NLD exhibit impaired visuospatial working memory, the cause could be deficits in the memory capacity of VSSP. Specifically, the storage function of VSSP is impaired; therefore, these children perform significantly lower on visuospatial working memory tests than normally developing children. However, one study indicated that impaired visuospatial working memory could not be explained solely by deficits in VSSP, if at all. Mammarella and Pazzaglia (2010) reported that children at risk of NLD show severe impairments in visuospatial working memory tests, and show impairments in perceptual tests in which memory processes are not involved. Because some studies indicate simply perceiving visual features and spatial configurations is impaired in children with NLD, there is the possibility that their impaired performance on visuospatial working memory tests is due to a problem in the encoding phase. However, there have been few studies to investigate the above problem. In this chapter, author's introduce a study conducted by Narimoto, Matsuura, Takezawa, Mitsuhashi, and Hiratani (2013) to show that difficulty encoding relational information between spatial locations presented in random positions simultaneously is responsible for impaired visuospatial working memory. Their results indicated that children with NLD indeed have difficulty in encoding relational information. Specifically, it was hard for children to encode a visual configuration formed by each spatial location. In other words, they seemed to encode each individual absolute position. It is important to understand the causal relationship between the encoding process and visuospatial working memory in order to further provide effective support to children with NLD.

Chapter 5 – Multiple diseases affect memory, but only in a few pathological processes, memory systems are discretely affected, allowing to study short and longterm - resilience and susceptibility of memory systems, in the absence of other background cognitive deficits. Idiopathic epilepsies (IE) are considered to have relatively good prognoses and normal or near normal developmental outcomes. Nevertheless, accumulating studies demonstrate memory and executive functions deficits in this population. The aim of this chapter is to describe in details memory systems in children with IE and to present a new structured cognitive group intervention protocol in children with mild memory deficits.

The intervention program is designed to improve auditory verbal short term and long term memory using strategic abilities in a specific manner. The program is composed of 5 weekly sessions in a group format. 33 children with IE, ages 9-14 years participated in the research protocol and were compared to 27 age and education matched healthy control. Initial results demonstrate that auditory verbal short term memory skills which were frequently deficient at baseline were improved as a result of the intervention. Further analysis indicated that executive functions mediated the intervention effect. The effects were such that participants with higher EF functioning gained less from the intervention and improved their auditory memory less than participants with lower baseline EF. Results suggest that group therapy for children with mild memory impairments such as children with IE may benefit from short term intervention which is specifically tailored to limit the degree of the persistent auditory verbal memory deficits. Based on these results, the chapter presents a theoretical model for memory intervention paths, designed for pediatric populations with mild memory deficits with emphasis on the role of executive functions in short term memory rehabilitation in these patients.

Future studies that will focus on pediatric populations with mild memory deficits and widen the knowledge on executive functions role in memory rehabilitation, utilization of retrieval strategies in memory intervention protocols and methods that help assimilate strategies learned are recommended in addition to examining long term effect and ecology of the model presented.

Chapter 6 – The self-reference effect in memory refers to the finding that performance on tests of episodic memory is better when information is encoded in relation to the self than when it is encoded in relation to another person. There have been many demonstrations of the self-reference effect in adults' memory, but its emergence in children's memory in less well understood. In this chapter the authors report three experiments in which they employed a self-reference paradigm to examine episodic memory in 4- to 6-year-old children. In the encoding phases of the three experiments, the items to be remembered were pictures of familiar objects which were presented along with a photo of the child's own face (self-reference condition) or a photo of another child's face (other-reference condition). In the test phase, memory for the items was assessed using free recall in Experiments 1 and 3, and recognition in Experiment 2. Memory for the encoding context (self versus other) was also assessed in the test phases of the three experiments using a 2-alternative forced choice task. Memory for the encoding context was tested for correctly recalled items in Experiment 1, and for correctly recognised items in Experiment 2. In Experiment 3, it was assessed for all items presented at encoding, irrespective of whether they were correctly recalled. The findings revealed significant self-reference effects on memory for the encoding context in all three experiments. That is, children were more accurate in identifying the encoding contexts in which photos of themselves rather than another child had been presented. The self-reference effect on memory for encoding context did not vary with age, indicating that 4-year-olds benefited as much from self-referent encoding as 5- and 6-year-olds did. The self-reference effect on item memory was not significant in any experiment. That is, children's recall and recognition of items did not differ when the items were encoded in relation to themselves as compared to another child. These findings extend their understanding of memory for encoding context and the role of the self in the development of episodic memory.

Chapter 7 – The authors developed models that can explain the working of the human brain. It is important to identify the source of memory. For example, it could be the distance, size, shape, or absorption capability of the neuron. Moreover, it may be multiple values or a single value memory. Considering the low density of neurons, the type of memory should be a multiple value memory. In their study, the authors employ a multiple value memory, whose source of information is distance. The distance information is defined as the distance between the neurons. Further, it is necessary to know how the brain processes the information stored in memory for thinking functions. The authors classify optical memory as temporary and long-term. The authors assigned long-term memory with the multiple value memory of distance. Fourier transforms are used to convert long-term memory into temporary memory.

The information stored in long-term memory is Fourier transformed into a hologram so that the brain can think associatively. Here, the hologram is a temporary image. The hologram has merit to explain easily the working of associative memory in the human brain. It is shown that the human brain is superior to a semiconductor computer especially in the field of associative memory. Further, a hologram is suitable for associative memory because it can easily recall total information from partial information. Finally, the authors explain the characteristics of the human brain by this model. A neuron can be representative of an image such as that of a grandmother and is therefore called a grandmother neuron. If one neuron represents an image, injury to the brain should destroy the memory of the image; however, it actually does not. The neuron is merely a tentative center to represent the image. The mechanism is as follows. The information is represented as the distance from the tentative center neuron to the other neurons. The memory consists of one center and other columns of redundant information. The center may stay at any position, as long as it is outside the corresponding neurons. If the tentative center is destroyed, another center takes over as an alternative center.

Chapter 8 – In the present study, participants had to rate words for their relevance in an ancestral survival scenario (e.g., is *bottle* relevant in the fictious scenario of being stranded in the grasslands of a foreign land without basic supplies) and for their pleasantness (e.g., is *bottle* a pleasant word?). A distractor task lasting a few minutes followed and the participants were then tested on their recall of the words. The authors used fNIRS to bilaterally monitor the dorsolateral-prefrontal cortex (DLPFC, known to be involved in strategic encoding) during the processing of verbal material in these two deep encoding situations. At the behavioral level, the authors replicated the survival processing advantage in recall rates, with the result that words processed for their survival value were better remembered than words processed for their pleasantness value. Importantly, at the neural level, the authors observed a lesser activation of the DLPFC during verbal encoding in the pleasantness condition compared to the survival condition, thus supporting the hypothesis that the survival processing advantage is underpinned by effortful processes, and more specifically relational processing.

Chapter 9 – The role of neuroplasticity, or the brain's ability to modify neural processes as a result of environmental changes, is crucial to normal memory functioning. Furthermore, this capacity of the central nervous system to adapt is essential for healthy aging and for recovery following trauma or disease states. In this chapter, the authors will identify the synaptic and structural mechanisms that drive plasticity, as well as describe the purported processes responsible for short- and long-term memory. The authors will then review the literature regarding the role of neuroplasticity in the aging brain and in recovery following various types of injury (e.g., traumatic brain injury and stroke). Particular focus will be placed on the implications of lifestyle factors, such as diet, exercise, and environmental enrichment, and formal cognitive training or rehabilitation strategies as potential methods for facilitating neuroplasticity and maintaining healthy memory functioning.

In: Spatial, Long-and Short-Term Memory
Editor: Edward A. Thayer
ISBN: 978-1-63484-148-1

Chapter 1

SPATIAL MEMORY ASSESSMENT: EXPERIMENTAL BEHAVIORAL TASKS IN RODENTS

Maite Solas**, Xabier Bengoetxea, Hilda Ferrero, Irene Muñoz-Cobo, Silvia Vela-Lumbreras, María J. Ramirez and Elena Puerta

Department of Pharmacology and Toxicology,
University of Navarra, Pamplona, Spain
IdiSNA, Navarra Institute for Health
Research, Navarra, Spain

ABSTRACT

Memory is one of the earliest cognitive functions to show decline during aging and some neurodegenerative diseases and this decline has a social and economic impact on individuals, families, the health care system, and society as a whole. Therefore, scientists have been experimenting to find methods to prevent the memory loss associated with neurodegeneration. The main strategy involved in these experiments is the use of animal models to assess hippocampal-based spatial memory. This kind of memory encodes, stores, recognizes and recalls spatial information about the environment and the agent's orientation within it and it is essential for independence, safety and a good quality of life.

In order to understand the pathophysiology of brain aging and to gain insight into the potential mechanisms underlying spatial memory dysfunctions many rodent behavioral tasks have been specifically designed, including Morris water maze (MWM), radial arm water maze (RAWM), Barnes maze or T-maze. Among them, the most widely employed spatial working memory test is MWM. Theoretically, preclinical rodent cognitive testing would assess identical cognitive domains to those examined through neuropsychological testing in human. However, researchers need to be aware of the advantages as well as of the potential weaknesses of the available behavioral models in terms of their ability to model cognitive changes observed in human.

* Corresponding author: Dr. Maite Solas. Department of Pharmacology and Toxicology, University of Navarra, C/ Irunlarrea, 1, 31008 Pamplona, Spain. Tel: +34 948425600 - ext: 806648, fax: +34 948425649, e-mail: msolaszu@unav.es.

The aim of this chapter is to discuss and detail several well-established spacial-memory behavioral tests, focusing specially on the MWM, describing the principal advantages or disadvantages of these memory tasks. Moreover it will review the most important studies demonstrating its accuracy and sensitivity to detect spatial memory dysfunction in different animal models of neurodegenerative and neuropsychiatric diseases. It is our hope that this review will assist researchers in selecting an appropriate behavioral paradigm to investigate different aspects of neurodegenerative pathology and disease progression.

1. INTRODUCTION

Over the last decades, the demographic transition has produced vast reductions in human mortality rates and roughly a doubling in the average length of life among advanced countries [1]. The size of the population aged 75 years and older is projected to grow to more than double in the next 20 years [2, 3] and a number of European countries such as Germany, Italy, Spain, Sweden, Greece, Austria and Japan are on the verge of serious social and economic problems due to historically unprecedented increases in their elderly demographics [4, 5].

This increase in life span reflects better health care, however, given that aging *per se* is one of the serious risk factors for many chronic, costly diseases such as cancer, Alzheimer's disease (AD), and type 2 diabetes, it also puts a pressure on governmental budgets on health and long-term care. Therefore, it is critical to better understand the fundamental mechanisms of aging and longevity and develop effective, affordable, anti-aging interventions to prevent those expensive diseases of aging.

1.1. Types of Memory

One of the most significant problems people deal with, as they get older is a decrease in memory function [6]. Memory can be defined as "the process by which experience-based information is encoded, stored and finally retrieved." The duration that a memory is stored is used to differentiate between short-term and long-term memory (Figure 1).

Short-term memory has a limited capacity and has a short-term temporal decay, usually defined between several seconds and one minute [7]. Often, short-term memory is confused with working memory, although the two concepts are generally believed to be distinct.

Working memory is a term that was used to refer to the type of memory that it is being used to plan and carry out behavior. Specifically, working memory is considered a cognitive process that includes attention, short-term memory and information processing [8]. Information stored in short-term memory can be transferred into long-term memory by a process called consolidation [9]. Contrary to short-term memory, long-term memory can store unlimited amounts of information for potentially unlimited duration [10]. Long-term memory is divided into non-declarative (or implicit) and declarative (or explicit) memory [11].

Non-declarative memory is the acquisition of motor skills and habits, for instance, procedural memories required for the execution of integrated procedures e.g., typing on the computer keyboard or riding a bicycle. It answers the question "how" and is mainly mediated by neostriatum and cerebellum [12-14].

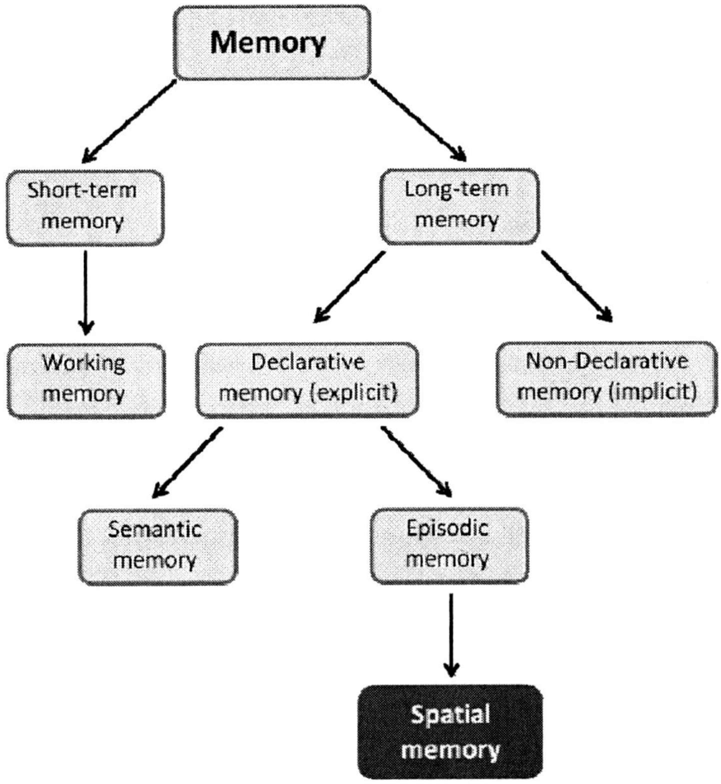

Figure 1. Types of memory.

Declarative memory, in contrast, answers the question "what." It is consciously activated and includes the knowledge or recollection of facts (places, things, people...) and the meaning of these facts. Declarative memory is further subdivided into semantic and episodic memories. Semantic memories store general factual knowledge independent of personal experience or the context in which they were learned [15, 16]. In contrast, episodic memories are recollections of personal experiences. Typically, spatial memory is conceptualized as a subtype of episodic memory because it stores information within the spatio-temporal frame [17]. It encompasses knowledge of location within an environmental context. Animal models of cognitive senescence confirm that spatial memory is enormously sensitive to age as it appears to be one of the earliest cognitive functions to decline [18-24]. In agreement with that observed in animal models, cognitive deficits are prominent when older human adults are tested for spatial memory [25-29]. The early onset and distinctive nature of cognitive decline, specific to spatial memory, suggests that specific neural systems involved in spatial navigation are exceptionally susceptible to aging.

1.2. Anatomical Substrate for Spatial Memory

The anatomical substrates for episodic and spatial memory are similar in animal models and humans. During the past decades strong evidence has emerged showing that the hippocampus plays a critical role in spatial memory [30-33].

Numerous studies have concluded that damage to the hippocampus results in impaired spatial memory in rodents [34-36], non-human primates [37-39], and humans [40-42]. Indeed, the progressive decline in memory during aging is associated with a decrease in hippocampal volume in humans [43-48], non-human primates [49], and rodents [22].

1.3. Spatial Memory Assessment

Impaired spatial ability can have a great impact on the quality of life with advancing age, since the capacity to acquire and recall the spatial features of a novel location is critical for adaptation to the environment and the ability to live independently. The rapidly growing population makes critical to develop new strategies to treat and prevent cognitive aging.

Cognitive aging can be studied in both human subjects and animal models. Without doubt, the best approach for cognitive aging studies is research with human populations. However, human studies have important constraints, particularly the limited ability to test hypotheses regarding neural substrates of age-related cognitive decline through experimental manipulations. Animal models are much better suited for these experiments, since they allow for neuropathological examination at different time points and for experimental manipulations that are not possible in human subjects. In this regard, scientists are utilizing animals to understand the pathophysiology of brain aging with the hope of finding ways to prevent or hopefully reverse memory loss.

Theoretically, preclinical rodent cognitive testing would assess identical cognitive domains to those examined through neuropsychological testing in human. Indeed, many rodent behavioral tasks have been specifically designed with this in mind. In the present chapter the main well-established spatial-memory behavioral tests will be described: T-Y maze, radial arm maze (RAM), Barnes maze and Morris water maze (MWM).

While the availability of tests for spatial memory in animal models poses tremendous opportunities, there are a variety of challenges and influencing factors to these studies that should be taken into account. In particular, there are many external variables that affect performance on these tests and must be carefully controlled to generate reliable and reproducible data.

One of those variables is the effect of diurnal variation and timing. By default, many investigators who study nocturnal rodents use a standard light dark cycle (LD) in synchrony with work schedules (12 h light starting around 6 am and 12 h dark starting around 6 pm).

Because rodents are in the inactive phase of their circadian rhythm during the daylight hours, some behavioral assays are better administered during the dark phase of the cycle [50].

To solve this problem inverted light cycles can be used, allowing the performance of nocturnal experiments during normal working hours. However, careful attention must be paid to maintaining darkness during dark cycle experiments to avoid disruption of the circadian rhythms with downstream effects on many neurophysiological parameters [51].

Another influential factor is the effect of pre-handling and test order. On some tests, naïve rodents behave differently than rodents that have been handled or have previously undergone other behavioral assays [52, 53]. Thus, protocols for pre-handling before testing and standardization of test order become important. The goal of animal pre-handling is to acclimatize the animals to being picked up, restrained, and placed in position.

Effects of single vs group housing is also an important factor. Rodents are social animals and the degree of social interactions can have a profound effect on cognitive parameters. For example, animals socially isolated after weaning can perform better in the MWM [54]. Therefore, the degree and timing of social isolation (single housing) should be clearly indicated.

Effects of housing conditions can be also crucial. Difficult to control issues such as noise levels and building vibrations can contribute to chronic stress and affect both the aging process and learning and memory. Controllable factors include frequency of cage changes, animal and cage density, chow, light cycle, and the use of ventilated cages.

Rodent experiments can be performed on different inbred and outbred background strains, which can vary considerably in their abilities on cognitive tasks [55] and therefore, effects of background strain is also an important variable when performing behavioral tasks.

This emphasizes the importance of a consistent genetic background. An important issue for cognitive studies is the identification of any sensory abnormalities (e.g., hearing or visual impairment) that might impair task performance independent of cognitive ability.

The animal species used is also essential, as cognitive aspects displayed in each task by different species do not need to be similar. In fact, memory tasks such as the MWM show consistent differences in the procedure protocol when applied to mice or rats. In this task, compared to rats, mice show lower learning capacity; therefore, mice MWM protocol is longer than rat protocol (10 days vs 5 days).

In addition to these general considerations, most tasks have specific aspects of the protocol that can affect results significantly, such as the number and spacing of trials. Therefore, key parameters for each task should be carefully analyzed when generating reliable data.

Finally, it is important to point out that in some cases, it can be challenging to relate certain findings in animal models to human disease. Obviously, these interpretive challenges are greater with tasks that have less relation to those used with human subjects.

2. T-Maze and Y-Maze

The T- and Y- mazes are simple behavioral paradigms based on the principle of natural alternation in rodents. The principle of alternation is based on the fact that the animal under observation will prefer to visit the less recently visited arm, thus implicating that it will need to recall which was the last arm visited [56].

The mazes are composed of three arms connected to form a T (with one central arm and two opposite arms) or a Y with an angle of 120° between two adjacent arms. In the case of the Y maze, the three arms have the same size, whereas in the case of the T maze, the central arm can be shorter or longer than the two opposite arms that have the same size (Figure 2a and 2b) [10].

The maze can be made from grey or black painted wood, medium-density fiberboard or a plastic such as PVC. The reason for painting the maze grey or black is that rodents avoid bright places, such as white painted floors. A white maze would provoke anxiety and habituation would be slower [57].

2.1. Experimental Design

Originally, the spontaneous alternation test was designed with the T maze. In the T maze, animals are placed at the dead-end of the central arm and can freely enter either the left or the right arm. Once the animal enters one of the two opposite arms, the animal is removed and placed once again at the starting position at the end of the central arm, whence it can start the next trial during which working memory is tested.

Based on the principle that animals would spontaneously visit unfamiliar places, they are expected to alternate. Because functional working memory is required to remember the arm that was last visited and thereby to alternate, an alternation is considered a correct choice, whereas a re-entry into a previously visited arm is counted as an error (Figure 2d). Because animals have a binary choice, values that are not higher than the chance level of 50% are interpreted as an indication of impaired working memory.

One of the main disadvantages of this task relies on the anxiety and stress caused by the constant handling of the animal. For this reason, the continuous spontaneous alternation test in the Y maze was proposed as an alternative paradigm in which animals freely move without being handled between trials. In this test animals are placed in the center of the Y maze and left to move until they perform a fixed number of transitions between arms. The parameters used to calculate working memory is the ratio (or percentage) of alternations among the total number of transitions. For instance, if we name the three arms A, B and C, an animal making a transition between arm A and B would be carrying out an alternation if it then entered arm C, whereas an entry into A is considered as an error. A limitation of the Y maze is that the inter-trial interval cannot be controlled, as animals freely decide when to make a transition. For this reason, the average time required to perform one transition is calculated by dividing the time to complete one session by the number of total transitions. Contrary to the Y maze, the inter-trial interval in the T maze test is defined by the experimenter by controlling the time between the end of one trial and the start of the next trial at which time-point the animals are placed once again in the starting arm. In this way, working memory can be challenged by increasing the inter-trial intervals (e.g., 5, 15, 30, or 60 s) [58]. To combine the advantages of the spontaneous alternation in the T maze (i.e., the control of the inter-trial interval) and Y maze (i.e., no handling and thereby reduced stress for the animals), a modified T maze test for the mouse that allows continuous spontaneous alternation has been proposed. In this case, sliding doors are placed at the entrance of the opposing arms and proximal to the dead-end of the central arm (Figure 2c). A session is started by placing a mouse at the dead-end of the central arm with the door closed. After 5 s, the door is opened and the mouse is allowed freely to enter one of the two opposing arms. Once the mouse has entered one arm, access to the opposite one is occluded by the sliding door and the mouse can only return into the dead-end of the central arm in which it is confined for a given period before starting the next trial. With this protocol, mice are not handled between trials but the inter-trial interval is defined by the duration that mice are confined at the starting position in the central arm between trials [10]. A general limitation of the spontaneous alternation test is that the performance is not only affected by working memory function but also by novelty seeking and the exploratory behavior of the animals. This problem can be solved by using the win-shift paradigm. In the T maze, mice must follow a win-shift criterion ("if you win, then shift") in order to get a reward (usually food) that is located in one dispenser at the end of the arm opposite to the arm in which it was previously found.

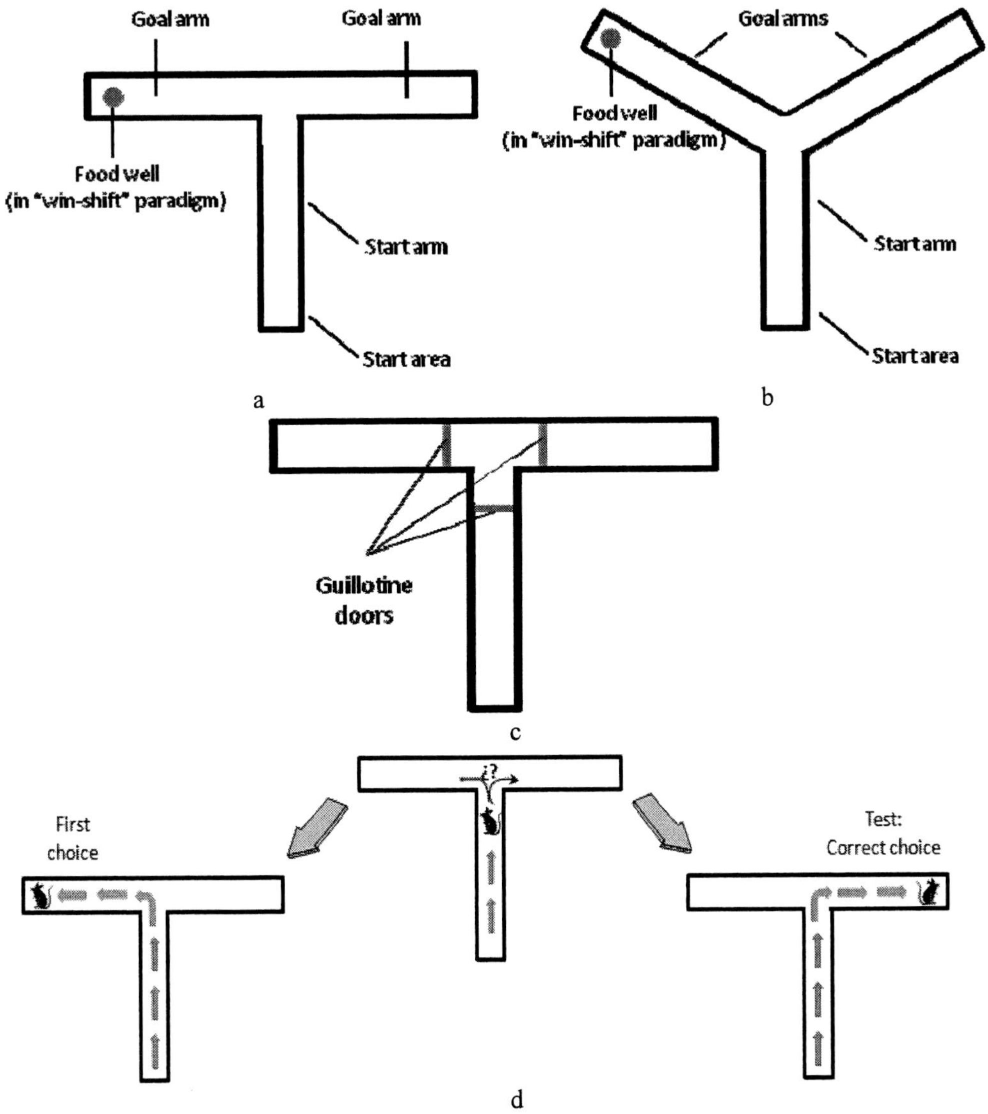

Figure 2. Experimental set-up of a) T-maze b) Y-maze and c) modified T-maze. In d) experimental design of T-maze: Once the animal enters one of the two opposite arms, the animal is removed and placed once again at the starting position at the end of the central arm, whence it can start the next trial during which working memory is tested. An alternation is considered a correct choice, whereas a re-entry into a previously visited arm is counted as an error.

In principle, the test runs similarly to the spontaneous alternation in the T maze, with the only difference being that an alternation is rewarded by food placed in dispensers at the end of the left and right arms. One limitation of the win-shift paradigm is that the performance is influenced by the motivation to obtain the food reward, so that animals are generally food-deprived to a level maintaining 80%-90% of their body weight under ad libitum feeding [59]. Recently, an aquatic version of the T-maze has been adapted and utilized.

Mice are required to locate the hidden platform beneath the water in one of the arms thus utilizing natural tendency of mice to escape to a safer place [60-62].

2.2. Brain Areas Involved

Alternation is very sensitive to dysfunction of the hippocampus, but other brain structures are also involved. It has been consistently demonstrated that, by comparison to sham-operated controls, spontaneous alternation rates in the T-maze procedure, decrease in rats with surgically-induced lesions of the hippocampus. For example, hippocampectomized animals notoriously adopt side preferences, e.g., always turning right on a T-maze [57]. In addition to the hippocampus, spontaneous T-maze alternation rates have consistently been shown to be decreased in rats with septal lesions. This supports the hypothesis that spontaneous alternation is dependent on a septo-hippocampal system [63-65]. Impairment in spontaneous alternation was also observed after lesions of the anterior thalamus in mice [66] and the medial part of the dorsal striatum in rats [67]. Another thalamic nucleus associated with alternation behaviors is the dorsomedial region [68]. Moreover, the influence of the prefrontal cortex in alternation behaviors has been demonstrated in rats and monkeys [67]. In addition, alternation rates were reduced in mutant mice with vestibular damage or medial raphe lesions [69, 70]. Finally, due to its well-recognized role in motor coordination, the cerebellum influences spatially oriented behaviors, as shown by the reduced spontaneous alternation rates in the forced-trial procedure by several mutant mice with cerebellar atrophy [71-74].

2.3. Limitations

T-mazes, and their variants Y-mazes, present the advantage of being simple devices useful for the assessment of spatial working memory, and also providing highly reproducible results. As a bonus, they do not require automated video-recording systems [75]. In contrast, the major disadvantage is that it has a single choice point with only two alternatives, which increases the possibilities of success (by default the probability of choosing the correct arm is 50%) or that the rodent may use a strategy other than spatial to solve the maze. Depriving the animal of food can be also a potential problem. Another disadvantage with using the T-maze is that it requires constant handling of animals, which may induce stress and affect the test result. However, habituating the animal and handling by the same experimenter reduce this stress [60]. Indeed, because of its simplicity of construction and use, combined with its sensitivity, T-maze alternation has almost universal applicability in detecting cognitive dysfunction. Moreover, alternation, whether rewarded or spontaneous, is very sensitive at detecting hippocampal dysfunction [57].

3. Radial Arm Maze

The radial arm maze (RAM) was developed by Olton and Samuelson in 1976 [76], and was originally designed to evaluate spatial working memory in rats.

The classic maze is comprised of eight equidistantly spaced arms radiating from a small circular central platform above the floor (Figure 3). The maze typically is made of wood and it has no cover or may have a clear acrylic cover. Traditionally, the most extensively studied species in the RAM are rodents. However, RAM has also demonstrated its validity across other species like pigeons, tortoises, dogs or even in humans [77]. The RAM has also been used to study age-related cognitive decline as well as gender differences in learning behavior in various mouse model [60, 78].

RAM is based on the idea that food-deprived animals (maintained at 85%–90% of body weight under ad libitum feeding conditions) use the distal cues to identify the arm that must be visited in order to receive the reward. At the end of each arm, a reward (food or water) can be available in a cup that hides it from sight. For RAM, two different versions have been described (Figure 3).

3.1. Experimental Design

In the most classic version task, all of maze arms are baited (Figure 3a). An animal is placed in the centre platform and is allowed to visit each arm until all the rewards have been collected. The optimum strategy for obtaining all the rewards in the least amount of time implies visit each arm only once during a trial. The index used for the analysis of memory is the number of re-entries into a previously visited arm that now is empty. This original version of RAM tests working memory and, more specially, spatial working memory because the principal cues to guide arm choice are visual cues. The location of reward is matched to a particular external cue so the animals use the information provided by the surrounding environment to recognize the arms previously visited.

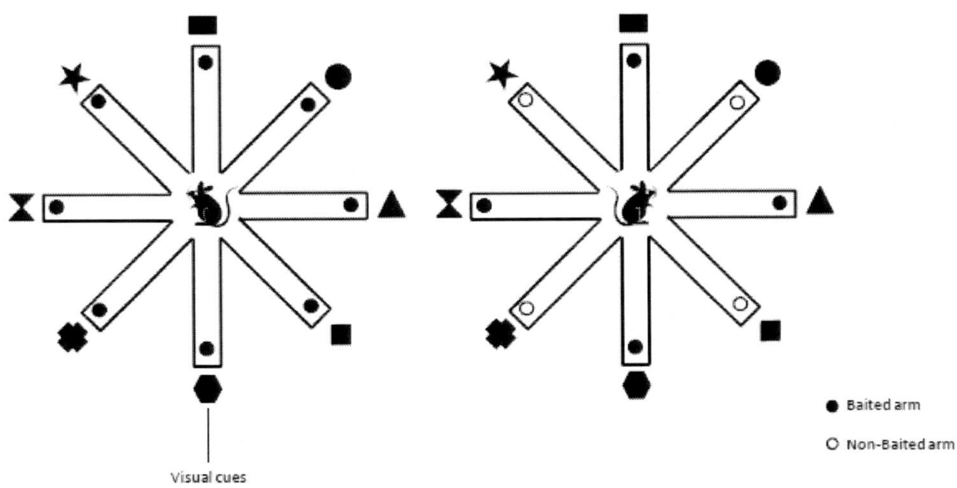

Figure 3. Experimental set-up of eight-arm radial maze test used for assessing reward-motivated spatial working memory and spatial reference memory. In a) classical RAM version where all arms are baited. In b) a variant of RAM where only four of eight maze arms are baited.

In a second variant of RAM only four of eight maze arms are baited. The same maze arms are baited each day, and across sessions, animals learn to ignore the remaining four baited arms without reward (Figure 3b). The entries into non-baited arms that never contained the reward are defined as errors and are used as an index of reference spatial memory. This version of RAM also allows assessing working memory by calculating the entries in a previously visited arm. Therefore entries into an arm more than once and entries into non-baited arms count as working memory errors and reference memory errors, respectively. In this second version of RAM, the reduced number of options or routes given represents a limitation for the assessment of working memory, which makes the sensitivity range even narrowed than performance in the first classic version of RAM. This has motivated the invention of radial arm mazes with 12, 17, 24 or even 48 arms.

The large number of arms is intended to make the task more difficult and to improve the method, especially when using the dual working/reference memory version.

3.2. Brain Areas Involved

Due to the spatial nature of this task, this maze is often used to assess the function of the hippocampus. In fact, hippocampectomised rats exhibits a delay-dependent impairment on this task [35]. In addition, mice with induced hippocampal lesions exhibited impaired memory in the RAM [79, 80].

3.3. Advantages and Limitations

This memory maze has some important limitations that have resulted in different modifications as described above. An important limitation of this protocol is that an animal can use an exploratory strategy like visiting adjacent arms to those visited previously either in a clockwise or anti-clockwise direction without using spatial cues. In order to eliminate this stereotypic behavior, the confinement was introduced by Olton [81]. When the animal achieves the reward and return to the central platform, it is confined by guillotine doors for a delay period. In this regard, some authors have showed that imposing an intertrial confinement interval prevents chaining [82, 83].

Other possible disadvantage is that in the RAM, olfactory cues can be used to detect those arms already visited, thereby modifying the behaviour of the animals [84]. To solve this problem, some research groups have used the aromatic saturation strategy allowing the animals to freely explore the maze before the test without any food with the aim to saturate the maze with aromatic cues [85]. Other strategies involve cleaning the device or/and rotating the arms while the location of the food reward [86]. It is important to mention also that, because food restriction is necessary, the experimenter should ensure that animals in control and experimental group are equally hungry and hence equally motivated to search for food, which are important issues in neuropharmacological and neurotoxicological experiments. Some drugs may induce anorexic episodes, also affecting regular behavior in the maze [87]. However, in order to eliminate the need for food-deprivation some alternative radial mazes have been developed in which the aversive stimulus is represented by open space and high luminosity; and their escape places are located at the end of some arms [88].

In this regard, an aquatic version of RAM, the Radial Water Maze (RWM) has been also developed [89]. As with the RAM, there are different versions of the RWM with different numbers of arms. There are also a variety of protocols. In RWM the stimulus driving behaviour is no longer linked to appetitive (food or water intake), but to aversive (water immersion) stimuli. In this aquatic version, one arm serves as the start and the other seven (or more) have submerged platforms at the ends.

On the first trial, the animal can enter any arm and find an escape platform, just as in the classic RAM where any choice leads to food. The animal is then removed for a specified length of time and the platform it found is also removed. On the second trial, if it remembers the arm it chose, it should not re-enter that arm but choose another one. This process continues until the animal finds all platforms. This can be adapted just like the appetitive RAM such that some arms have platforms at the start of each new trial and others never have platforms. The RWM requires about 10 days for rats or mice to become proficient [87].

Although the RAM and RWM both assess spatial memory they also possess some fundamental differences. In the RAM, once the reward has been consumed from an arm, the animal has no incentive to search that arm again, whereas in the RWM there is an incentive to return to the last arm visited because it found an escape there.

Different versions of this radial maze offered advantages that overcome initial limitations. The training protocol and data interpretation of the basic version is simple.

Another advantage is that the scientific literature validating and supporting its use in mice and rats is considerable, since it has been widely employed to test the effects of an important number of drugs, including anticholinergic agents, cannabinoids, dopaminergic agents, dopaminergic blockers, barbiturics, glutamatergic agonists or endogenous modulators [88-95]. Indeed, the opportunity to simultaneously test both spatial reference memory and spatial working memory is considered a typical advantage of RAM [96-99]. Moreover, this maze only generates a moderate level of stress in the animals during testing [97].

It is important to note that although some studies indicate that radial devices are not sensitive enough to spot differences between animal strains or genders [95], the RAM has been used in both male and female mice to detect gender differences in learning behavior [78].

4. Barnes Maze

The Barnes maze was developed by Carol Barnes [100]. It is a dry-land maze, consisting of a large white elevated round platform with about 20 holes around its perimeter under one of which is placed an escape tunnel leading to a dark compartment (Figure 4a) [101-104]. The model is based on the fact that rodents tend to avoid open, bright and exposed areas [105-107].

4.1. Experimental Design

Mice are placed in the center of the maze and the search begins [104]. External and internal visual cues may be used to help the animal to solve the maze.

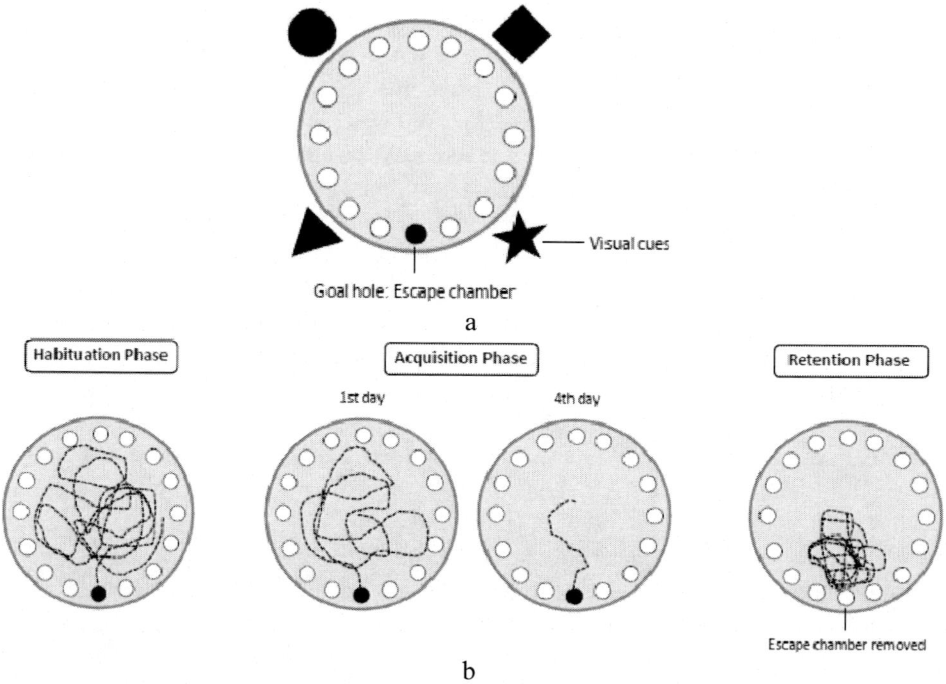

Figure 4. In a) experimental set-up of Barnes maze. In b) experimental protocol of Barnes maze consisting in habituation, acquisition and retention phases and the expected behaviour of a healthy wild type rodent. For detailed explanation, please check point 4.1.

During the test, rodents should learn the spatial location of the target hole. Training for this test is usually divided into three phases [103, 108] (Figure 4b):

1. Habituation phase: the test animal is introduced for one minute in the maze in the experimental room. Then it is placed in the start box located in the center of the maze for 30 seconds and finally into the target box where it is allowed to remain for 30 seconds before returning to its cage.
2. Acquisition phase: the animal is placed in the box in the center of the maze. After 30 seconds the box is removed and the animal is allowed to freely explore the illuminated platform for 4 minutes until it finds the target compartment [108]. If the rodent is not able to find it, the researcher must place it into the target box leaving it stay there for 30 seconds before starting a new test.

Although there is a great variation at the consulted protocols [100, 101, 108, 109] most consider that four training for four consecutive days are enough for proper learning the task. Appropriate learning can be checked by the quick reduction in errors and escape time.

3. Probe trial or retention phase: some authors perform one day after the acquisition phase, which is on the fifth day (short-term retention phase) and on the twelfth day (long-term retention phase). During probe trial the tunnel leading to the target box is closed and rodents are allowed to explore the maze for a minute [107].

In both acquisition and retention phases, the main parameters measured are latency to escape, path length used and number of errors [103, 108]. Mistakes are animal attempts to pass through non-escape holes. Escape time is the time it takes the animal to solve the maze. Usually animals are able to learn the location of the escape hole with 2-4 trials/day over 2-5 days. It is also interesting to record the speed and type of search strategy.

Several studies have shown that rodents mainly take three kinds of escape strategies: direct, random and peripheral [104]:

- Random escape strategy: animals move back and forth across the platform without definite pattern until the escape compartment is found.
- Peripheral escape strategy: animals sequentially check each opening at the periphery of the maze until they find the correct one.
- Direct or also called spatial strategy [107]: animals directly travel to and escape through the circular opening leading into the escape compartment, consistent with the use of a spatial strategy. Animal strains with normal vision are expected to use the spatial search strategy to locate the escape hole [103].

Animals reduce the use of the random one increasingly choosing the two remaining escape strategies. Barnes maze construction and testing methodologies can differ for small rodents, such as mice, and large rodents, such as rats.

For example, while extra-maze cues are effective for rats, smaller wild rodents may require intra-maze cues with a visual barrier around the maze [104]. Other studies show that mice not only use spatial cues to learn the location of the escape hole in the Barnes maze but they also use discrete proximal cues if are available [108].

4.2. Brain Areas Involved

Taking into account that damage in the CA1 and CA3 areas in hippocampus leads to deficits in performance of the task [110-112] the validity of this test to study spatial memory is confirmed. In addition, some authors have correlated lower spatial learning in this maze with lower number of Purkinge neurons in cerebellum, but not with less hippocampal volume [113].

4.3. Advantages and Limitations

Sometimes it has been detected a lack of motivation in animals when they perform the Barnes maze. Although they know the position of the escape hole, they continue exploring the maze due to lack of positive or negative reinforcement. Further maze exploration leads them to an increased number of mistakes and to a longer path length [104, 108]. To solve this problem it has been suggested to focus on the latency, path length and number of errors from the first encounter of the escape hole, called primary latency, primary path length and primary errors respectively [108]. Although no explanation has been given for differences founded between animal strains, it has been suggested that stress-related or anxiety-related behaviour strongly influences the performance of the maze. Patil et al. [107] observed a better performance by the C57BL/6J mice than the CD1 mice, which made more total mistakes compared to the C57BL/6J mice.

The Barnes maze is considered less aversive, less anxiogenic and less stressful than other mazes. Its performance is not influenced by differences in motivation due to hunger or physical effort. Therefore it's becoming increasingly popular for testing visuospatial learning and memory as well as spatial navigational abilities [103, 104]. Due to all different details and variations found in the many reviewed papers, it would be highly advisable to adapt parameters such as the size of the platform, the cues used and the protocol itself to fit better each species of experimental rodent [101, 103, 104, 114-116]. It should be also noticed that, compared to other mazes, the learning process in the Barnes maze may be slow, and will require more experiments due to the weak nature of motivational stimuli [109].

5. Morris Water Maze

Morris Water Maze (MWM) was first used by Richard Morris in 1981 for evaluating spatial memory in rats [117]. At that time, other procedures were already established for the same purpose (for instance, the RAM). However, MWM showed to be more reliable and reproducible than other previous methods [118]. Nowadays, MWM turns out to be the "gold standard" for spatial memory assessment in rodents.

5.1. Description

The apparatus for rats consist in a round pool of ~2 m in diameter and ~50 cm depth. This pool is placed in a room with 4 spatial clues in the walls surrounding. These positions labeled with clues are named as cardinal points (north, south, east and west). Attached to the ceiling, a camera records the animal's performance inside the pool (Figure 5a). Mouse equipment is very similar, but the pool tends to be smaller (~1.22 m in diameter). Either for rat or mouse, it is important to mention that pools cannot be excessively small, as it increases the chances of casually finding the platform. A circular platform of ~12 cm in diameter is placed in the pool in any of the cardinal points, far enough from the wall of the pool. The high of the platform is so that it is covered by only some millimeters of water, making it not visible for the animal (~40 cm should be enough). The color of the platform and the pool should be as close as possible to make the platform invisible. The animal tracing software uses contrast to detect animals in the pool, so black pools and platforms should be used with albino rodents and white pools for black and hooded rodents. Opacifying agents in the water (i.e., black/white paint, milk…) might be useful to either increase the contrast of the animal with the water and/ or hide better the platform. Water temperature is a critical point [119].

Some authors recommend to have 26° in the water [120] but other authors consider room temperature acceptable (20-22°) [121]. It is important to mention that mice are more prone to hypothermia than rats, so water temperature is likely more critical for them. In any case, during the performance hypothermia sings should be checked frequently, as it could decrease the exploratory behavior of rodents.

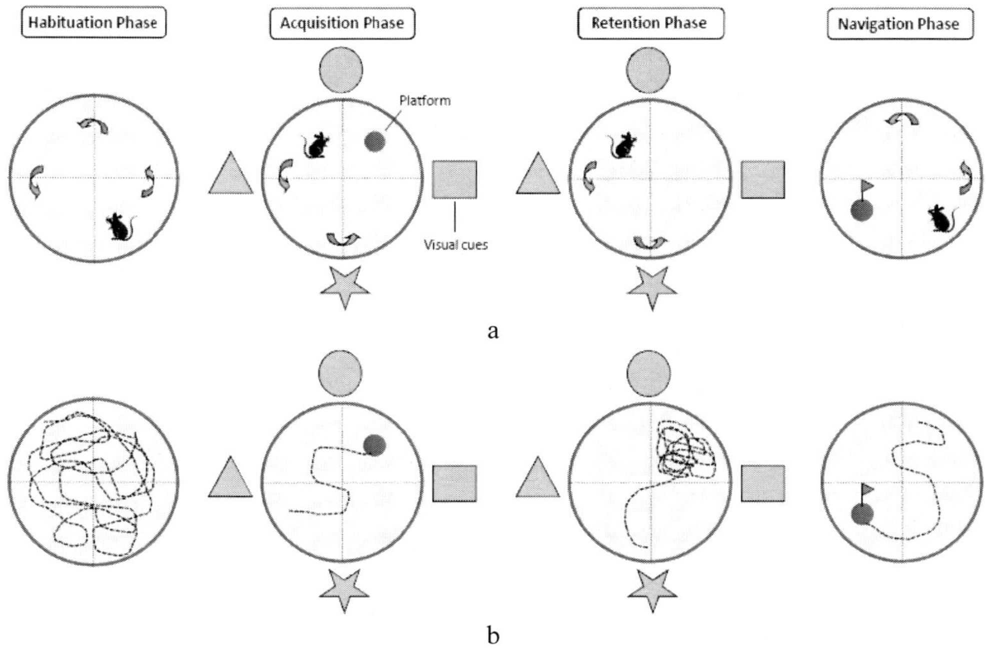

Figure 5. In a) experimental set-up of MWM. In b) experimental protocol of MWM consisting in habituation, acquisition, retention and navigation phases and the expected behaviour of a healthy wild type rodent. For detailed explanation, please check point 5.2.

5.2. Experimental Design

The protocol of the MWM could be summarize as following [120] (Figure 5b):

1. Habituation phase: animals are placed in the water without platform for a short time (1 min) to recognize the swimming pool.
2. Acquisition phase: rats are placed 4 to 6 times per day, letting them search for the platform in the apparatus. The number of days could vary between 2 and 5 days. Each trial lasts 1-2 minutes. If the animal does not find the platform, the researcher should gently guide it to the platform and let it there for 20 seconds. Along the trials, escape latency will decrease.

The number of trials varies considerably between different methodologies in the bibliography. This is because number of trials and its distribution along the days is a critical point. The acquisition schema should be carefully chosen so that animals achieve a plateau level in the learning curve (i.e., animals do not reduce the escape latency anymore).

3. Retention phase: after removing the platform, animals are again placed in the pool for 1 minute. Competent animals will swim preferentially in the area surrounding the position of the platform. It is important to execute this phase one day after the last

acquisition trial. Otherwise, short-term memory will be evaluated rather that long-term memory.

4. Navigation phase: The platform is place in a new position, but making it visible (for instance, with flag standing out of the water). Animals should find the platform quickly independently of their spatial learning capabilities. This phase confirms the visual and motor competencies of the animals.

5.3. Specific Issues When Performing MWM Task

Rodents are in general good swimmers, but they always try to avoid water if possible. In fact, this impulse in the animals makes this test work appropriately. However, putting the animals in such adverse conditions will presumably lead to some stress to the animals.

Stress leads to a poor performance in the MWM [122]. Therefore, excessive stress should be avoided. Animals should be carefully let in the pool without dropping them into the water, facing the wall if possible. Concerns about water temperature have been already addressed (see above). There are also some reports of overtraining [123]. Overtraining could lead to overlooking an existing cognitive impairment, likely due to a long acquisition phase (i.e., too many acquisition trials). Therefore, it is important to adapt the protocol to the concrete conditions of the experimental design. MWM was firstly proposed for rats, but it has been successfully applied to mice too. Although the performance of MWM does not differ substantially between mouse and rat, there are some differences that are important to take into account. Frick et al. [124] showed that strategies for searching the platform differ between these two species. Rats use a pure spatial strategy whereas mice use other non-spatial strategies too. In general, mice need more trials than rats to achieve the competency in the task, so these differences could explain the divergences that exist between protocols.

5.4. Derivations

Since the development of MWM, some derivation and improvements have been introduce [118]. Here are some of them. Some authors have tried to evaluate not only learning, but also the abilities to adapt to a new learned concept. This task can be achieved by changing the place of the platform after the retention phase, and performing again an acquisition and a retention phase [125]. This is the so called "reversal procedure," and not only spatial memory can be evaluated, but also the re-adaptation to the new rules for the escape. After changing the position of the platform animals firstly swim towards the old position of the platform, but they change the strategy along the different trials. Therefore, changes in re-learning capacities could be detected. One issue in the MWM is the fact of finding the platform just by chance. In order to ameliorate this factor one improvement is the introduction on demand platforms (also known as Atlantis platform) in the MWM [126]. This platform is mechanically programmed to stay inaccessible during the first 10 seconds of the trial. After that time, a mechanic pump pushes the platform up to an accessible level (but still hidden). This system has shown to avoid the casual finding of the platform during the first most erratic seconds of swimming, when presumably no spatial orientation strategy can be followed yet.

5.5. Brain Regions Involved

Spatial memory is a complex ability that depends of the integrity of many structures in the brain. Therefore, many local brain lesions have shown to induce impairment in MWM performance. One of the most important structures for the spatial memory is the hippocampus [127]. In fact, first efforts of Dr. Morris in the development of the MWM was to evaluate the effects of lesions at this level [123], showing that damaging the hippocampus leads to a poor performance in the MWM.

Some aspects of the cholinergic system appear to be necessary for the competent performance in the MWM. Lesions in the area surrounding the ventral septum induced depletion of cholinergic activity in the hippocampus and subsequently a cognitive impairment in the MWM. Interestingly, lesions in the cholinergic structure called nucleus basalis magnocellularis, which projects mainly to the anterior cortex, does not lead to such an impairment in MWM [128].

MWM performance is a complex task, and although it strongly depends in spatial memory, other non-spatial memory components may be involved too [87]. Therefore, some authors found relationship of areas involved with non-spatial memory, such as striatum or anterior thalamus [129].

Along these 30 years of use and development, MWM has proven its reliability in detecting cognitive impairment many fields. Cognitive aspects concerning aging [130], stroke [131], AD [132] and potentially nootropic agents [133] have been successfully evaluated with this test. Its wide acceptance between the scientific community will make this test still widely used in the future.

5.6. Advantages and Limitations

Water mazes in general and the MWM in particular, have advantages over other learning and memory tasks.

First, water is an equal-opportunity motivator that balances motivation to escape over a wide range of body weight differences among groups of animals [134], an effect that does not apply to appetitive tasks that are inherently problematic when a treatment causes differences in body weight, appetite, or the reward value of the reinforcement. Moreover, by assessing swim speed during learning one can determine whether animals in all groups are equal in their ability to swim and motivation to escape.

Second, in the MWM, 100% of control rats and nearly 100% of mice (in most strains) master the task; this aspect of the task is important because flat or shallow learning curves may not only prevent one from detecting group differences, but they also raise concerns about the validity of the test.

Third, the training required for the MWM and water mazes in general are minimal. Because rodents are natural swimmers, only a few trials are needed for animals to learn that active searching leads to escape and, once found, leads to removal from the pool.

A fourth advantage is that water is as motivating on the last trial as it is on the first, whereas appetitive tasks are subjected to satiation effects. The more trials given during a test session, the more rewards the animal consumes, which reduces hunger and motivation.

On the other hand, the most often stated criticism of the MWM (and all swimming mazes) is that they are stressful. The implication is that stress is always negative and should be avoided. In this sense, it is worth noting that food restriction and exposure to novel environments have also been shown to activate stress responses in animals [135-137]. In any case, taking into account that most rodents show high levels of learning in the MWM and high levels of retention of platform location, it is difficult to suggest that the task is overly stressful. In weighing the pros and cons of different methods of assessing spatial memory in rodents, MWM has demonstrated to possess many advantages and few disadvantages compared with other methods. All these features may explain at least part of why the MWM is the most widely used test of learning and memory [87].

Table 1. Progression of cognitive déficits in mouse models of AD

Strain	T/Y maze		RAM		Barnes Maze	MWM		Age (months)
	= [139]							1-2
	↓ [140]	= [138]	= [142]			↓ [144]		3-5
	↓ [141]	= [142]	↓ [144]	= [142]	↓ [146]	↓ [147]	= [142]	6-8
Tg2576 [138]	↓ [138,139]					↓ [138]	= [140]	9-11
						↓ [147]	= [140]	12-14
	↓ [143]	= [142]	↓ [145]		↓ [146]	↓ [147]		15-18
	↓ [140]					↓ [147]	= [140]	≥19
								1-2
			↓ [151]			↓ [154]		3-5
			↓ [152]			↓ [155]		6-8
J20 [148]	↑ [149]		↓ [153]			↓ [149]		9-11
	= [150]		↓ [152]			↓ [156]		12-14
								15-18
			↓ [152]					≥19
								1-2
			↓ [160]					3-5
	= [158, 159]		= [138]		↓ [162]	↓ [159]		6-8
APP/PS1 [157]			↓ [161]			↓ [163]		9-11
			↓ [160]			↓ [142]		12-14
					↓ [144]	↓ [142]		15-18
								≥19
	= [164]							1-2
	↓ [164]	= [165]				↓ [167]		3-5
	↓ [165, 166]					↓ [167]		6-8
5xFAD [164]	↓ [165]					↓ [168]		9-11
	↓ [165, 166]							12-14
								15-18
								≥19
						= [173]		1-2
	= [170]					↓ [173]	= [174]	3-5
	↓ [171]					↓ [175]		6-8
3xTgAD [169]	↓ [170]					= [176]		9-11
	↓ [170]				↓ [172]	↓ [174]		12-14
						↓ [176]		15-18
								≥19

↓ Represents impairment, = represents no impairment compared to control and ↑ represents increases vs control. White cells represent time points where no data are available for the respective behaviour. Adapted from [116].

CONCLUSION

Impaired spatial ability can have a great impact on the quality of life with advancing age. In addition, certain brain diseases, such as AD, are well known to affect episodic memory during an early stage of its progression. One value of working with animals is to develop models of human diseases with a view to understanding them better and developing appropriate therapeutic strategies. Therefore, using appropriate animal models and behavioral tests of learning and memory is essential for the correct interpretation of the results and their translation to humans. Rodent experiments can be performed on different inbred and outbred background strains, which can vary considerably in their abilities on cognitive tasks [55].

For each specific mouse model the temporal time course and progression of cognitive deficits in each cognitive domain can be different. In addition, in some models, cognitive deficits can be detected prior to the appearance of significant neuropathology.

As an example, an overview of the progressive cognitive deficits detected in some of the commonly used mouse models of AD by using the memory tests explained in this chapter is presented in Table 1.

Animal behavior evaluation has become a fundamental tool in multiple areas of translational neuroscience and is useful for studying (i) the physiological mechanisms underlying neurological disorders, (ii) the functional modifications induced by genetic manipulation or chemical treatment, and (iii) the efficacy of novel drugs in reversing phenotypes in disease models. Although cognitive assays of rodent models can provide important information on the validity and efficacy of targets and compounds, it is important to keep in mind that these tasks are incomplete analogs of human cognition. However, it is our hope that this comprehensive chapter of the spectrum of behavioral tasks commonly used for the assessment of spatial learning will assist investigators in selecting an appropriate test to investigate different aspects of neurological pathologies and disease progression, as well as the potential utility of new drugs and compounds.

REFERENCES

[1] Lee, R. D. The demographic transition: Three centuries of Fundamental Change. *Journal of Economic Perspectives* 2003;17: 167-190.

[2] Hewitt, J., Refshauge, K. M., Goodall, S., Henwood, T., Clemson, L. Does progressive resistance and balance exercise reduce falls in residential aged care? Randomized controlled trial protocol for the SUNBEAM program. *Clin. Interv. Aging* 2014;9: 369-376.

[3] *Statistics ABo*. Household and Family Projections, Australia, 2006 to 2031. http://www.abs.gov.au/ausstats/abs@.nsf/mf/3236.0. 2013.

[4] Carone, G. C., D. Can Europe afford to grow old?. *Finance and Development*. Vol. 43. International Monetary Fund 2006.

[5] Hewitt, P. Depopulation and ageing in Europe and Japan: The hazardous transition to a labor shortage economy. *Global Action on Aging*. 2002.

[6] Albert, M. S. F. H. The effects of age: normal variation and its relation to disease. In: Asbury, A. K., McDondald, W. I., McKhann, G. M. (Eds.), *Diseases of the Nervous System: Clinical Neurobiology*. Saunders, Philadelphia. 1992;598-611.
[7] Eysenck, M. W. Models of memory: information processing. *Psychopharmacol. Ser.* 1988;6: 3-11.
[8] Becker, J. T., Morris, R. G. Working memory(s). *Brain Cogn.* 1999;41: 1-8.
[9] Wang, S. H., Morris, R. G. Hippocampal-neocortical interactions in memory formation, consolidation, and reconsolidation. *Annu. Rev. Psychol.* 2010;61: 49-79, C41-44.
[10] Morellini, F. Spatial memory tasks in rodents: what do they model? *Cell Tissue Res.* 2013;354: 273-286.
[11] JR. A. *Learning and Retention. Language, Memory and Thought.* Lawrence Erlbaum Associates Inc, New Jersey. 1976;378-437.
[12] Bechara, A., Tranel, D., Damasio, H., Adolphs, R., Rockland, C., Damasio, A. R. Double dissociation of conditioning and declarative knowledge relative to the amygdala and hippocampus in humans. *Science* 1995;269: 1115-1118.
[13] Knowlton, B. J., Mangels, J. A., Squire, L. R. A neostriatal habit learning system in humans. *Science* 1996;273: 1399-1402.
[14] Salmon, D. P., Butters, N. Neurobiology of skill and habit learning. *Curr. Opin. Neurobiol.* 1995;5: 184-190.
[15] Miller, G. A. The magical number seven plus or minus two: some limits on our capacity for processing information. *Psychol. Rev.* 1956;63: 81-97.
[16] E. T. (1972) *Episodic and semantic memory*, Academic Press, New York.
[17] Nadel, L., MacDonald, L. Hippocampus: cognitive map or working memory? *Behav. Neural Biol.* 1980;29: 405-409.
[18] Davis, S., Markowska, A. L., Wenk, G. L., Barnes, C. A. Acetyl-L-carnitine: behavioral, electrophysiological, and neurochemical effects. *Neurobiol. Aging* 1993;14: 107-115.
[19] Lindner, M. D. Reliability, distribution, and validity of age-related cognitive deficits in the Morris water maze. *Neurobiol. Learn. Mem.* 1997;68: 203-220.
[20] Blalock, E. M., Chen, K. C., Sharrow, K., Herman, J. P., Porter, N. M., Foster, T. C., Landfield, P. W. Gene microarrays in hippocampal aging: statistical profiling identifies novel processes correlated with cognitive impairment. *J. Neurosci.* 2003;23: 3807-3819.
[21] Foster, T. C., Sharrow, K. M., Kumar, A., Masse, J. Interaction of age and chronic estradiol replacement on memory and markers of brain aging. *Neurobiol. Aging* 2003; 24: 839-852.
[22] Driscoll, I., Howard, S. R., Stone, J. C., Monfils, M. H., Tomanek, B., Brooks, W. M., Sutherland, R. J. The aging hippocampus: a multi-level analysis in the rat. *Neuroscience* 2006;139: 1173-1185.
[23] Adams, M. M., Shi, L., Linville, M. C., Forbes, M. E., Long, A. B., Bennett, C., Newton, I. G., Carter, C. S., Sonntag, W. E., Riddle, D. R., Brunso-Bechtold, J. K. Caloric restriction and age affect synaptic proteins in hippocampal CA3 and spatial learning ability. *Exp. Neurol.* 2008;211: 141-149.
[24] Bizon, J. L., LaSarge, C. L., Montgomery, K. S., McDermott, A. N., Setlow, B., Griffith, W. H. Spatial reference and working memory across the lifespan of male Fischer 344 rats. *Neurobiol. Aging* 2009;30: 646-655.

[25] Park, D. C., Puglisi, J. T., Lutz, R. Spatial memory in older adults: effects of intentionality. *J. Gerontol.* 1982;37: 330-335.
[26] Park, D. C., Puglisi, J. T., Sovacool, M. Memory for pictures, words, and spatial location in older adults: evidence for pictorial superiority. *J. Gerontol.* 1983;38: 582-588.
[27] Evans, G. W., Brennan, P. L., Skorpanich, M. A., Held, D. Cognitive mapping and elderly adults: verbal and location memory for urban landmarks. *J. Gerontol.* 1984;39: 452-457.
[28] Zelinski, E. M., Light, L. L. Young and older adults' use of context in spatial memory. *Psychol. Aging* 1988;3: 99-101.
[29] Uttl, B., Graf, P. Episodic spatial memory in adulthood. *Psychol. Aging* 1993;8: 257-273.
[30] Abrahams, S., Pickering, A., Polkey, C. E., Morris, R. G. Spatial memory deficits in patients with unilateral damage to the right hippocampal formation. *Neuropsychologia* 1997;35: 11-24.
[31] Astur, R. S., Taylor, L. B., Mamelak, A. N., Philpott, L., Sutherland, R. J. Humans with hippocampus damage display severe spatial memory impairments in a virtual Morris water task. *Behav. Brain Res.* 2002;132: 77-84.
[32] Feigenbaum, J. D., Polkey, C. E., Morris, R. G. Deficits in spatial working memory after unilateral temporal lobectomy in man. *Neuropsychologia* 1996;34: 163-176.
[33] Rosenbaum, R. S., Priselac, S., Kohler, S., Black, S. E., Gao, F., Nadel, L., Moscovitch, M. Remote spatial memory in an amnesic person with extensive bilateral hippocampal lesions. *Nat. Neurosci.* 2000;3: 1044-1048.
[34] Schenk, F., Morris, R. G. Dissociation between components of spatial memory in rats after recovery from the effects of retrohippocampal lesions. *Exp. Brain Res.* 1985;58: 11-28.
[35] Jarrard, L. E. On the role of the hippocampus in learning and memory in the rat. *Behav. Neural Biol.* 1993;60: 9-26.
[36] Devan, B. D., Goad, E. H., Petri, H. L. Dissociation of hippocampal and striatal contributions to spatial navigation in the water maze. *Neurobiol. Learn. Mem.* 1996;66: 305-323.
[37] Murray, E. A., Davidson, M., Gaffan, D., Olton, D. S., Suomi, S. Effects of fornix transection and cingulate cortical ablation on spatial memory in rhesus monkeys. *Exp. Brain Res.* 1989;74: 173-186.
[38] Banta Lavenex, P., Lavenex, P. Spatial memory and the monkey hippocampus: not all space is created equal. *Hippocampus* 2009;19: 8-19.
[39] Lavenex, P. B., Amaral, D. G., Lavenex, P. Hippocampal lesion prevents spatial relational learning in adult macaque monkeys. *J. Neurosci.* 2006;26: 4546-4558.
[40] Bohbot, V. D., Kalina, M., Stepankova, K., Spackova, N., Petrides, M., Nadel, L. Spatial memory deficits in patients with lesions to the right hippocampus and to the right parahippocampal cortex. *Neuropsychologia* 1998;36: 1217-1238.
[41] Holdstock, J. S., Mayes, A. R., Cezayirli, E., Isaac, C. L., Aggleton, J. P., Roberts, N. A comparison of egocentric and allocentric spatial memory in a patient with selective hippocampal damage. *Neuropsychologia* 2000;38: 410-425.

[42] Parslow, D. M., Morris, R. G., Fleminger, S., Rahman, Q., Abrahams, S., Recce, M. Allocentric spatial memory in humans with hippocampal lesions. *Acta Psychol.* (Amst.) 2005;118: 123-147.

[43] Mungas, D., Harvey, D., Reed, B. R., Jagust, W. J., DeCarli, C., Beckett, L., Mack, W. J., Kramer, J. H., Weiner, M. W., Schuff, N., Chui, H. C. Longitudinal volumetric MRI change and rate of cognitive decline. *Neurology* 2005;65: 565-571.

[44] Kramer, J. H., Mungas, D., Reed, B. R., Wetzel, M. E., Burnett, M. M., Miller, B. L., Weiner, M. W., Chui, H. C. Longitudinal MRI and cognitive change in healthy elderly. *Neuropsychology* 2007;21: 412-418.

[45] Mueller, S. G., Stables, L., Du, A. T., Schuff, N., Truran, D., Cashdollar, N., Weiner, M. W. Measurement of hippocampal subfields and age-related changes with high resolution MRI at 4T. *Neurobiol. Aging* 2007;28: 719-726.

[46] Head, D., Rodrigue, K. M., Kennedy, K. M., Raz, N. Neuroanatomical and cognitive mediators of age-related differences in episodic memory. *Neuropsychology* 2008;22: 491-507.

[47] Reuter-Lorenz, P. A., Park, D. C. Human neuroscience and the aging mind: a new look at old problems. *J. Gerontol. B Psychol. Sci. Soc. Sci.* 2010;65: 405-415.

[48] Sexton, C. E., Mackay, C. E., Lonie, J. A., Bastin, M. E., Terriere, E., O'Carroll, R. E., Ebmeier, K. P. MRI correlates of episodic memory in Alzheimer's disease, mild cognitive impairment, and healthy aging. *Psychiatry Res.* 2010;184: 57-62.

[49] Picq, J. L., Aujard, F., Volk, A., Dhenain, M. Age-related cerebral atrophy in nonhuman primates predicts cognitive impairments. *Neurobiol. Aging* 2012;33: 1096-1109.

[50] Hossain, S. M., Wong, B. K., Simpson, E. M. The dark phase improves genetic discrimination for some high throughput mouse behavioral phenotyping. *Genes Brain Behav.* 2004;3: 167-177.

[51] Reiter, R. J. Pineal gland interface between the photoperiodic environment and the endocrine system. *Trends Endocrinol. Metab.* 1991;2: 13-19.

[52] Holmes, A., Rodgers, R. J. Responses of Swiss-Webster mice to repeated plus-maze experience: further evidence for a qualitative shift in emotional state? *Pharmacol. Biochem. Behav.* 1998;60: 473-488.

[53] Voikar, V., Vasar, E., Rauvala, H. Behavioral alterations induced by repeated testing in C57BL/6J and 129S2/Sv mice: implications for phenotyping screens. *Genes Brain Behav.* 2004;3: 27-38.

[54] Wongwitdecha, N., Marsden, C. A. Effects of social isolation rearing on learning in the Morris water maze. *Brain Res.* 1996;715: 119-124.

[55] Crawley, J. N., Belknap, J. K., Collins, A., Crabbe, J. C., Frankel, W., Henderson, N., Hitzemann, R. J., Maxson, S. C., Miner, L. L., Silva, A. J., Wehner, J. M., Wynshaw-Boris, A., Paylor, R. Behavioral phenotypes of inbred mouse strains: implications and recommendations for molecular studies. *Psychopharmacology* (Berl.) 1997;132: 107-124.

[56] C. T-B. Exploration and spatial knowledge. Animal Spatial Cognition. *Behavioral and Neural Approaches* 1996; 1st ed. Singapore: Word Scientific: 1-42.

[57] Deacon, R. M., Rawlins, J. N. T-maze alternation in the rodent. *Nat. Protoc.* 2006;1: 7-12.

[58] Morellini, F., Schachner, M. Enhanced novelty-induced activity, reduced anxiety, delayed resynchronization to daylight reversal and weaker muscle strength in tenascin-C-deficient mice. *Eur. J. Neurosci.* 2006;23: 1255-1268.

[59] Morellini, F., Sivukhina, E., Stoenica, L., Oulianova, E., Bukalo, O., Jakovcevski, I., Dityatev, A., Irintchev, A., Schachner, M. Improved reversal learning and working memory and enhanced reactivity to novelty in mice with enhanced GABAergic innervation in the dentate gyrus. *Cereb. Cortex.* 2010;20: 2712-2727.

[60] Sharma, S., Rakoczy, S., Brown-Borg, H. Assessment of spatial memory in mice. *Life Sci.* 2010;87: 521-536.

[61] Guariglia, S. R., Chadman, K. K. Water T-maze: a useful assay for determination of repetitive behaviors in mice. *J. Neurosci. Methods* 2013;220: 24-29.

[62] Murray, C., Sanderson, D. J., Barkus, C., Deacon, R. M., Rawlins, J. N., Bannerman, D. M., Cunningham, C. Systemic inflammation induces acute working memory deficits in the primed brain: relevance for delirium. *Neurobiol. Aging* 2012;33: 603-616 e603.

[63] Johnson, C. T., Olton, D. S., Gage, F. H., 3rd, Jenko, P. G. Damage to hippocampus and hippocampal connections: effects on DRL and spontaneous alternation. *J. Comp. Physiol. Psychol.* 1977;91: 508-522.

[64] Clody, D. E., Carlton, P. L. Behavioral effects of lesions of the medial septum of rats. *J. Comp. Physiol. Psychol.* 1969;67: 344-351.

[65] Douglas, R. J., Raphelson, A. C. Spontaneous alternation and septal lesions. *J. Comp. Physiol. Psychol.* 1966;62: 320-322.

[66] Celerier, A., Ognard, R., Decorte, L., Beracochea, D. Deficits of spatial and non-spatial memory and of auditory fear conditioning following anterior thalamic lesions in mice: comparison with chronic alcohol consumption. *Eur. J. Neurosci.* 2000;12: 2575-2584.

[67] Divac, I. W. R., Gade, A. Spontaneous alternation in rats with lesions in the frontal lobes: an extension of the frontal lobe syndrome. *Physiol. Psychol.* 1975;3: 39-42.

[68] Wikmark, R. G., Divac, I., Weiss, R. Retention of spatial delayed alternation in rats with lesions in the frontal lobes. Implications for a comparative neuropsychology of the prefrontal system. *Brain Behav. Evol.* 1973;8: 329-339.

[69] Lalonde, R. The neurobiological basis of spontaneous alternation. *Neurosci. Biobehav. Rev.* 2002;26: 91-104.

[70] Douglas, R. J., Clark, G. M., Erway, L. C., Hubbard, D. G., Wright, C. G. Effects of genetic vestibular defects on behavior related to spatial orientation and emotionality. *J. Comp. Physiol. Psychol.* 1979;93: 467-480.

[71] Lalonde, R. Delayed spontaneous alternation in weaver mutant mice. *Brain Res.* 1986; 398: 178-180.

[72] Lalonde, R., Botez, M. I., Boivin, D. Spontaneous alternation and habituation in a t-maze in nervous mutant mice. *Behav. Neurosci.* 1986;100: 350-352.

[73] Lalonde, R., Manseau, M., Botez, M. I. Spontaneous alternation and exploration in staggerer mutant mice. *Behav. Brain Res.* 1988;27: 273-276.

[74] Lalonde, R., Manseau, M., Botez, M. I. Spontaneous alternation and habituation in Purkinje cell degeneration mutant mice. *Brain Res.* 1987;411: 187-189.

[75] Carrillo-Mora, P. G. M., Santamaría, A. Spatial memory: Theoretical basis and comparative review on experimental methods in rodents. *Behav. Brain Res.* 2009;203 (2): 151-164.

[76] Olton, D. S. Spatial memory. *Sci. Am.* 1977;236: 82-84, 89-94, 96, 98.

[77] Astur, R. S., St Germain, S. A., Baker, E. K., Calhoun, V., Pearlson, G. D., Constable, R. T. fMRI hippocampal activity during a virtual radial arm maze. *Appl. Psychophysiol. Biofeedback* 2005;30: 307-317.

[78] LaBuda, C. J., Mellgren, R. L., Hale, R. L. Sex differences in the acquisition of a radial maze task in the CD-1 mouse. *Physiol. Behav.* 2002;76: 213-217.

[79] Olton, D. S., Papas, B. C. Spatial memory and hippocampal function. *Neuropsychologia* 1979;17: 669-682.

[80] Olton, D. S. The use of animal models to evaluate the effects of neurotoxins on cognitive processes. *Neurobehav. Toxicol. Teratol.* 1983;5: 635-640.

[81] Olton, D. S. C. C., Werz, M. A. Spatial memory and radial arm maze performance of rats. *Learn. Motiv.* 1977;8(3): 289-314.

[82] Suzuki, S. A. G., Black, A. H. Stimulus control of spatial behavior on the eight-arm maze in rats. *Learn. Motiv.* 1980;11(1): 1-18.

[83] Dubreuil, D., Tixier, C., Dutrieux, G., Edeline, J. M. Does the radial arm maze necessarily test spatial memory? *Neurobiol. Learn. Mem.* 2003;79: 109-117.

[84] Wasserman, E. A., Jensen, D. D. Olfactory stimuli and the "pseudo-extinction" effect. *Science* 1969;166: 1307-1309.

[85] Roullet, P., Lassalle, J. M., Jegat, R. A study of behavioral and sensorial bases of radial maze learning in mice. *Behav. Neural Biol.* 1993;59: 173-179.

[86] Dudchenko, P. A. An overview of the tasks used to test working memory in rodents. *Neurosci. Biobehav. Rev.* 2004;28: 699-709.

[87] Vorhees, C. V., Williams, M. T. Assessing spatial learning and memory in rodents. *ILAR J.* 2014;55: 310-332.

[88] Paganelli, R. A., Benetolli, A., Lima, K. C., Cestari-Junior, L. A., Favero Filho, L. A., Milani, H. A novel version of the 8-arm radial maze: effects of cerebral ischemia on learning and memory. *J. Neurosci. Methods* 2004;132: 9-18.

[89] Hyde, L. A., Hoplight, B. J., Denenberg, V. H. Water version of the radial-arm maze: learning in three inbred strains of mice. *Brain Res.* 1998;785: 236-244.

[90] Avila-Costa, M. R., Fortoul, T. I., Nino-Cabrera, G., Colin-Barenque, L., Bizarro-Nevares, P., Gutierrez-Valdez, A. L., Ordonez-Librado, J. L., Rodriguez-Lara, V., Mussali-Galante, P., Diaz-Bech, P., Anaya-Martinez, V. Hippocampal cell alterations induced by the inhalation of vanadium pentoxide (V(2)O(5)) promote memory deterioration. *Neurotoxicology* 2006;27: 1007-1012.

[91] Beatty, W. W., Bierley, R. A. Scopolamine degrades spatial working memory but spares spatial reference memory: dissimilarity of anticholinergic effect and restriction of distal visual cues. *Pharmacol. Biochem. Behav.* 1985;23: 1-6.

[92] Brown, M. F. Does a cognitive map guide choices in the radial-arm maze? *J. Exp. Psychol. Anim. Behav. Process* 1992;18: 56-66.

[93] Chess, A. C., Simoni, M. K., Alling, T. E., Bucci, D. J. Elevations of endogenous kynurenic acid produce spatial working memory deficits. *Schizophr. Bull.* 2007;33: 797-804.

[94] Jonasson, Z. Meta-analysis of sex differences in rodent models of learning and memory: a review of behavioral and biological data. *Neurosci. Biobehav. Rev.* 2005;28: 811-825.

[95] Seymoure, P. D. H., Juraska, J. M. Sex differences in radial maze performance: influence of rearing environment and room cues. *Psychobiology* 1996;24: 33-37.

[96] Belotti, M., Galey, D. Consequences of selective blockade of septal noradrenergic afferents on anxiety and spatial working memory performance in mice. *Pharmacol. Biochem. Behav.* 1996;53: 541-547.
[97] Hodges, H. Maze procedures: the radial-arm and water maze compared. *Brain Res. Cogn. Brain Res.* 1996;3: 167-181.
[98] Schmitt, W. B., Deacon, R. M., Seeburg, P. H., Rawlins, J. N., Bannerman, D. M. A within-subjects, within-task demonstration of intact spatial reference memory and impaired spatial working memory in glutamate receptor-A-deficient mice. *J. Neurosci.* 2003;23: 3953-3959.
[99] Zhang, J. X., Chen, X. Q., Du, J. Z., Chen, Q. M., Zhu, C. Y. Neonatal exposure to intermittent hypoxia enhances mice performance in water maze and 8-arm radial maze tasks. *J. Neurobiol.* 2005;65: 72-84.
[100] Barnes, C. A. Memory deficits associated with senescence: a neurophysiological and behavioral study in the rat. *J. Comp. Physiol. Psychol.* 1979;93: 74-104.
[101] Harrison, F. E., Hosseini, A. H., McDonald, M. P. Endogenous anxiety and stress responses in water maze and Barnes maze spatial memory tasks. *Behav. Brain Res.* 2009;198: 247-251.
[102] O'Leary, T. P., Brown, R. E. The effects of apparatus design and test procedure on learning and memory performance of C57BL/6J mice on the Barnes maze. *J. Neurosci. Methods* 2012;203: 315-324.
[103] O'Leary, T. P., Savoie, V., Brown, R. E. Learning, memory and search strategies of inbred mouse strains with different visual abilities in the Barnes maze. *Behav. Brain Res.* 2011;216: 531-542.
[104] Rosenfeld, C. S., Ferguson, S. A. Barnes maze testing strategies with small and large rodent models. *J. Vis. Exp.* 2014;e51194.
[105] Koopmans, G., Blokland, A., van Nieuwenhuijzen, P., Prickaerts, J. Assessment of spatial learning abilities of mice in a new circular maze. *Physiol. Behav.* 2003;79: 683-693.
[106] Kuc, K. A., Gregersen, B. M., Gannon, K. S., Dodart, J. C. Holeboard discrimination learning in mice. *Genes Brain Behav.* 2006;5: 355-363.
[107] Patil, S. S., Sunyer, B., Hoger, H., Lubec, G. Evaluation of spatial memory of C57BL/6J and CD1 mice in the Barnes maze, the Multiple T-maze and in the Morris water maze. *Behav. Brain Res.* 2009;198: 58-68.
[108] Harrison, F. E., Reiserer, R. S., Tomarken, A. J., McDonald, M. P. Spatial and nonspatial escape strategies in the Barnes maze. *Learn. Mem.* 2006;13: 809-819.
[109] Attar, A., Liu, T., Chan, W. T., Hayes, J., Nejad, M., Lei, K., Bitan, G. A shortened Barnes maze protocol reveals memory deficits at 4-months of age in the triple-transgenic mouse model of Alzheimer's disease. *PLoS One* 2013;8: e80355.
[110] Fox, G. B., Fan, L., LeVasseur, R. A., Faden, A. I. Effect of traumatic brain injury on mouse spatial and nonspatial learning in the Barnes circular maze. *J. Neurotrauma* 1998;15: 1037-1046.
[111] Fedor, M., Berman, R. F., Muizelaar, J. P., Lyeth, B. G. Hippocampal theta dysfunction after lateral fluid percussion injury. *J. Neurotrauma* 2010;27: 1605-1615.
[112] Amador-Arjona, A., Elliott, J., Miller, A., Ginbey, A., Pazour, G. J., Enikolopov, G., Roberts, A. J., Terskikh, A. V. Primary cilia regulate proliferation of amplifying

progenitors in adult hippocampus: implications for learning and memory. *J. Neurosci.* 2011;31: 9933-9944.

[113] Kennard, J. A., Woodruff-Pak, D. S. Age sensitivity of behavioral tests and brain substrates of normal aging in mice. *Front. Aging Neurosci.* 2011;3: 9.

[114] Holmes, A., Wrenn, C. C., Harris, A. P., Thayer, K. E., Crawley, J. N. Behavioral profiles of inbred strains on novel olfactory, spatial and emotional tests for reference memory in mice. *Genes Brain Behav.* 2002;1: 55-69.

[115] Yoshida, M., Goto, K., Watanabe, S. Task-dependent strain difference of spatial learning in C57BL/6N and BALB/c mice. *Physiol. Behav.* 2001;73: 37-42.

[116] Webster, S. J., Bachstetter, A. D., Nelson, P. T., Schmitt, F. A., Van Eldik, L. J. Using mice to model Alzheimer's dementia: an overview of the clinical disease and the preclinical behavioral changes in 10 mouse models. *Front. Genet.* 2014;5: 88.

[117] Morris, R. Developments of a water-maze procedure for studying spatial learning in the rat. *J. Neurosci. Methods* 1984;11: 47-60.

[118] Vorhees, C. V., Williams, M. T. Morris water maze: procedures for assessing spatial and related forms of learning and memory. *Nat. Protoc.* 2006;1: 848-858.

[119] Lindner, M. D., Gribkoff, V. K. Relationship between performance in the Morris water task, visual acuity, and thermoregulatory function in aged F-344 rats. *Behav. Brain Res.* 1991;45: 45-55.

[120] Nunez, J. Morris Water Maze Experiment. *J. Vis. Exp.* 2008.

[121] Bromley-Brits, K., Yu Deng and Weihong Song. Morris Water Maze Test for Learning and Memory Deficits in Alzheimer's Disease Model Mice. *Journal of Visualized Experiments: JoVE* 2011;53: doi:10.3791/2920.

[122] Holscher, C. Stress impairs performance in spatial water maze learning tasks. *Behav. Brain Res.* 1999;100: 225-235.

[123] Morris, R. G., Schenk, F., Tweedie, F., Jarrard, L. E. Ibotenate Lesions of Hippocampus and/or Subiculum: Dissociating Components of Allocentric Spatial Learning. *Eur. J. Neurosci.* 1990;2: 1016-1028.

[124] Frick, K. M., Stillner, E. T., Berger-Sweeney, J. Mice are not little rats: species differences in a one-day water maze task. *Neuroreport* 2000;11: 3461-3465.

[125] Lipp, H. P., Wolfer, D. P. Genetically modified mice and cognition. *Curr. Opin. Neurobiol.* 1998;8: 272-280.

[126] Spooner, R. I., Thomson, A., Hall, J., Morris, R. G., Salter, S. H. The Atlantis platform: a new design and further developments of Buresova's on-demand platform for the water maze. *Learn. Mem.* 1994;1: 203-211.

[127] O'Keefe, J., Burgess, N. Dual phase and rate coding in hippocampal place cells: theoretical significance and relationship to entorhinal grid cells. *Hippocampus* 2005;15: 853-866.

[128] Hagan, J. J., Salamone, J. D., Simpson, J., Iversen, S. D., Morris, R. G. Place navigation in rats is impaired by lesions of medial septum and diagonal band but not nucleus basalis magnocellularis. *Behav. Brain Res.* 1988;27: 9-20.

[129] Mendez-Couz, M., Conejo, N. M., Gonzalez-Pardo, H., Arias, J. L. Functional interactions between dentate gyrus, striatum and anterior thalamic nuclei on spatial memory retrieval. *Brain Res.* 2015;1605: 59-69.

[130] Gallagher, M., Rapp, P. R. The use of animal models to study the effects of aging on cognition. *Annu. Rev. Psychol.* 1997;48: 339-370.

[131] Ji, S., Kronenberg, G., Balkaya, M., Farber, K., Gertz, K., Kettenmann, H., Endres, M. Acute neuroprotection by pioglitazone after mild brain ischemia without effect on long-term outcome. *Exp. Neurol.* 2009;216: 321-328.
[132] Lord, A., Englund, H., Soderberg, L., Tucker, S., Clausen, F., Hillered, L., Gordon, M., Morgan, D., Lannfelt, L., Pettersson, F. E., Nilsson, L. N. Amyloid-beta protofibril levels correlate with spatial learning in Arctic Alzheimer's disease transgenic mice. *FEBS J.* 2009;276: 995-1006.
[133] Lelong, V., Dauphin, F., Boulouard, M. RS 67333 and D-cycloserine accelerate learning acquisition in the rat. *Neuropharmacology* 2001;41: 517-522.
[134] Cravens, R. W. Effects of maternal undernutrition on offspring behavior: incentive value of a food reward and ability to escape from water. *Dev. Psychobiol.* 1974;7: 61-69.
[135] Johansson, A., Fredriksson, R., Winnergren, S., Hulting, A. L., Schioth, H. B., Lindblom, J. The relative impact of chronic food restriction and acute food deprivation on plasma hormone levels and hypothalamic neuropeptide expression. *Peptides* 2008; 29: 1588-1595.
[136] Marinkovic, P., Pesic, V., Loncarevic, N., Smiljanic, K., Kanazir, S., Ruzdijic, S. Behavioral and biochemical effects of various food-restriction regimens in the rats. *Physiol. Behav.* 2007;92: 492-499.
[137] Pesic, V., Marinkovic, P., Janac, B., Ignjatovic, S., Popic, J., Kanazir, S., Ruzdijic, S. Changes of behavioral parameters during long-term food restriction in middle-aged Wistar rats. *Physiol. Behav.* 2010;101: 672-678.
[138] Hsiao, K., Chapman, P., Nilsen, S., Eckman, C., Harigaya, Y., Younkin, S., Yang, F., Cole, G. Correlative memory deficits, Abeta elevation, and amyloid plaques in transgenic mice. *Science* 1996;274: 99-102.
[139] Chapman, P. F., White, G. L., Jones, M. W., Cooper-Blacketer, D., Marshall, V. J., Irizarry, M., Younkin, L., Good, M. A., Bliss, T. V., Hyman, B. T., Younkin, S. G., Hsiao, K. K. Impaired synaptic plasticity and learning in aged amyloid precursor protein transgenic mice. *Nat. Neurosci.* 1999;2: 271-276.
[140] King, D. L., Arendash, G. W., Crawford, F., Sterk, T., Menendez, J., Mullan, M. J. Progressive and gender-dependent cognitive impairment in the APP(SW) transgenic mouse model for Alzheimer's disease. *Behav. Brain Res.* 1999;103: 145-162.
[141] Ohno, M., Sametsky, E. A., Younkin, L. H., Oakley, H., Younkin, S. G., Citron, M., Vassar, R., Disterhoft, J. F. BACE1 deficiency rescues memory deficits and cholinergic dysfunction in a mouse model of Alzheimer's disease. *Neuron* 2004;41: 27-33.
[142] Arendash, G. W., Gordon, M. N., Diamond, D. M., Austin, L. A., Hatcher, J. M., Jantzen, P., DiCarlo, G., Wilcock, D., Morgan, D. Behavioral assessment of Alzheimer's transgenic mice following long-term Abeta vaccination: task specificity and correlations between Abeta deposition and spatial memory. *DNA Cell Biol.* 2001; 20: 737-744.
[143] Corcoran, K. A., Lu, Y., Turner, R. S., Maren, S. Overexpression of hAPPswe impairs rewarded alternation and contextual fear conditioning in a transgenic mouse model of Alzheimer's disease. *Learn. Mem.* 2002;9: 243-252.
[144] Arendash, G. W., Lewis, J., Leighty, R. E., McGowan, E., Cracchiolo, J. R., Hutton, M., Garcia, M. F. Multi-metric behavioral comparison of APPsw and P301L models for

Alzheimer's disease: linkage of poorer cognitive performance to tau pathology in forebrain. *Brain Res*. 2004;1012: 29-41.

[145] Morgan, D., Diamond, D. M., Gottschall, P. E., Ugen, K. E., Dickey, C., Hardy, J., Duff, K., Jantzen, P., DiCarlo, G., Wilcock, D., Connor, K., Hatcher, J., Hope, C., Gordon, M., Arendash, G. W. A beta peptide vaccination prevents memory loss in an animal model of Alzheimer's disease. *Nature* 2000;408: 982-985.

[146] Yassine, N., Lazaris, A., Dorner-Ciossek, C., Despres, O., Meyer, L., Maitre, M., Mensah-Nyagan, A. G., Cassel, J. C., Mathis, C. Detecting spatial memory deficits beyond blindness in tg2576 Alzheimer mice. *Neurobiol. Aging* 2013;34: 716-730.

[147] Westerman, M. A., Cooper-Blacketer, D., Mariash, A., Kotilinek, L., Kawarabayashi, T., Younkin, L. H., Carlson, G. A., Younkin, S. G., Ashe, K. H. The relationship between Abeta and memory in the Tg2576 mouse model of Alzheimer's disease. *J. Neurosci*. 2002;22: 1858-1867.

[148] Mucke, L., Masliah, E., Yu, G. Q., Mallory, M., Rockenstein, E. M., Tatsuno, G., Hu, K., Kholodenko, D., Johnson-Wood, K., McConlogue, L. High-level neuronal expression of abeta 1-42 in wild-type human amyloid protein precursor transgenic mice: synaptotoxicity without plaque formation. *J. Neurosci*. 2000;20: 4050-4058.

[149] Murakami, K., Yokoyama, S., Murata, N., Ozawa, Y., Irie, K., Shirasawa, T., Shimizu, T. Insulin receptor mutation results in insulin resistance and hyperinsulinemia but does not exacerbate Alzheimer's-like phenotypes in mice. *Biochem. Biophys. Res. Commun*. 2011;409: 34-39.

[150] Karl, T., Bhatia, S., Cheng, D., Kim, W. S., Garner, B. Cognitive phenotyping of amyloid precursor protein transgenic J20 mice. *Behav. Brain Res*. 2012;228: 392-397.

[151] Lustbader, J. W., Cirilli, M., Lin, C., Xu, H. W., Takuma, K., Wang, N., Caspersen, C., Chen, X., Pollak, S., Chaney, M., Trinchese, F., Liu, S., Gunn-Moore, F., Lue, L. F., Walker, D. G., Kuppusamy, P., Zewier, Z. L., Arancio, O., Stern, D., Yan, S. S., Wu, H. ABAD directly links Abeta to mitochondrial toxicity in Alzheimer's disease. *Science* 2004;304: 448-452.

[152] Du, H., Guo, L., Zhang, W., Rydzewska, M., Yan, S. Cyclophilin D deficiency improves mitochondrial function and learning/memory in aging Alzheimer disease mouse model. *Neurobiol. Aging* 2011;32: 398-406.

[153] Fang, F., Chen, X., Huang, T., Lue, L. F., Luddy, J. S., Yan, S. S. Multi-faced neuroprotective effects of Ginsenoside Rg1 in an Alzheimer mouse model. *Biochim. Biophys. Acta* 2012;1822: 286-292.

[154] Cheng, I. H., Scearce-Levie, K., Legleiter, J., Palop, J. J., Gerstein, H., Bien-Ly, N., Puolivali, J., Lesne, S., Ashe, K. H., Muchowski, P. J., Mucke, L. Accelerating amyloid-beta fibrillization reduces oligomer levels and functional deficits in Alzheimer disease mouse models. *J. Biol. Chem*. 2007;282: 23818-23828.

[155] Palop, J. J., Jones, B., Kekonius, L., Chin, J., Yu, G. Q., Raber, J., Masliah, E., Mucke, L. Neuronal depletion of calcium-dependent proteins in the dentate gyrus is tightly linked to Alzheimer's disease-related cognitive deficits. *Proc. Natl. Acad. Sci. US* 2003; 100: 9572-9577.

[156] Galvan, V., Gorostiza, O. F., Banwait, S., Ataie, M., Logvinova, A. V., Sitaraman, S., Carlson, E., Sagi, S. A., Chevallier, N., Jin, K., Greenberg, D. A., Bredesen, D. E. Reversal of Alzheimer's-like pathology and behavior in human APP transgenic mice by mutation of Asp664. *Proc. Natl. Acad. Sci. US* 2006;103: 7130-7135.

[157] Games, D., Adams, D., Alessandrini, R., Barbour, R., Berthelette, P., Blackwell, C., Carr, T., Clemens, J., Donaldson, T., Gillespie, F. et al. Alzheimer-type neuropathology in transgenic mice overexpressing V717F beta-amyloid precursor protein. *Nature* 1995; 373: 523-527.

[158] Dodart, J. C., Bales, K. R., Gannon, K. S., Greene, S. J., DeMattos, R. B., Mathis, C., DeLong, C. A., Wu, S., Wu, X., Holtzman, D. M., Paul, S. M. Immunization reverses memory deficits without reducing brain Abeta burden in Alzheimer's disease model. *Nat. Neurosci.* 2002;5: 452-457.

[159] Chen, G., Chen, K. S., Knox, J., Inglis, J., Bernard, A., Martin, S. J., Justice, A., McConlogue, L., Games, D., Freedman, S. B., Morris, R. G. A learning deficit related to age and beta-amyloid plaques in a mouse model of Alzheimer's disease. *Nature* 2000;408: 975-979.

[160] Nilsson, L. N., Arendash, G. W., Leighty, R. E., Costa, D. A., Low, M. A., Garcia, M. F., Cracciolo, J. R., Rojiani, A., Wu, X., Bales, K. R., Paul, S. M., Potter, H. Cognitive impairment in PDAPP mice depends on ApoE and ACT-catalyzed amyloid formation. *Neurobiol. Aging* 2004;25: 1153-1167.

[161] Dineley, K. T., Xia, X., Bui, D., Sweatt, J. D., Zheng, H. Accelerated plaque accumulation, associative learning deficits, and up-regulation of alpha 7 nicotinic receptor protein in transgenic mice co-expressing mutant human presenilin 1 and amyloid precursor proteins. *J. Biol. Chem.* 2002;277: 22768-22780.

[162] Hartman, R. E., Izumi, Y., Bales, K. R., Paul, S. M., Wozniak, D. F., Holtzman, D. M. Treatment with an amyloid-beta antibody ameliorates plaque load, learning deficits, and hippocampal long-term potentiation in a mouse model of Alzheimer's disease. *J. Neurosci.* 2005;25: 6213-6220.

[163] Dodart, J. C., Meziane, H., Mathis, C., Bales, K. R., Paul, S. M., Ungerer, A. Behavioral disturbances in transgenic mice overexpressing the V717F beta-amyloid precursor protein. *Behav. Neurosci.* 1999;113: 982-990.

[164] Prut, L., Abramowski, D., Krucker, T., Levy, C. L., Roberts, A. J., Staufenbiel, M., Wiessner, C. Aged APP23 mice show a delay in switching to the use of a strategy in the Barnes maze. *Behav. Brain Res.* 2007;179: 107-110.

[165] Lalonde, R., Dumont, M., Staufenbiel, M., Sturchler-Pierrat, C., Strazielle, C. Spatial learning, exploration, anxiety, and motor coordination in female APP23 transgenic mice with the Swedish mutation. *Brain Res.* 2002;956: 36-44.

[166] Chishti, M. A., Yang, D. S., Janus, C., Phinney, A. L., Horne, P., Pearson, J., Strome, R., Zuker, N., Loukides, J., French, J., Turner, S., Lozza, G., Grilli, M., Kunicki, S., Morissette, C., Paquette, J., Gervais, F., Bergeron, C., Fraser, P. E., Carlson, G. A., George-Hyslop, P. S., Westaway, D. Early-onset amyloid deposition and cognitive deficits in transgenic mice expressing a double mutant form of amyloid precursor protein 695. *J. Biol. Chem.* 2001;276: 21562-21570.

[167] Kelly, P. H., Bondolfi, L., Hunziker, D., Schlecht, H. P., Carver, K., Maguire, E., Abramowski, D., Wiederhold, K. H., Sturchler-Pierrat, C., Jucker, M., Bergmann, R., Staufenbiel, M., Sommer, B. Progressive age-related impairment of cognitive behavior in APP23 transgenic mice. *Neurobiol. Aging* 2003;24: 365-378.

[168] Hyde, L. A., Kazdoba, T. M., Grilli, M., Lozza, G., Brusa, R., Zhang, Q., Wong, G. T., McCool, M. F., Zhang, L., Parker, E. M., Higgins, G. A. Age-progressing cognitive

impairments and neuropathology in transgenic CRND8 mice. *Behav. Brain Res.* 2005; 160: 344-355.

[169] Hanna, A., Iremonger, K., Das, P., Dickson, D., Golde, T., Janus, C. Age-related increase in amyloid plaque burden is associated with impairment in conditioned fear memory in CRND8 mouse model of amyloidosis. *Alzheimers Res. Ther.* 2012;4: 21.

[170] Gortz, N., Lewejohann, L., Tomm, M., Ambree, O., Keyvani, K., Paulus, W., Sachser, N. Effects of environmental enrichment on exploration, anxiety, and memory in female TgCRND8 Alzheimer mice. *Behav. Brain Res.* 2008;191: 43-48.

[171] Janus, C. Search strategies used by APP transgenic mice during navigation in the Morris water maze. *Learn. Mem.* 2004;11: 337-346.

[172] Saura, C. A., Chen, G., Malkani, S., Choi, S. Y., Takahashi, R. H., Zhang, D., Gouras, G. K., Kirkwood, A., Morris, R. G., Shen, J. Conditional inactivation of presenilin 1 prevents amyloid accumulation and temporarily rescues contextual and spatial working memory impairments in amyloid precursor protein transgenic mice. *J. Neurosci.* 2005; 25: 6755-6764.

[173] Ambree, O., Richter, H., Sachser, N., Lewejohann, L., Dere, E., de Souza Silva, M. A., Herring, A., Keyvani, K., Paulus, W., Schabitz, W. R. Levodopa ameliorates learning and memory deficits in a murine model of Alzheimer's disease. *Neurobiol. Aging* 2009; 30: 1192-1204.

[174] Richter, H., Ambree, O., Lewejohann, L., Herring, A., Keyvani, K., Paulus, W., Palme, R., Touma, C., Schabitz, W. R., Sachser, N. Wheel-running in a transgenic mouse model of Alzheimer's disease: protection or symptom? *Behav. Brain Res.* 2008;190: 74-84.

[175] Lovasic, L., Bauschke, H., Janus, C. Working memory impairment in a transgenic amyloid precursor protein TgCRND8 mouse model of Alzheimer's disease. *Genes Brain Behav.* 2005;4: 197-208.

[176] Hanna, A., Horne, P., Yager, D., Eckman, C., Eckman, E., Janus, C. Amyloid beta and impairment in multiple memory systems in older transgenic APP TgCRND8 mice. *Genes Brain Behav.* 2009;8: 676-684.

In: Spatial, Long-and Short-Term Memory
Editor: Edward A. Thayer

ISBN: 978-1-63484-148-1

Chapter 2

AMPA RECEPTOR SUBUNIT CONTRIBUTION TO HIPPOCAMPAL-MEDIATED SPATIAL MEMORY

Niko Tzakis* and Matthew R. Holahan
Department of Neuroscience, Carleton University, Ottawa, ON, Canada

ABSTRACT

The ability to acquire and utilize spatial memory representations in the brain is key for successful navigation through novel and familiar environments. This ability is critically dependent on cellular, synaptic and systems mechanisms within medial temporal lobe structures of the mammalian brain. One such structure, the hippocampus, appears to play an important role in integrating relationships amongst stimuli in the environment, forming neural representations of those relationships and utilizing that information to navigate seamlessly through a variety of surroundings. For efficient navigation, synaptic responses within the hippocampus should show potentiated responses when presented with either novel or familiar spatial cues. A key feature underlying this ability, and an important cellular mechanism of memory and spatial memory specifically, is long-term potentiation (LTP). LTP describes a process whereby increases in the strength of synapses lead to highly efficient signal transmission between neurons and through neural networks. The induction of LTP nominally requires the interplay between N-methyl-D-aspartate receptors (NMDAr) and α-amino-3-hydroxy-5-methylisoxazole-4-propionic acid receptors (AMPAr) while the expression of LTP appears to be largely dependent on changes in AMPAr composition. The current chapter examines the importance of the AMPAr and its specific subunits (GluR1 – GluR4) in LTP processes as well as the formation and utilization of spatial memory representations. A summary of *in vitro* work will be provided to examine how different subunit compositions of the AMPAr contribute to the induction and expression of LTP. This will be compared and contrasted with work examining *in vivo* hippocampal AMPAr subunit manipulations and outcomes on spatial behavioral processes.

* Corresponding author: Niko Tzakis. Carleton University, 1125 Colonel By Drive, 325 Life Sciences Research Building, Ottawa, ON K1S 5B6 Canada. Tel: 613-520-2600 ext 1543, fax: 613-520-3667, e-mail: nikolaostzakis@cmail.carleton.ca.

INTRODUCTION

Overview of Consolidation

Synaptic consolidation involves neural and biochemical processes that work to reorganize synapses once learning has taken place. Consolidation involving cellular events, known as cellular consolidation, has been hypothesized to be responsible for transforming an initially labile memory to a more permanent representation (McGaugh 2000). Once this has taken place, memories undergo what is classified as systems consolidation whereby a memory, for example, initially begins as being hippocampus-dependent to one that is hippocampus-independent (Meeter and Murre 2004, Rudy and Sutherland 2008). In this model, systems consolidation theory is based on the idea that the hippocampus serves only as a temporary repository of memories (Frankland and Bontempi 2005). The systems consolidation model posits that after some time has elapsed (months to years), the memory initially processed within the hippocampus is "transferred" to the neocortex via hippocampal-neocortical connections. Although no exact timeframe is known outlining the amount of time required for a memory to transfer from one brain region to another, it appears that remotely stored memories come to be stored in and retrieved by neural circuits in the frontal lobe (Frankland and Bontempi 2005). Within the frontal lobe circuits, cellular consolidation stabilizes the memory and strengthens both the memory representation within the frontal lobe circuits and connections made with the hippocampus in order to facilitate retrieval of the memory (Meeter and Murre 2004). As the memory trace stored in the neocortical region strengthens, the memory representation weakens within the hippocampus (Meeter and Murre 2004).

Cellular Consolidation

Cellular consolidation, also known as synaptic consolidation, is a process through which synapses are strengthened, and memory representations are stabilized, by cellular and molecular processes within the hippocampus and other brain regions (Mednick et al. 2011, Rudy and Sutherland 2008). The conversion of short-term memories into long-term ones involves the synthesis of new proteins, which allow for persistent modifications in synaptic functions (Debiec et al. 2002). Dudai (2004) explains synaptic consolidation as being triggered by receptor activation leading to a series of intracellular signal transduction cascades such as the upregulation of adenylate cyclase that activates cyclic adenosine monophosphate (cAMP).

The initiation of intracellular signal transduction cascades that lead to the expression of certain transcription factors occurs during and immediately after training, which corresponds to synaptic consolidation (Dudai, 2004). cAMP-dependent kinases initiate phosphorylating and activating isoforms of cAMP-response element binding proteins (CREBs). CREBs then allow for a modification of the cAMP response element (CRE) – regulated genes, including transcription factors that regulate the expression of genes whose products are induced after a few hours, known as late-response genes (Dudai 2004). In general, these cascades modulate long-term synaptic proteins and synaptic modeling and growth, along with regulating gene expression through the activation of transcription factors (Dudai 2004).

In addition to structural modifications of the synapse, the synthesis of neuronal proteins appears to be required for functional changes to the synapse.

Newly modified synaptic proteins tag the activated synapse, which attract new proteins from the cell through a reorganization of the synapse (Dudai 2004). In addition, proteins synthesized in the synapse may function to enhance and fortify the synaptic tagging, while acting as retrograde messages that inform the nucleus of the change.

The tagged synapses also receive newly synthesized messenger RNAs and proteins via modulation of gene expression in the nucleus. This coordination between the synapse and the nucleus is thought to enhance the specificity of the consolidation process (Dudai 2004).

Systems Consolidation

One hypothesis of systems consolidation suggests a transformation of memories from being hippocampus-dependent to hippocampus-independent. Specifically, systems consolidation posits that, initially, new memories are temporarily stored in the hippocampus and neocortical regions that it projects to. The hippocampus strengthens the initially weak connections within the hippocampal-neocortical network, and after continuous activation of those connections, the new memory trace integrates with pre-existing memories within the neocortex, and the memory storage or retrieval becomes independent from the hippocampus (Mednick et al. 2011, Wang and Morris 2010, Rudy and Sutherland 2007).

As opposed to cellular consolidation, which is achieved within minutes to hours, systems consolidation processes are achieved over a period of weeks, months, or even years (Dudai 2004). Research supporting the systems consolidation theory includes functional magnetic resonance imaging studies, which have shown that blood flow to the hippocampus appears to be higher for semantic memory recall of news events within the past 3 years compared to older news events (Smith and Squire 2009, Wang and Morris 2010). Additionally, Takashima et al. (2006) found reduced hippocampal activity during memory recall tasks for memories that were 90 days old compared to memories that were 1 day old (Wang and Morris 2010). These results indicate that the hippocampus is responsible for the storage and/or retrieval of the initial memory, but then storage/retrieval is mediated by other brain structures.

Systems consolidation begins with the initial encoding of the memory within the hippocampal and neocortical system, with the hippocampal system possessing the stronger initial memory trace.

Through memory recall, the hippocampal-neocortical traces become successively activated and reactivated, which leads to the strengthening of existing neocortical memory, either through adjustments of neocortical connections involving cellular consolidation, or through the establishment of new connections within the neocortex. This strengthening allows the memory trace to integrate with pre-existing memories within the neocortex (Dudai 2004, Frankland and Bontempi 2005).

Concurrently, the memory traces within the hippocampal system gradually degrade, resulting in the traces becoming independent from the hippocampus. In this view of systems consolidation, the hippocampus can be seen as ‘teaching’ the neocortex about the information stored in the memory, while freeing up space through degradation to allow for rapid learning of new information without disrupting the memory reservoirs within the neocortex (Dudai 2004).

Memory Retrieval

Memory retrieval involves the expression and reactivation of a memory trace, usually triggered by some external stimulus or cue (Cai 1990, Lopez et al. 2015). It was previously thought that memory retrieval was a passive process, but a recent study has shown that it is, in fact, a very dynamic process (Lopez et al. 2015). Memory retrieval has been shown to be dependent on the activation of α-amino-3-hydroxy-5-methylisoxazole-4-propionic acid (AMPA) and metabotropic glutamate (mGluR) receptors, but not N-methyl-D-aspartate (NMDA) receptors. Evidently, inactivating AMPA receptors before undergoing a memory retrieval task has been shown to diminish recall. In addition to AMPA receptor blockade, the use of mGluR antagonists has also prevented the retrieval of contextual fear memories (Szapiro et al. 2002). Systemically injecting rapamycin or anisomycin, which act to inhibit protein synthesis, impaired auditory fear memory recall, and decreased postsynaptic AMPA receptor GluA1 levels. This suggests that, in addition to glutamatergic receptor activation, ongoing protein synthesis is required for memory recall (Lopez et al. 2015).

From a systems view, memory retrieval involves the coordination and activation of different regions in the brain. Positron emission tomography (PET) studies have revealed the involvement of several brain regions including the right prefrontal cortex, the hippocampus and parahippocampus, the anterior and posterior cingulate cortices, the inferior parietal cortex, and the left side of the cerebellum during an episodic retrieval word recognition task (Cabeza et al. 1997, Nyberg et al. 1995). These results suggest the presence of a general episodic retrieval network, composed of the aforementioned brain regions (Nyberg et al. 1995). Although the specific contribution that each of these regions make to the retrieval of memory is unclear, the role of certain brain regions has been postulated. The right prefrontal cortex has been shown to contribute to retrieval attempts, while the hippocampus allows for conscious recollection, and the cerebellum plays a role in self-initiated retrieval (Cabeza et al. 1997).

Spatial Memory

The ability for humans and animals to navigate around their environment, record information about their spatial orientation, and remember any event that may have occurred within that environment has been credited to spatial memory. Integrating and processing sensory cues from the environment to facilitate navigation through that environment requires spatial working memory processes. A number of factors contribute to spatial memory and successful navigation. Factors such as dimensionality (knowledge of the 3-dimensional elements of the environment), orientation, and self-motion, which informs the individual of any changes in the orientation of spatial representation of the environment all need to be integrated for successful navigation (Burgess et al. 2002).

Though a resilient and dynamic process, spatial memory is not impervious to impairment. In fact, one of the first symptoms presented by patients with pathologies such as Alzheimer's has been shown to be impairments of spatial and episodic memory, brought about by cumulative damage to medial temporal lobe structures (Burgess et al. 2002).

One of the more popular approaches to measuring spatial memory and spatial navigation in rats and humans has been the Morris Water Maze.

Conceived by Richard Morris in the 1980s, the water maze procedure was used to understand the fundamental basis of spatial and working memory and to differentiate spatial learning from other forms of associative learning (Morris 1984). Implementing the water maze has given new insight into the neurobiology of spatial learning and memory. Although rodents are natural swimmers, the motivation to escape from water can be used as an incentive for learning (Morris 1984). The basic procedure of the water maze involves an acquisition training phase, where the spatial memory is acquired, and a testing phase, which tests the retention of that memory. The training phase begins with a circular pool filled with water and a platform hidden just beneath the surface of the water, enough so that the surface of the platform is accessible but not visible to the rodent. The subject is then placed into the pool and allowed to swim freely about the pool. The goal is for the subject to locate the platform by learning the spatial position of the platform relative to distal cues. Although the subject initially finds the platform 'accidentally' by swimming randomly, learning becomes evident when the subject is able to swim directly towards the platform from any starting position (Morris 1984). The testing phase implements the same procedure as the training phase, but the platform is removed from the pool. An intact memory is assessed based on the spatial accuracy of the subject, represented by the amount of time the subject spends in the area associated with the platform location (Morris 1984, D'Hooge and De Deyn 2001). A subject that has successfully acquired and retained the spatial memory will show a high preference for the area associated with the platform, spending an average of 50% or more of its swimming time in the target area (D'Hooge and De Deyn 2001). The use of more sophisticated tracking devices allows for a measurement and quantification of thigmotaxis, speed, latency, and direction.

Hippocampal Contribution to Spatial Memory

While many brain regions have been implicated in spatial memory acquisition and retention, the hippocampus appears to be the region most involved in those processes. O'Keefe and Nadel (1978) postulated the existence of a cognitive map and identified it within the hippocampus. According to them, the cognitive map is made up of a place system, which contains information about places and objects in the environmental surroundings of the organism, along with their spatial relation within that environment, and a misplace system, which signals changes within the environment. The place system allows an organism to explore and locate itself within a familiar environment independent of particular cues, while the misplace system builds maps of new environments and incorporates new information into existing maps (O'Keefe and Nadel 1978). This model suggests that animals formulate and test hypotheses to find solutions to a problem, which may involve approaching or avoiding places in their environment based on information processed in their hippocampal cognitive mapping system (O'Keefe and Nadel 1978). The hippocampus possesses specialized pyramidal cells, known as place cells, which encode the location of an organism within their environment (Muir and Bilkey 2001). These place cells increase their firing rate when the individual enters a particular place in the environment, known as the place field. The location of the place field of a place cell remains stable in a familiar environment, even when the individual is removed from that environment for extended periods of time. Thus, activation of place cells may indicate that the individual perceives the environment as familiar (Muir and Bilkey 2001).

Place cells where first discovered by O'Keefe and Dostrovsky (1971) while recording hippocampal cells. They found that the only time the cells produced any activity was when the rat was pointing in a particular direction, and that both the orientation and specific stimuli in that direction were required to produce a response. Any other stimulus in that same direction produced no cellular response (O'Keefe and Dostrovsky 1971). Rats with hippocampal damage showed difficulty navigating their way around mazes and tasks which required alteration of responses on successive trials, which may be due to the loss of these places cells (O'Keefe and Dostrovsky 1971). They concluded that the hippocampus provided the rest of the brain with a spatial reference map, and that the activity of the place cells would specify the orientation that the subject was in based on the landmarks that were present in the environment and the presentation of stimuli while facing in that direction. Further, they postulated that the spatial memory deficits experienced by rats with hippocampal lesions were attributed to the loss of their spatial reference map (O'Keefe and Dostrovsky 1971).

In addition to place cells, hippocampal-dependent spatial memory requires the activation of *c-fos*, an immediate early gene that is part of the activator protein-1 transcription factor (Fleischmann et al. 2003). *c-fos* has been shown to be involved in the molecular mechanisms of learning and memory, such as synaptic plasticity (Fleischmann et al. 2003). These genes also play a role in the consolidation of short-term memory into long-term stores based on the fact that they are expressed during acquisition and the early phases of memory consolidation (Tischmeyer and Grimm 1999). Several pharmacological studies have further strengthened the correlation between *c-fos* expression and memory formation. One study implementing a post-training application of apamine, a toxin that facilitates memory processing, showed an increase in training-induced *c-fos* expression (Tischmeyer and Grimm 1999, Messier et al. 1991). Similarly, Zhou et al. (1995) saw enhanced *c-fos* expression in the hippocampus of rats after injecting them with AVP (4–8), a metabolite of arginine-vasopressin that facilitates the acquisition of memory. Conversely, mice with a nervous system-specific *c-fos* knock-out showed impairments in various hippocampal-dependent spatial memory tasks, which were correlated with a reduction of long-term potentiation (LTP). These results suggest a role for *c-fos* in spatial memory formation (Fleischmann et al. 2003).

Further evidence for hippocampal contribution to spatial memory can be found in hippocampal lesion studies. Morris et al. (1982) performed a study where they removed the entire dorsal and ventral hippocampus by aspiration lesion in rats then subjected them to the Morris water maze task. In doing so, they discovered that the hippocampal-lesioned rats showed a highly significant impairment in the task measured by longer routes to find the hidden platform, compared to control rats. They concluded that hippocampal lesions caused a severe place-navigational impairment (Morris et al. 1982).

Additionally, Lavenex et al. (2006) performed bilateral hippocampal ibotenic acid lesions on macaque monkeys, who then performed various spatial relational tasks. They discovered that monkeys that received hippocampal lesions were unable to discriminate between different food locations in the absence of local cues.

This indicated that the hippocampal lesion impaired their ability to use spatial relational representations of their environment to discriminate between the different food locations (Lavenex et al. 2006). Studies involving hippocampal inactivation can also give insight into the hippocampal contribution to spatial memory. Poe et al. (2000) used tetracaine, a potent local anesthetic, to inactivate one or both hippocampal hemispheres in aged and young rats, before putting them through the radial arm maze task.

They discovered that bilateral and unilateral left hippocampal inactivation impaired the performance of the rats on the task, while unilateral right hippocampal inactivation had no effect on performance (Poe et al. 2000). Because inactivation of both hippocampal hemispheres caused a dysfunction in spatial memory processing, it suggested that the hippocampus plays a significant role in those processes. Additionally, the asymmetrical response of the hippocampal impairment indicates that the left hippocampus may be more involved in spatial working memory processes (Poe et al. 2000).

Anatomy of the Hippocampus

The hippocampal structure as a whole does not work as one cohesive unit, but instead may be split up into different subunits with various functions. The two major units of the hippocampus are the dorsal hippocampus and the ventral hippocampus. There remains some debate, however, as to which part of the hippocampus is more important for spatial memories, the dorsal or the ventral. One hypothesis suggests that the dorsal hippocampus is more involved in the memory process due to the fact that place fields in this region are more confined, as opposed to the ventral hippocampus, where the place fields are more dispersed (Jung et al. 1994, Faneslow and Dong 2010).

A study completed by Moser et al. (1993) supports this theory. After performing localized hippocampal aspiration lesions and testing rats in the Morris water maze, they observed an impaired acquisition rate and precision on the probe test in the rats that received lesions in their dorsal hippocampus, ultimately leading to diminished spatial learning. The rats that received lesions in their ventral hippocampus, however, experienced no such impedance in their spatial learning abilities.

Based on these results, they concluded that the dorsal hippocampus is more important for the encoding of new spatial information than the ventral aspect (Moser et al. 1993, Riedel and Micheau 2001).

Further evidence to support this theory comes from studies completed by Moser et al. (1995) and Pothuizen et al. (2004), who observed that hippocampal-dependent learning is impeded if the dorsal portion of the hippocampus is lesioned, and, interestingly, that dorsal hippocampal lesions were just as effective as complete hippocampal lesions in disrupting working memory, as opposed to lesions in the ventral hippocampus, which showed no effect on working memory.

Subregions of the Dorsal Hippocampus

The dorsal hippocampus consists of three major regions; the dentate gyrus, the cornu ammonis (CA) fields, which consist of pyramidal cells and are subdivided into four regions (CA1 – CA4), and the parahippocampal gyrus (Amaral 1993, Cohen et al. 1999, Wible 2013). The parahippocampal gyrus can be further broken down into three subregions, which include the subiculum, the entorhinal cortex, and the perirhinal cortex. The perirhinal and parahippocampal cortices are the first structures to receive input, generally from the temporal, frontal, and parietal lobes (Lavenex and Amaral 2000). They then integrate and process sensory information and transmit it to the second stage of processing, in the entorhinal cortex.

The entorhinal cortex is thought to process sensory information with a higher level of associativity, allowing for an increase in the level of integration of information (Lavenex and Amaral 2000).

The perforant pathway begins with the entorhinal cortex sending glutamatergic projections to the dentate gyrus, which has an abundance of both NMDA and AMPA receptors, resulting in the activation of the trisynaptic pathway in the hippocampus. The first synapse in this pathway bypasses the dentate gyrus and sends direct inputs from the entorhinal cortex to the CA3 region, which contains numerous kainate receptors (Naber et al. 1999). The second synapse in the pathway projects from the dentate gyrus to the dendrites of CA3 pyramidal cells via mossy fibres. The third synapse projects glutamatergic inputs from pyramidal cells in the CA3 region to pyramidal cells in the CA1 region via Schaffer collaterals (Neves et al. 2008).

In addition to receiving input from cortical regions, the entorhinal cortex receives output from the CA1 layer via the subiculum, which then projects to other brain regions, such as the mamillary nuclei, the thalamus, and the nucleus accumbens (Amaral 1993, Wible 2013).

The Occurrence of LTP in the Hippocampus

Some neurons are able to continuously form new, stronger connections while simultaneously eliminating weaker connections in response to information processing demands. As a result of these constant changes, neurons must garner the ability to adapt, but also remain somewhat stable, in response to intrinsic and extrinsic signals, a process known as neural plasticity (Wainwright and Galea 2013). This plasticity permits adaptability in a network, regulates future experience-dependent plasticity, and, most importantly for memory, contributes to the formation of a memory trace within the brain (Sehgal et al. 2013). Santiago Ramon y Cajal was the first to postulate that the changes in the strength of synaptic connections between active neurons form the basis of the coding and storage of memories (Lynch 2004). Later, this came to be known as "Hebbian plasticity," which suggests that memory formation results from strengthening synaptic connections between pre- and post-synaptic neurons that are activated simultaneously (Hebb 1949, Bliss and Collingridge 1993, Johansen et al. 2014).

One important cellular mechanism of learning and memory, and a feature of neural plasticity, is LTP. The occurrence of LTP has been observed in several brain regions, from subcortical to cortical regions, and from brain regions involved in basic survival mechanisms, to those underlying higher cognitive and perceptual processes (Lynch 2004). First described in 1973, LTP describes how increased efficiency of synaptic transmission results from the concurrent activation of both pre- and post-synaptic elements (Bliss and Lomo 1973, Bliss and Collingridge 1993, Cooke and Bliss 2006). LTP is usually induced by a series of high-frequency stimuli, known as tetani, at 100 Hz or more. There is an intensity threshold that must be reached in order to induce LTP; failure to reach that threshold will not trigger LTP. However, Kelso et al. (1986), found that a weak stimulus can induce LTP as long as it is active at the same time as a strong tetanus, and as long as they converge on the same input. Gustaffson et al. (1987) also performed an experiment whereby they paired an excitatory postsynaptic potential (EPSP) formed by a weak stimulus (0.15-0.1 Hz) in the stratum radiatum with depolarizing current pulses. They found that potentiation occurred, as long as the EPSP and current pulse occurred no more than 100 milliseconds apart from each other and that no potentiation occurred if the EPSP came after the pulse. This property of LTP, known as the 'associative' property, suggests that LTP is a possible neuronal underpinning for learning and memory, as it allows associations to be made at the cellular level (Gustaffson et al. 1987, Cooke and Bliss 2006).

LTP is known to have two phases; an early phase, which lasts 2 to 3 hours and is protein synthesis independent, and a long-lasting phase, which can last several hours *in vitro* and weeks *in vivo* and requires protein synthesis.

Interestingly, it has been shown that the retention of long-term memories requires gene expression, protein synthesis, and new synaptic connections (Lynch 2004).

Excitatory Connections in Hippocampal Subregions

The importance of the associative property of LTP becomes evident when examining the role of NMDA receptors in the induction of LTP. One feature of NMDA receptors is that their channels are blocked by a voltage-dependent Mg^{+2} ion. When a single, weak stimulus is applied, it is typically not sufficient to depolarize the membrane and displace the Mg^{+2} block. If, however, a strong stimulus is applied via activation of multiple inputs, there will be a depolarization of the membrane releasing the Mg^{+2} block. The coincident release of the Mg^{+2} block and glutamate binding causes Ca^{+2} to enter the cell. The subsequent influx of Ca^{+2} induces LTP and activates a series of intracellular signaling cascades. Those cascades lead to the activation of immediate early genes, such as *c-fos*, which, among other processes, regulate synaptic protein synthesis (Fleischmann et al. 2003).

Using the competitive NMDA receptor antagonist DL-2-amino-5-phosphonovalerate (AP5) lead to the discovery of the involvement of the NMDA receptor in the induction of LTP (Collingridge et al. 1983, Harris et al. 1984, Monaghan et al. 1989).

A study completed by Morris et al. (1986) blocked NMDA receptors in the hippocampus using AP5, which ultimately prevented the induction of hippocampal LTP. They discovered that preventing LTP impaired place learning, adding further support to the involvement of LTP in learning (Morris et al. 1986). Additional studies have confirmed these findings by inhibiting NMDA receptors with noncompetitive antagonists, such as phencyclidine (PCP) and ketamine (Stringer et al. 1983, Monaghan et al. 1989).

In order to assess the potential role of NMDA receptors in memory expression, Steele and Morris (1999) infused the hippocampus of rats with the NMDA receptor antagonist, D-AP5, before a retrieval test on a Morris Water Maze. They discovered that NMDA receptor blockade did not seem to impede memory retrieval, indicating that, although there is strong evidence for the involvement of NMDA receptors in acquiring and consolidating memories, they do not seem to be involved in memory retrieval (Steele and Morris 1999, Szapiro et al. 2002).

The CA1 region of the hippocampus possesses the highest concentration of NMDA receptors in the brain (Wible 2013). These receptors are permeable to Ca^{+2}, sodium, and potassium ions, but it is the increase in intracellular Ca^{+2} ions that is thought to be responsible for NMDA receptor-induced plasticity in the brain (Monaghan et al. 1989). Although NMDA receptors are extensively studied for their role in learning and memory, they are not the only receptor types that contribute to those processes.

Kainate receptors, as well as quisqualate receptors, which are now known as AMPA receptors, also have an important function in mediating information processing in the hippocampus. NMDA and AMPA receptors are colocalized, and thus like NMDA receptors, one of the highest areas of concentration of AMPA receptor binding sites is in the CA1 stratum radiatum region of the hippocampus, an area that contains Schaffer collaterals and is one of the main sites for observing LTP (Cotman et al. 1988, Monaghan et al. 1989).

AMPA Contribution to LTP

While NMDA receptors are important during the induction phase of LTP, activation of AMPA receptors seem to be critical during both the induction and expression phases of LTP. As previously mentioned, the influx of Ca^{+2} through the NMDA receptors activates a series of intracellular signaling cascades, which act as secondary messengers. Those secondary messengers include Ca^{+2}-calmodulin-dependent protein kinase II (CAMKII), which function to phosphorylate the AMPA receptors, increasing their sensitivity to glutamate, while inserting more AMPA receptors into the post-synaptic membrane.

In mature hippocampal pyramidal cells, AMPA receptors are made up of four homologous subunits, from GluR1 to GluR4, with GluR1 and GluR2 or GluR2 and GluR3 being the predominate combination of subunits (Song and Huganir 2002, Malinow and Malenka 2002). Of the four different subunits, studies have provided evidence to suggest that the GluR1 subunit is the most important in terms of the expression of LTP. Studies that have used genetic knockout mice lacking the GluR1 subunit have shown that, while glutamatergic synaptic transmission is unaffected, these mice do not express LTP in the Schaffer collateral region of the hippocampus, indicating the importance of AMPA receptors in LTP expression (Jensen et al. 2003).

Additional evidence supporting this finding comes from a study by Sanderson et al. (2010), who found that spatial working memory was hindered in knockout mice lacking the GluR1 subunit, suggesting that hippocampal synaptic plasticity was impaired and that the GluR1 subunit of the AMPA receptor is required for short-term spatial working memory tasks. Szapiro et al. (2000) antagonized AMPA receptors 10 minutes before testing subjects on a memory recall task. They found that the pre-test blocking of AMPA receptors resulted in impaired retrieval, suggesting that AMPA receptors played a role in the expression of long-term memories. Similarly, Riedel et al. (1999) antagonized AMPA receptors during training and before testing, or before testing alone on the Morris Water Maze. They discovered that rats whose AMPA receptors were blocked during training and before testing performed poorly during both occasions and the rats whose receptors were blocked before testing spent less time in the quadrant associated with the platform, even though they were trained with fully functioning AMPA receptors. These results indicate that the AMPA receptors play a role in the encoding, consolidating, and retrieval of memories (Meeter and Murre 2004, Szapiro et al. 2002, Riedel et al. 1999).

As previously mentioned, the underlying mechanism that mediates AMPA GluR1 subunit function and importance in terms of generating LTP lies in its ability to be phosphorylated, which enhances the function of the AMPA receptor ion channel. The GluR1 subunit possesses two sites that can be phosphorylated, Serine 831 (Ser831) and Serine 845 (Ser845), which are found at the intracellular C-terminus.

Ser831 is phosphorylated by Ca^{+2}-calmodulin-dependent protein kinase II (CaMKII) and protein kinase C (PKC), while Ser845 is phosphorylated by cAMP-dependent protein kinase A (PKA). Once the receptor sites are phosphorylated, the AMPA receptor shows increased conductance during LTP expression (Lee et al., 2003, Song and Huganir 2002, Malinow and Malenka 2002). Out of the two phosphorylation sites, an increase in Ser831 phosphorylation is most probably associated with LTP expression, while long-term depression (LTD) is associated more so with the dephosphorylation of the Ser845 site.

In addition, Lee et al. (2000) observed that, upon expression of LTP, there was a significant increase in Ser831 phosphorylation, while there was no significant increase in Ser845 phosphorylation. These findings are consistent with the notion that GluR1 phosphorylation is responsible for the expression of LTP and LTD, as well spatial memory retention (Lee et al. 2000, Lee et al. 2003).

Not only does the phosphorylation of the AMPA GluR1 receptor subunit mediate LTP and LTD expression, but it has also been found to contribute to the retention of spatial memories. Genetically substituting the Ser831 and Ser845 sites with alanine in mice prevented phosphorylation of these sites, which inhibited both LTD and LTP. However, in addition to blocking LTP and LTD expression, these mutations interrupted the retention of a spatial memory task; the mice were able to remember the new location of the platform in the Morris water maze task after a short delay, but were unable to retain that memory in the long-term. These results suggest that the phosphorylation of the GluR1 subunit may be necessary for the retention and consolidation of spatial memories (Lee et al. 2003).

Along with GluR1, GluR2 subunits play a role in the induction of LTP. While AMPA receptors composed of GluR1, GluR3, and/or GluR4 are Ca^{+2} permeable, GluR2-containing AMPA receptors are impermeable to divalent cations, including Ca^{+2} (Isaac et al. 2007). Jia et al. (1996) further investigated the role that GluR2 played in the induction of LTP. Using mice with a GluR2 knockout mutation, they observed a 9-fold increase in Ca^{+2} permeability, which coincided with a 2-fold increase in LTP in the CA1 region of the hippocampus. These results suggest a possible modulatory role of GluR2 subunits for synaptic plasticity and behavior (Jia et al. 1996). GluR2 subunits are also thought to be important in the expression of cortical LTD, a component of learning, memory, and development. Toyoda et al. (2007) tested GluR2 knockout mice and observed an absence of LTD in adult cingulate slices of the mutant mice. Meng et al. (2003) reported similar impairments in basal synaptic transmission in mice with the GluR2 mutation, but also noted that, despite their mutation, LTD and other forms of long-lasting synaptic changes in the CA1 region of the hippocampus could still be induced in the mice. These results suggest that, while GluR2 subunits may be important in the expression of LTD, there exist GluR2-independent mechanisms of LTD expression that are activated in the wake of their absence (Meng et al. 2003).

Unlike the GluR1 and GluR2 receptor subunits, research on the GluR3 and GluR4 subunits is scarce. While it is known that GluR3 and GluR4 are involved in cognitive processes, including learning and memory, the extent of their involvement is largely unknown. One study observed a decrease in GluR3 receptor complex levels in mice that were trained on a multiple T-maze, and concluded that GluR3 complex levels cannot be linked to spatial memory (Falsafi et al. 2012). The same study found an increase in GluR4 complex levels in the hippocampus after training, which correlated with significant increases in performance on the spatial memory task, linking the GluR4 subunit to spatial memory performance (Falsafi et al. 2012).

Sagata et al. (2010) examined the role of the GluR4 subunit in synaptic plasticity by generating GluR4 knockout mice. They found that the mutant mice showed normal LTP in the CA1 region of the hippocampus, along with slight improvements in spatial working memory in the T-maze test. They also found impaired acquisition of spatial reference memory in the Barnes circular maze test, despite normal retention of that memory, suggesting the involvement of the GluR4 subunit in learning and memory processes (Sagata et al. 2010).

Conclusion

Learning and memory processes involve an interplay between cortical regions and subcortical regions, including the anterior cingulate cortex and the hippocampus, coupled with the activation of multiple neural and biochemical pathways that function to acquire, consolidate, and store the memory. The hippocampus remains the predominate brain region of interest in studies involving learning and memory, largely due to its abundance of excitatory glutamate receptors, specifically AMPA and NMDA, which are critical to the induction and expression of LTP. While GluR1 and GluR2 AMPA receptor subunits have been investigated for their role in LTP induction, further research is required to understand the contribution of GluR3 and GluR4 to learning and memory processes. Comprehending the cellular foundations of learning and memory, in conjunction with the systems that mediate those processes, allows for a greater appreciation of the intricateness of one of the most fundamental cognitive processes that exists in humans and animals alike.

References

Amaral, D. G. (1993). Emerging principles of intrinsic hippocampal organization. *Current Opinion in Neurobiology*, 3, pp. 225–229.

Bliss, T. V. and Lomo, T. (1973). Long-lasting potentiation of synaptic transmission in the dentate area of the anaesthetized rabbit following stimulation of the perforant path. *J. Physiol.*, 232(2), pp. 331–356.

Bliss, T. V. P. and Collingridge, G. L. (1993). A synaptic model of memory: long-term potentiation in the hippocampus. *Nature*, 361, pp. 31–39.

Burgess, N., Maguire, E. A. and O'Keefe, J. (2002). The human hippocampus and spatial and episodic memory. *Neuron*, 35(4), pp. 625–641.

Cabeza, R., Kapur, S., Craik, F. I. M., McIntosh, A. R., Houle, S. et al. (1997). Functional neuroanatomy of recall and recognition: a PET study of episodic memory. *Journal of Cognitive Neuroscience*, 9(2), pp. 254–265.

Cai, Z.-J. (1990). Memory consolidation and retrieval: a hypothesis. *Neuroscience and Biobehavioral Reviews*, 14, pp. 295–304.

Cohen, N. J., Ryan, J, Hunt, C., Romine, L., Wszalek, T. et al. (1999). Hippocampal system and declarative (relational memory): summarizing the data from functional neuroimaging studies. *Hippocampus*, 9, pp. 83–98.

Collingridge, G. L., Kehl, S. J. and McLennan, H. (1983). Excitatory amino acids in the Schaeffer collateral-commisural pathway of the rat hippocampus. *J. Physiol.*, 334(1), pp. 33–46.

Cooke, S. F. and Bliss, T. V. P. (2006). Plasticity in the human central nervous system. *Brain*, 129, pp. 1659–1673.

Cotman, C. W., Monaghan, D. T. and Ganong, A. H. (1988). Excitatory amino acid neurotransmission: NMDA receptors and Hebb-type synaptic plasticity. *Ann. Rev. Neurosci.*, 11, pp. 61–80.

D'Hooge, R. D. and De Deyn, P. P. (2001). Applications of the Morris water maze in the study of learning and memory. *Brain Research Reviews*, 36, pp. 60–90.

Debiec, J., LeDoux, J. E. and Nader, K. (2002). Cellular and systems reconsolidation in the hippocampus. *Neuron*, 36, pp. 527–538.

Dudai, Y. (2004). The neurobiology of consolidations, or, how stable is the engram? *Annu. Rev. Psychol.*, 55, pp. 51–86.

Falsafi, S. K., Ghafari, M., Pollak, A., Hoger, H. and Lubec, G. (2012). Hippocampal AMPA-type receptor complexes containing GluR3 and GluR4 are paralleling training in the multiple T-maze. *Neurochemistry International*, 60, pp. 425–430.

Faneslow, M. S. and Dong, H.-W. (2010). Are the dorsal and ventral hippocampus functionally distinct structures? *Neuron*, 65(1), pp. 1–25.

Fleischmann, A., Hvalby, O., Jensen, V., Strekalova, T., Zacher, C. et al. (2003). Impaired long-term memory and NR2A-type NMDA receptor-dependent synaptic plasticity in mice lacking c-Fos in the CNS. *Journal of Neuroscience*, 23(27), pp. 9116–9122.

Frankland, P. W. and Bontempi, B. (2005). The organization of recent and remote memories. *Nature Reviews Neuroscience*, 6, pp. 119–130.

Harris, E. W., Ganong, A. H. and Cotman, C. W. (1984). Long-term potentiation in the hippocampus involves activation of N-methyl-D-aspartate receptors. *Brain Research*, 323 (1), pp. 132–137.

Isaac, J. T. R., Ashby, M. C. and McBain, C. J. (2007). The role of the GluR2 subunit in AMPA receptor function and synaptic plasticity. *Neuron*, 54(6), pp. 859–871.

Jensen, V., Kaiser, K. M. M., Borchardt, T., Adelmann, G., Rozov, A. et al. (2003). A juvenile form of postsynaptic hippocampal long-term potentiation in mice deficient for the AMPA receptor subunit GluR-A. *J. Physiol.*, 553(3), pp. 843–856.

Jia, Z., Agopyan, N., Miu, P., Xiong, Z., Henderson, J. et al. (1996). Enhanced LTP in mice deficient in the AMPA receptor GluR2. *Neuron*, 17, pp. 945–956.

Johansen, J. P., Diaz-Mataix, L., Hamanaka, H., Ozawa, T., Ycu, E. et al. (2014). Hebbian and neuromodulatory mechanisms interact to trigger associative memory formation. *Proc. Natl. Acad. Sci. US*, 111(51), pp. 5584–5592.

Jung, M. W., Weiner, S. I. and McNaughton, B. L. (1994). Comparison of spatial firing characteristics of units in dorsal and ventral hippocampus of the rat. *Journal of Neuroscience*, 14(12), pp. 7347–7356.

Kelso, S. R., Ganong, A. H. and Brown, T. H. (1986). Hebbian synapses in hippocampus. *Proc Natl Acad Sci US*, 83, pp. 5326–5330.

Lavenex, P. and Amaral, D. G. (2000). Hippocampal-neocortical interaction: a hierarchy of associativity. *Hippocampus*, 10, pp. 420–430.

Lavenex, P. B., Amaral, D. G. and Lavenex, P. (2006). Hippocampal lesion prevents spatial relational learning in adult macaque monkeys. *Journal of Neuroscience*, 26(17), pp. 4546–4558.

Lee, H.-K., Barbarosie, M., Kameyama, K., Bear, M. F. and Huganir, R. L. (2000). Regulation of distinct AMPA receptor phosphorylation sites during bidirectional synaptic plasticity. *Nature*, 405, pp. 955–959.

Lee, H.-K., Takamiya, K., Han, J.-S., Man, H., Kim, C.-H. et al. (2003). Phosphorylation of the AMPA receptor GluR1 subunit is required for synaptic plasticity and retention of spatial memory. *Cell*, 112(5), pp. 631–643.

Lopez, J., Gamache, K., Schneider, R. and Nader, K. Memory retrieval requires ongoing protein synthesis and NMDA receptor activity-mediated AMPA receptor trafficking. *Journal of Neuroscience*, 35(6), pp. 2465–2475.

Lynch, M. A. (2004). Long-term potentiation and memory. *Physiol. Rev.*, 84, pp. 87–136.

Malinow, R. and Malenka, R. C. (2002). AMPA receptor trafficking and synaptic plasticity. *Annu. Rev. Neurosci.*, 25, pp. 103–126.

McGaugh, J. L. (2000). Memory – a century of consolidation. *Science*, 287(5451), pp. 248–251.

Mednick, S. C., Cai, D. J., Shuman, T., Anagnostaras, S. and Wixted, J. (2011). An opportunistic theory of cellular and systems consolidation. *Trends In Neuroscience*, 34 (10), pp. 504–514.

Meeter, M. and Murre, J. M. J. (2004). Consolidation of long-term memory: evidence and alternatives. *Psychological Bulletin*, 130(6), pp. 843–857.

Meng, Y., Zhang, Y. and Jia, Z. (2003). Synaptic transmission and plasticity in the absence of AMPA glutamate receptor GluR2 and GluR3. *Neuron*, 39(1), pp. 163–176.

Messier, C., Mourre, C., Bontempi, B., Sif, J., Lazdunski, M. et al. (1991). Effect of apamin, a toxin that inhibits Ca^{+2}-depndent K^{+} channels, on learning and memory processes. *Brain Research*, 551, pp. 322–326.

Monaghan, D. T., Bridges, R. J. and Cotman, C. W. (1989) . The excitatory amino acid receptors: their classes, pharmacology, and distinct properties in the function of the central nervous system. *Annu. Rev. Pharmacol. Toxicol.*, 29, pp. 365–402.

Morris, R. (1984). Developments of a water-maze procedure for studying spatial learning in the rat. *Journal of Neuroscience Methods*, 11, pp. 47–60.

Morris, R. G. M., Anderson, E., Lynch, G. S. and Baudry, M. (1986). Selective impairment of learning and blockade of long-term potentiation by an *N*-methyl-D-aspartate receptor antagonist, AP5. *Nature*, 319, pp. 774–776.

Morris, R. G. M., Garraud, P., Rawlins, J. N. P., and O'Keefe, J. (1982). Place navigation impaired in rats with hippocampal lesions. *Nature*, 297, pp. 681–683.

Moser, E., Moser, M. B. and Andersen, P. (1993). Spatial learning impairment parallels the magnitude of dorsal hippocampal lesions, but is hardly present following ventral lesions. *Journal of Neuroscience*, 13(9), pp. 3916–3925.

Moser, M. B., Moser, E. L., Forrest, E., Andersen, P. and Morris, R. G. (1995). Spatial learning with a minislab in the dorsal hippocampus. *Proc. Natl. Acad. Sci. US*, 92(21), pp. 9697–9701.

Muir, G. M. and Bilkey, D. K. (2001). Instability in the place field location of hippocampal place cells after lesions centered on the perirhinal cortex. *Journal of Neuroscience*, 21 (11), pp. 4016–4025.

Naber, P. A., Witter, M. P. and Lopes da Silva, F. H. (1999). Perirhinal cortex input to the hippocampus in the rat: evidence for parallel pathways, both direct and indirect. A combined physiological and anatomical study. *European Journal of Neuroscience*, 11, pp. 4119–4133.

Neves, G., Cooke, S. F. and Bliss, T. V. P. (2008). Synaptic plasticity, memory and the hippocampus: a neural network approach to causality. *Nature Reviews Neuroscience*, 9, pp. 65–75.

Nyberg, L., Tulving, E., Habib, E., Nilsson, L.-G., Kapur, S. et al. (1995). Functional brain maps of retrieval mode and recovery of episodic information. *NeuroReport*, 7, pp. 249–252.

O'Keefe, J. and Dostrovsky, J. (1971). The hippocampus as a spatial map. Preliminary evidence from unit activity in the freely-moving rat. *Brain Research*, 34, pp. 171–175.

O'Keefe, J. and Nadel, L. (1978). *The hippocampus as a cognitive map*. Oxford: Clarendon Press.

Poe, G. R., Teed, R. G., Insel, N., White, R., McNaughton, B. L. et al. (2000). Partial hippocampal inactivation: effects on spatial memory performance in aged and young rats. *Behavioral Neuroscience*, 114(5), pp. 940–949.

Pothuizen, H. H., Zhang, W. N., Jongen-Relo, A. L., Feldon, J. and Yee, B. K. (2004). Dissociation of function between the dorsal and the ventral hippocampus in spatial learning abilities of the rat: a within-subject, within-task comparison of reference and working spatial memory. *Eur. J. Neurosci.*, 19(3), pp. 705–712.

Riedel, G. and Micheau, J. (2001) Function of the hippocampus in memory formation: desperately seeking resolution. *Prog. Neuro-Psychopharmacol. and Biol. Psychiat.*, 25, pp. 835–853.

Riedel, G., Micheau, J., Lam, A. G. M., Roloff, E. V. L., Martin, S. J., et al. (1999). Reversible neural inactivation reveals hippocampal participation in several memory processes. *Nature Neuroscience*, 2(10), pp. 898–905.

Rudy, J. W. and Sutherland, R. J. (2008). Is it systems or cellular consolidation? Time will tell. An alternative interpretation of the Morris Group's recent science paper. *Neurobiology of Learning and Memory*, 89(4), pp. 366–369.

Sagata, N., Iwaki, A., Aramaki, T., Takao, K., Kura, S. et al. (2010). Comprehensive behavioral study of GluR4 knockout mice: implication in cognitive function. *Genes, Brain and Behavior*, 9, pp. 899–909.

Sanderson, D. J., McHugh, S. B., Good, M. A., Sprengel, R., Seeburg, P. H. et al. (2010). Spatial working memory deficits in GluA1 AMPA receptor subunit knockout mice reflect impaired short-term habituation: evidence for Wagner's dual-process memory model. *Neuropsychologia*, 48(8), pp. 2303–2315.

Sehgal, M., Song, C., Ehlers, V. L. and Moyer, J. R. (2013). Learning to learn – intrinsic plasticity as a metaplasticity mechanism for memory formation. *Neurobiology of Learning and Memory*, 105, pp. 186–199.

Smith, C. N. and Squire, L. R. (2009). Medial temporal lobe activity during retrieval of semantic memory is related to the age of the memory. *Journal of Neuroscience*, 29, pp. 930–938.

Song, I. and Huganir, R. L. (2002). Regulation of AMPA receptors during synaptic plasticity. *Trends in Neurosciences*, 25(11), pp. 578–588.

Steele, R. J. and Morris, R. G. M. (1999). Delay-dependent impairment of a matching-to-place task with chronic and intrahippocampal infusion of the NMDA-antagonist D-AP5. *Hippocampus*, 9, pp. 118–136.

Stringer, J. L., Greenfield, L. J., Hackett, J. T. and Guyenet, P. G. (1983). Blockade of long-term potentiation by phencyclidine and σ opiates in the hippocampus in vivo and in vitro. *Brain Research*, 280(1), pp. 127–138.

Szapiro, G., Galante, J. M., Barros, D. M. Levi de Stein, M., Vianna, M. R. M. et al. (2002). Molecular mechanisms of memory retrieval. *Neurochemical Research*, 27(11), pp. 1491–1498.

Szapiro, G., Izquierdo, L. A., Alonso, M., Barros, D., Paratcha, G. et al. (2000). Participation of hippocampal metabotropic glutamate receptors, protein kinase A and mitogen-activated protein kinases in memory retrieval. *Neuroscience*, 99(1), pp. 1–5.

Takashima, A., Petersson, K. M., Rutters, F., Tendolkar, I., Jensen, O. et al. (2006). Declarative memory consolidation in humans: a prospective functional magnetic resonance imaging study. *Proc. Natl. Acad. Sci. US*, 103, pp. 756–761.

Tischmeyer, W. and Grimm, R. (1999). Activation of immediate early genes and memory formation. *Cellular and Molecular Life Sciences*, 55, pp. 564–574.

Toyoda, H., Wu, L.-J., Zhao, M.-G., Xu, H., Jia, Z. et al. (2007). Long-term depression requires postsynaptic AMPA GluR2 receptor in adult mouse cingulate cortex. *Journal of Cellular Physiology*, 211(2), pp. 336–343.

Wainwright, S. R. and Galea, L. A. M. (2013). The Neural Plasticity Theory of Depression: Assessing the Roles of Adult Neurogenesis and PSA-NCAM within the Hippocampus. *Neural Plasticity*, 2013, pp. 1–14.

Wang, S.-H. and Morris, G. M. (2010). Hippocampal-neocortical interactions in memory formation, consolidation, and reconsolidation. *Annu. Rev. Psychol.*, 61, pp. 49–79.

Wible, C. G. (2013). Hippocampal physiology, structure and function and the neuroscience of schizophrenia: a unified account of declarative memory deficits, working memory deficits and schizophrenic symptoms. *Behav. Sci.*, 3(2), pp. 298–315.

Zhou, A. W., Guo, J., Wang, H. Y., Gu, B. X. and Du, Y. C. (1995). Enhancement of NGF gene expression in rat brain by the memory-enhancing peptide AVP (4–8). *Peptides*, 16, pp. 581–586.

In: Spatial, Long-and Short-Term Memory
Editor: Edward A. Thayer
ISBN: 978-1-63484-148-1

Chapter 3

MANIPULATING SPATIAL AND VISUAL CUES IN A WIN-STAY FORAGING TASK IN CAPTIVE GRIZZLY BEARS (*URSUS ARCTOS HORRIBILUS*)

Jennifer Vonk[1,*], Stephanie Allard[2], Lauri Torgerson-White[2], Cynthia Bennett[2], Moriah Galvan[1], Molly McGuire[1], Jennifer Hamilton[1], Zoe-Johnson-Ulrich[1] and Jennifer M. Lieb[1]

[1]Oakland University, Rochester, MI, US
[2]Detroit Zoological Society, Royal Oak, MI, US

ABSTRACT

We wished to determine the efficacy of cues from different modalities in order to better understand the cues that grizzlies may utilize to recall the location of food. In this study, two captive grizzly bears (*Ursus arctos horribillis*; one male juvenile and one adult female) at the Detroit Zoological Society were tested for the use of spatial memory under two testing conditions; spatial and visual. The female completed only the spatial condition whereas the male completed first visual and then spatial cue testing. The bears were presented with three of six baited sites in their outdoor habitat. In the spatial condition, the same sites were always baited. In the visual condition, differently colored containers varied by location but the same colors consistently predicted food. Neither bear utilized spatial or visual cues in order to reduce time spent foraging at unbaited sites, and no learning was demonstrated across the course of 12 to 36 sessions. We conclude that the reduced cost of foraging in captive environments mitigates against motivation to use the most efficient foraging strategies for animals with large home ranges.

[*] Corresponding author: Jennifer Vonk. Department of Psychology, Oakland University, 2200 N. Squirrel Rd., Rochester MI, 48309. E-mail: vonk@oakland.edu.

INTRODUCTION

Remembering the location of resources such as food, shelter and potential mates is an important cognitive ability for species in the wild – particularly those with large home ranges, such as grizzly bears (*Ursus arctos horribilus*). It is expected that animals evolve optimal foraging behavior to better cope with selection pressures such as diminishing food resources, scarcity of mates, competition from conspecifics and other predators, which necessitates memory for the location of resources. Researchers have investigated the use of spatial memory in captive environments using win-stay and win-shift tasks where animals find food in previously baited or unbaited locations respectively. Non-human primates have been extensively studied in such paradigms (Gibeault and MacDonald 1998, MacDonald 1994, MacDonald and Agnes 1999, MacDonald, Pang and Gibeault 1994, MacDonald and Wilkie 1990) but researchers have also more recently investigated spatial memory in bears and other carnivores (Perdue, Snyder, Pratte, Marr and Maple 2009, Perdue, Snyder, Zhihe, Marr and Maple 2011, Tarou 2004, Zamisch and Vonk 2012). Bears should exhibit good spatial memory because, in addition to their large brain size, they inhabit large home ranges and exploit unpredictable food sources (Gittleman 1986). However, at least one study found little evidence for the use of spatial memory in captive American black bears (*Ursus americanus,* Zamisch and Vonk 2012), which raised the question of whether an omnivorous diet or captive environment affects the use or expression of spatial memory in bears. The current work was thus motivated by a desire to test the spatial memory of another omnivorous bear species – the grizzly bear – in captivity.

In Zamisch and Vonk (2012), four adult captive American black bears participated in four spatial memory experiments modelled after previous work with primates. Each experiment included two phases, an exploration and a search phase. The first experiments tested the use of a win-stay foraging strategy and consisted of an individual foraging alone. In the first experiment, four of eight sites were baited and there was a delay interval of two hours between the two phases. The bears showed a preferred travel route to adjacent sites similar to that seen with giant pandas and spectacled bears in a previous study (Tarou 2004), but they did not learn the location of the baited sites. In attempts to increase the probability of observing the use of spatial memory, the experimenters reduced the latency between exploration and search phases to 5-15 minutes and the number of baited sites to three out of five – also increasing the proportion of baited sites. The bears still failed to demonstrate an efficient search strategy – preferring three sites to visit first regardless of whether they had been baited in the previous phase.

Subsequently, the experimenters increased the cost of foraging and added an uninformed competitor to the search phase with two baited sites and two non-baited sites. The same sites were baited over the course of 12 days. The bears continued to evidence chance accuracy. The final experiment involved all of the bears foraging together at the same baited sites with a 2-3 day interval between test days. It was thought that a longer delay interval may actually be more likely to evoke the use of a win-stay strategy because food may not be expected to replenish over shorter intervals. However, it is important to note that none of the bears had exhibited a win-shift strategy in the earlier studies. In this final test, one of the female bears now demonstrated some use of spatial memory. We adopted a similar procedure for the current study except that we tested only one bear at a time. We also wished to extend the previous findings by examining which cues might be given priority; spatial or visual.

Only one previous study examined the type of cues used by different bear species to locate food. Tarou (2003) tested giant pandas (*Ailuropoda melanoleuca*) and spectacled bears (*Tremarctos ornatus*) using foraging tasks consisting of exploratory and search phases. She used a spatial task with a reversal of the location of baited sites, and a visual discrimination task also with a reversal of baited sites. The reversal phases constituted a win-shift test. Three male and four female giant pandas and one female and one male spectacled bear participated in the tasks. The bears were required to lift the Plexiglas lids off of PVC containers in order to find food at four of eight sites. In the exploratory task similar to a previous test with orangutans (MacDonald and Agnes 1999), working memory was tested to determine if the bears would recall which of eight sites were depleted over a period of 15 sessions. Revisits to depleted sites by both bear species decreased over the 15 sessions, but, for the spectacled bears, revisits were lower from the beginning and remained consistently lower. Thus, the spectacled bears outperformed the giant pandas, although, with experience, the giant pandas' performance did improve. Also, an increase in preference for adjacent sites was seen in the giant pandas as they became more experienced with the location of sites, while the spectacled bears consistently visited adjacent sites from the beginning. This use of preferred travel routes was observed throughout subsequent experiments as well (Tarou 2004).

Tarou's spatial tasks were set up based on a win-stay strategy to determine if the bears visited only baited sites and ignored the non-baited sites. If three baited sites were visited out of the first four visits on four or five consecutive sessions, then a reversal task was conducted to further determine whether the bears could use a win-shift as well as a win-stay strategy. Criterion was met by five of the seven giant pandas tested in the win-stay phase. In the spatial reversal, only four of the giant pandas reached the criterion and spent more time learning the reversal as compared to the previous spatial task. Only one of the spectacled bears, the female, met the criterion for reversal. A decrease in the female spectacled bear's performance in the reversal task was seen with only one correct site visit. These findings emphasize the fact that foraging ecologies of different species may dictate the use of different foraging strategies. In primate studies, marmosets were shown to prefer a win-stay strategy (MacDonald et al. 1994), whereas yellow-nosed monkeys successfully used both win-stay and win-shift strategies (MacDonald and Wilkie 1999).

In addition to comparing strategies, Tarou also manipulated the cues that were available to signal the presence of food. In the third experimental task, both bear species were tested for the ability to use color as a cue to the location of baited and non baited sites. Previous research had shown American black bears to discriminate food sites based on the hue of visual signals (Bacon and Burghardt 1974), and giant pandas to discriminate other hues from grey (Kelling et al. 2006), making it reasonable to use color as a cue in studies with bears. In Tarou's experiment four baited feeders had white lids and four non baited feeders were covered with black lids. The spectacled bears met criterion on this task while the giant pandas failed to do so. In a reversal of cue for the spectacled bears, black lids were used for the baited sites and the white lids were used for non baited sites. After this reversal, the female spectacle bear's performance was higher than the male's performance. However, with such small samples, it is difficult to draw firm conclusions regarding species or sex differences, thus calling for the need for further studies of spatial memory in bears.

Because some bears, along with non-human primates who also experience patchy and unpredictable food sources, rely on spatial memory and adjust their foraging strategy accordingly, it is possible that grizzly bears could also demonstrate the ability to correctly remember and distinguish between baited sites and non-baited sites, using spatial and visual memory. Based on this assumption we wanted to determine which cues take priority when foraging for food. Two grizzly bears, one adult female and one juvenile male participated in this study involving a spatial condition and a visual condition. We wanted to determine based on indications from MacDonald and Agnes (1999), Tarou (2003) and Zamisch and Vonk (2012), if grizzly bears, like other species tested, could utilize a win-stay foraging strategy to learn to locate baited sites and avoid non-baited sites. From the findings of these two conditions insight could be offered as to which cues are used more often in locating food. In addition, based on Zamisch and Vonk's (2012) finding that captive black bears did not appear to recall the location of baited sites, it was important to assess spatial memory in another omnivorous bear species housed in a captive environment.

METHOD

Participants

Two captive grizzly bears participated in this study, an adult female named Kintla and a juvenile male named Thor, both of whom reside at the Detroit Zoological Society (DZS). Kintla, who was rescued from the wild in 1986 at approximately 2 and ½ years of age, was housed with an adult male grizzly and Thor was housed with his two brothers. Thor and his brothers were rescued from the wild at around a year of age in Oct. 2011. Neither bear had previously participated in cognitive studies.

Kintla participated in the spatial memory condition and was tested between September and October of 2012. Thor participated in the visual condition between September and October 2012 and resumed testing from June until early September of 2013, when he also completed 21 sessions of the spatial condition. Testing was then halted due to the possibility of stress to one of the juvenile males during separation for testing, and the desire to allocate time to computerized test training with the bears (Vonk et al., in preparation).

Testing Area

All testing was conducted in the bears' outdoor habitats at the DZS. The habitats are depicted in aerial view in Figure 1 (Kintla) and 2 (Thor). The participants were released individually from their indoor to their outdoor habitats with a gate controlling access between habitats during testing. Each habitat contained six foraging locations, half of which were baited with desirable food. Thor's habitat included a large pond and both habitats included climbing walls.

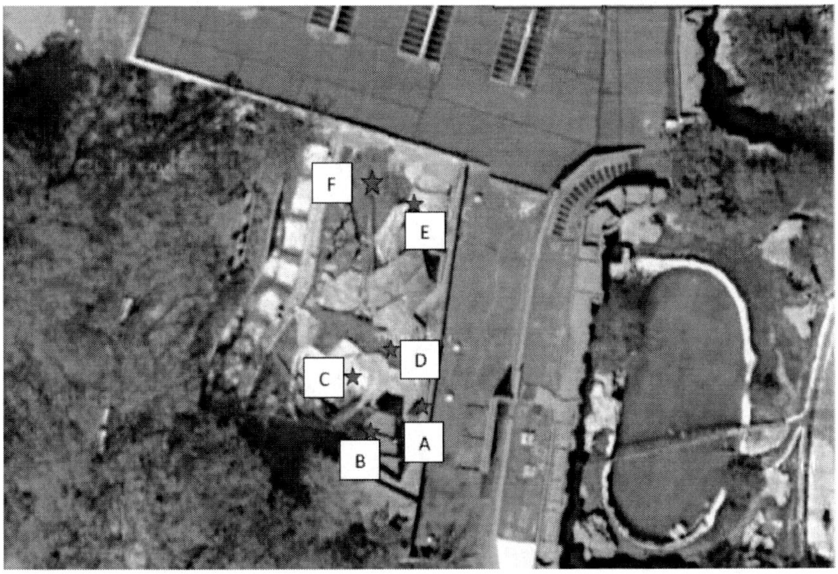

Figure 1. An aerial view of Kintla's habitat indicating the location of the foraging sites.

Materials

Six large PVC pipes that were placed in designated locations labeled A, B, C, D, E, and F were evenly distributed throughout the habitat. The pipes were attached to straps that were hooked on to permanent metal brackets affixed to the walls of the enclosure, such that manipulation was required to extract the food. The food within the pipes was not visible upon approach. Each pipe was painted a different solid color: red, blue, gray, black, white and green.

Given that a prior study had found that black bears had the most difficulty discriminating green from red (Bacon and Burghardt 1973), a black stripe was painted across the green pipe to distinguish the green and red pipes. The spatial condition that Kinta participated in utilized all white PVC pipes.

Meatballs were used for bait for the first 12 sessions for both bears. Almonds and almond extract were used for all testing sessions after session 12 for Thor. A cap was added to the pipes with holes for the almonds to fall out so as to create a more challenging extraction task. It was hoped that this added challenge would increase motivation to use spatial memory rather than wasting time at unbaited sites. Almond extract or meat juice was placed into the unbaited pipes to control for scent cues.

A stopwatch was used to record the timing of visits to the sites. A Sony camcorder was used to record each testing session. A set of data sheets were used to record the order and timing of visits, duration of time the bear spent at each site, weather conditions and the date. An independent rater viewed the sessions on video and recorded the same information for reliability.

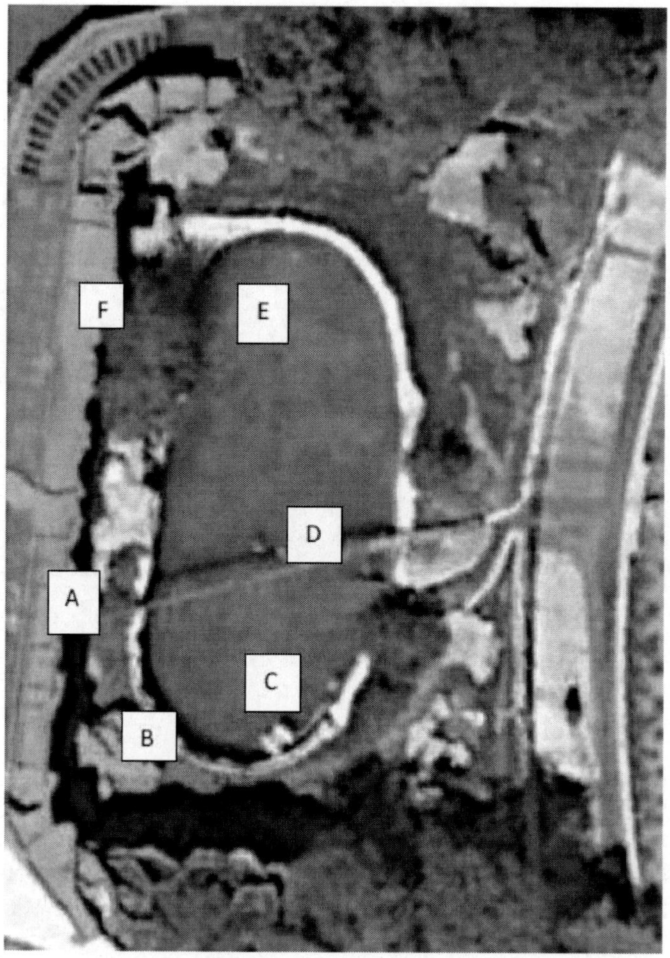

Figure 2. An aerial view of Thor's habitat indicating the location of the foraging sites.

Procedure

Testing began at 08:30 hrs three days of the week. A period of 2-3 days passed between testing days to allow for a consistent delay interval and each bear was tested only once per testing day. The locations of the baited pipes remained consistent for every day of testing and the experimenter followed the same path when hanging PVC pipes; A, B, C, F, E and then D. Location of the bait was randomly determined, with the location held constant for the spatial condition across sessions, and varied for each session for the visual condition. Experimenters confirmed the location of bait as they placed the pipes with a second experimenter who was responsible for filming the sessions.

Once the pipes had been placed, an animal caretaker released the subject bear into the habitat. A researcher filmed the bear's movements until the bear went inside and out of sight. This researcher also recorded each visit to a site and the time that each visit began and ended, and whether food was consumed.

Revisits were also recorded. Except for the first six sessions that lasted ten minutes, each session lasted four minutes, at which point an animal caretaker called the subject back into the indoor habitat and the session was terminated. Sessions were shortened when it was realized that the bears needed only about four minutes to investigate all of the sites fully.

At the end of each session the presence of any leftover food was recorded and the pipes were removed and cleaned. All bears were then released back into their habitats.

The original plan was to reverse the location of the baits once a bear met the criterion, which consisted of four consecutive sessions in which a bear visited the three baited sites without first visiting any non-baited sites. However, neither bear met the criterion within a maximum of 36 sessions (3 counterbalanced blocks). After failing to demonstrate any learning after 36 sessions of the visual condition, Thor began testing in the spatial condition.

Spatial Condition

The spatial condition included blocks of 12 sessions with each baited site labeled either A, B, C, D, E or F. For Thor the same sites (B, D, E) were always baited, but different colored PVC pipes were placed at each location on a counterbalanced schedule such that there was one relevant cue (spatial location) and one irrelevant cue (color).

For Kintla, the same sites (A, C, E) were always baited with white PVC pipes such that only spatial location served as a cue.

Visual Condition

A total of 36 sessions were conducted with Thor. The bait was always placed in three designated pipes, which were colored grey, black, and white. The red, green, and blue pipes were never baited.

The spatial location of each colored pipe was determined with a counterbalanced schedule such that each color appeared equally often (twice) at each of the six sites across blocks of twelve sessions. In this manner color was always a relevant cue and spatial location was irrelevant.

RESULTS

An independent rater coded the data from video and those codings were compared to the data recorded live during the sessions. Raters agreed on the first three sites visited for 191 of the 198 sessions coded, for an agreement of 96.5%. Coded data from the video was used for all analyses and figures.

The sessions were analyzed in six session blocks to examine changes in accuracy over time. Accuracy of the bears' search strategy was defined as the probability of visiting the baited sites first before visiting any unbaited sites. Thus, proportion of visits to baited sites out of the first three visits for each session were calculated and compared to chance probabilities using one sample t-tests. Given that half of the sites were baited, chance was set to .50. Proportions of accurate visits within each block of six sessions were compared to chance for each bear to determine if and when searching accuracy was significantly different from chance.

Spatial Condition

Kintla completed only 12 sessions (two 6-session blocks). Kintla's performance for the first block was not significantly above chance, ($t_5 = .79, p = .47$), but was significantly above chance on the second block, ($t_5 = 9.51, p < .001$). See Figure 3. Thor completed only 21 sessions (three complete and one partial 6-session block). Thor's performance on the spatial condition was above chance only for the first session block, ($t_5 = 9.51, p < .001$). Performance was at chance on all other testing blocks (all t's < 2.0). There was no evidence of learning across session blocks. See Figure 3.

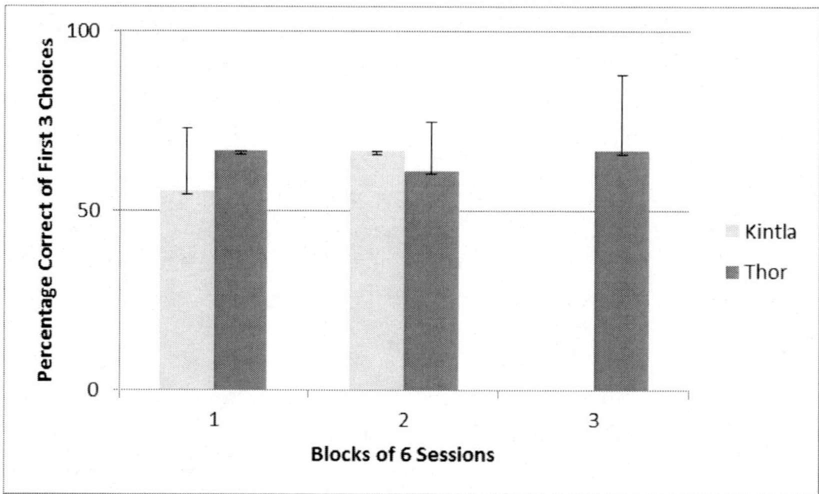

Figure 3. Percentage of visits to baited sites within the first three visits during six session blocks for the spatial condition.

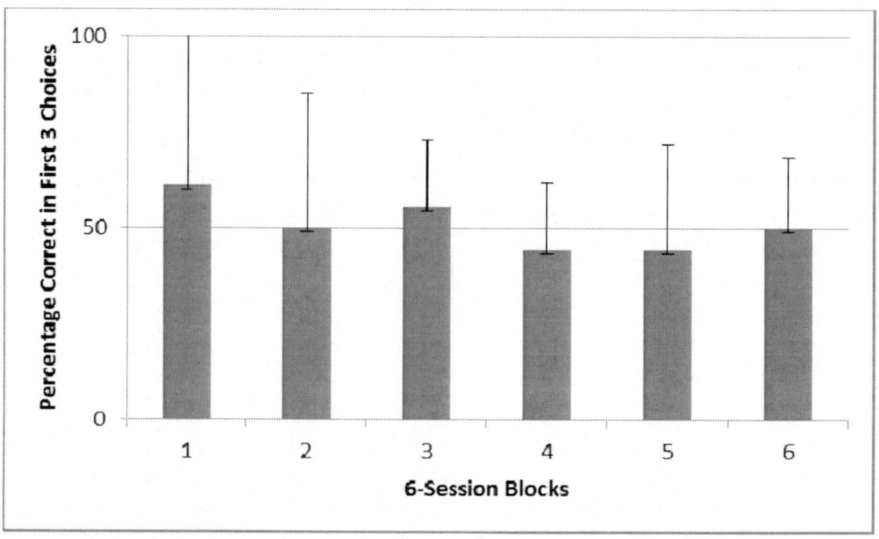

Figure 4. Percentage of visits to baited sites within the first three visits during six session blocks for the visual condition.

Visual Condition

Thor completed 36 sessions (six testing blocks). Thor's performance for the visual condition was not significantly above chance for any of the six session blocks (all *t's* < 1.0, *p's* > .05), and there was no evidence of learning. See Figure 4. Overall, Thor performed better in the spatial condition, but given the order of testing it is impossible to determine whether this improvement was due to the type of cue used or to order effects.

Re-Visits

Figure 5 displays the number of revisits by bear as a function of whether the site was originally baited and the type of test (spatial, visual). A paired t-test reveals that Kintla re-visited the baited sites (M = 2.82, SD = .98) significantly more often than the unbaited sites (M = 1.36, SD = 1.57) in the spatial test, (t = 4.66, p = .001) indicating working memory for the presence of food.

Thor revisited less than Kintla and showed the opposite pattern; he re-visited unbaited sites (M = .28, SD = .46) more than he re-visited baited sites (M = 0, SD = 0) in the spatial test, (t = -2.56, p = .02). This pattern was likely due to the fact that Thor often checked the unbaited site closest to the door on his way back into the indoor habitat at the end of the session. There was no significant difference in his re-visits to baited and unbaited sites in the visual test, although he tended to re-visit baited (M = .60, SD = .95) more than unbaited sites (M = .34, SD = .80).

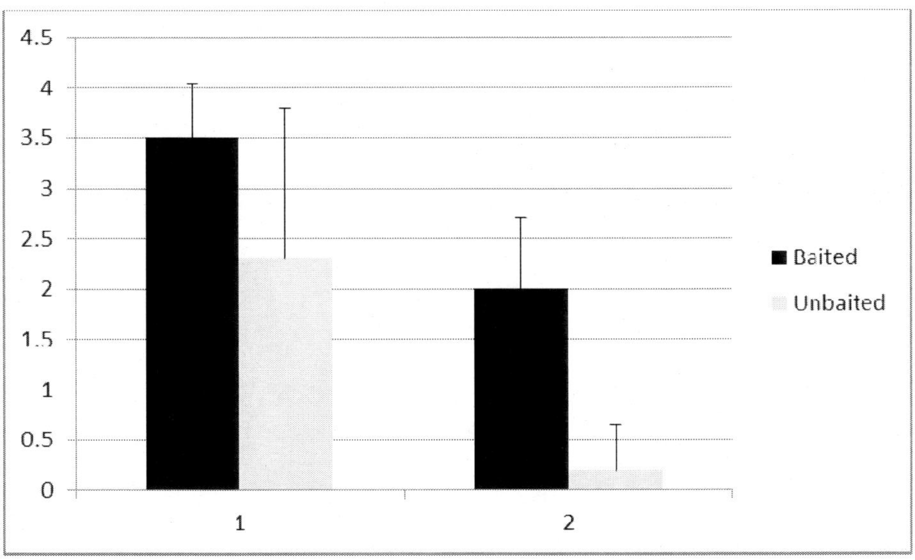

Figure 5. (Continued).

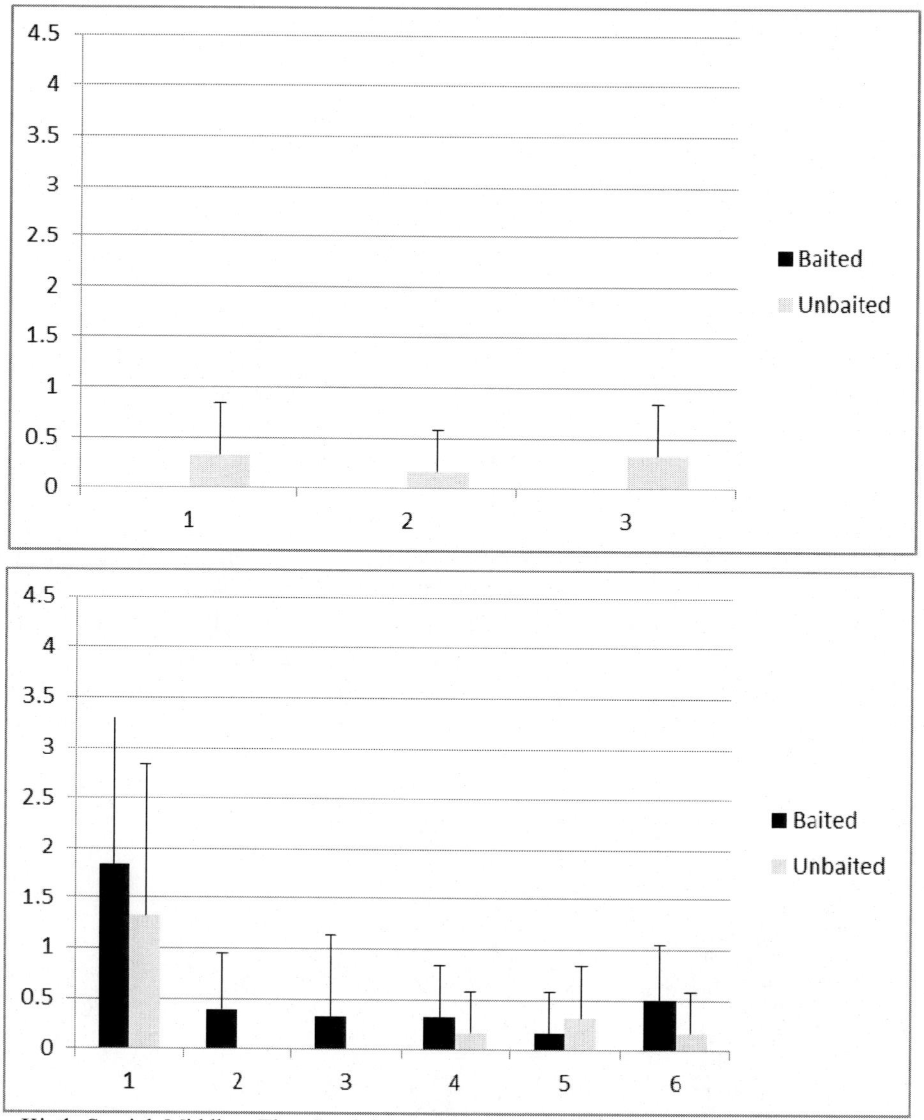

Top = Kintla Spatial, Middle = Thor Spatial, Bottom = Thor Visual.

Figure 5. Number of revisits by bear as a function of whether the site was originally baited and the type of test (spatial, visual).

DISCUSSION

Although we were not able to test each bear across multiple tests involving different cues as to the location of hidden food, the preliminary results presented here are consistent with prior research in which captive American black bears failed to demonstrate evidence for the use of spatial memory in a win-stay foraging task (Zamisch and Vonk 2012). As with the previous research, the grizzly bears tested here did not learn to ignore the non-baited sites and visited them equally often prior to visiting the baited sites, even after multiple sessions (up to 12 for Kintla and up to 36 for Thor). We did not observe any evidence for learning across sessions, suggesting that the bears may not have been motivated to reduce time spent foraging in their captive environments. As Zamisch and Vonk (2012) concluded, captive environments are much smaller than natural home ranges and food is not scarce, thus minimizing the energetic costs required to investigate unbaited sites. The bears may have found it enriching to investigate all sites and in fact, were quite accustomed to finding treats scattered throughout their outdoor habitat – sometimes within similar hanging devices. Anecdotally, we ironically observed Thor often make his first visit to one particular site, which was a site favored by keepers when placing enrichment food items in the habitat outside of testing. This practice demonstrates that Thor did in fact remember where food had been discovered previously, but did not discriminate between sites in the current experiment. Given our failure to obtain evidence of spatial memory we were also unable to determine which cues were more likely to be used by the bears.

This is unfortunate as only one previous study (Tarou 2004) investigated the use of various cues by different bear species but her study included only giant pandas and spectacled bears. Spectacled bears were found to use more visual cues and make fewer revisits to depleted sites. Their frugivorous diet was postulated as an explanation for their superior performance. Examining the use of specific cues in an omnivorous species like the grizzly could make a nice addition to the literature and further explain the evolution of foraging strategies across diverse foraging ecologies. Overall, performance did appear to be better in the spatial condition, which is consistent with evidence that animals readily use spatial cues in various tasks (Healy 1998, Thorpe, Hallett and Wilkie 2007). However, Kintla's performance may have been artificially inflated due to the fact that two of her three randomly determined baited sites were within the first three to be encountered when she exited from the indoor habitat into the testing habitat. Given the design of the habitats it was not possible to create arrays where all six sites were equidistant or equally visible from the entrance into the habitat. Thor's performance in the spatial condition was quite variable. It is possible that given more sessions and added cost to manipulating unbaited sites, that his accuracy may have increased. Future studies should increase the costs associated with visiting unbaited sites. Zamisch and Vonk (2012) added the cost of competition by releasing four bears at once into the testing habitat but did not observe any increase in foraging accuracy for the single informed bears in their study. In fact, the mother bear was observed to actively defend unbaited sites and bears did not actively avoid sites that other bears were feeding at.

Foraging in a captive environment clearly differs in important ways from foraging in the wild. In captivity, competitors are well-known and often related conspecifics and costs of "errors" are minimal. The cost of locating food in captivity is low because of scheduled feeding times, the small size of the habitat, and the short travel distance to each baited and non-baited site. There is no risk of predation. Furthermore, animals are well-fed in captivity and not food adjusted in order to take part in experiments, whereas, in the wild, animals are often hungry and well-motivated to seek food.

Another limitation of the study was our small sample size. Perdue et al. (2011) observed sex differences in working memory but we did not have a large enough sample size to observe potential sex differences in spatial memory. The question is an interesting one because male grizzly bears have a larger home range compared to female grizzly bears and therefore may rely more heavily on working memory (Perdue et al. 2011). Perdue's study was the first to find evidence of sex differences that were reliant on home range size.

In addition to the small habitat size, zoo habitats sometimes do not allow for multiple possible routes between sites. In our study, this may have been especially problematic in Thor's habitat – a large portion of which is taken up with a pool. Thor and Kintla traveled a fixed route when released into the habitat for each testing day, which was also observed in Tarou (2004). In her study, the giant pandas and spectacled bears preferred visiting adjacent sites during sessions, as did the grizzly bears. This behavior might indicate a preference for a fixed foraging pathway that might not be easily reversed.

Overall the lack of accuracy or learning does not lead to the conclusion that captive bears lack spatial memory. There was some evidence for working memory for sites that had been baited during a session as Kintla more often re-visited sites that had been baited in the spatial condition, and Thor showed a similar trend in the visual condition. Number of re-visits also tended to decline across sessions suggesting that bears learned that sites did not replenish and remembered where they had been.

The use of spatial memory might also be demonstrated if tests were conducted in a larger habitat or a greater cost was incurred by visiting unbaited sites. Costs could be added by reducing time allowed to forage, increasing competition, or adding an aversive outcome to the manipulation of unbaited sites. However, it is difficult to insist that bears cut short visits into outdoor habitats, thus making option one untenable. Option two has proven to be unsuccessful in previous studies with bears (Zamisch and Vonk 2012) and orangutans (MacDonald and Agnes 1999), and option three is unappealing from an animal welfare standpoint. Future studies should test captive bears in much larger habitats, ideally with a comparison to their wild counterparts under conditions in which inaccurate choices impose significant delays or energy expenditures – perhaps by making containers very difficult to access. Bears that receive their entire daily ration in the context of foraging and are not permitted to visit all sites would most likely quickly learn to demonstrate spatial memory skills. Future studies should also provide cues that make use of all of the bears' senses. For instance, providing an odor trail to food sites might encourage encoding of relevant information. Of course odor trails would have to be arbitrary and distinct from trails to unbaited sites such that bears would have to rely on memory rather than simply following observable cues to the location of food, which makes odor cues more difficult to implement in experimental settings. We would advocate for animals to be challenged and have problems to solve even in captive environments. We are delighted to see an increase in studies of bear cognition (Dungl, Schratter and Huber 2008, Keen et al. 2014, Kelling et al. 2006, Vonk and Beran 2012, Vonk, Jett and Mosteller 2012, Vonk and Johnson-Ulrich 2014, West, Jett, Beckman and Vonk 2010) as they indicate an increase in attention to the need to stimulate and enrich the bears in our care.

References

Bacon, E. S., Burghardt, G. M. (1974). Learning and color discrimination in the American black bear. *Third international conference on Bears*, 3, 27-36.

Dungl, E., Schratter, D. and Huber, L. (2008). Discrimination of face-like patterns in the giant panda (*Ailuropoda melanoleuca*). *Journal of Comparative Psychology*, 122, 335-343, doi:10.1037/0735-7036.122.4.335.

Gibeault, S. and MacDonald, S. E. (1998). Spatial memory and foraging behavior in captive western lowland gorillas (*Gorilla gorilla gorilla*). *Primates*, 41, 147-170.

Gittleman, J. L. (1986). Carnivore brain size, behavioral ecology, and phylogeny. *Journal of Mammalogy*, 67, 23-36.

Healy, S. (1998). *Spatial representation in animals*. Oxford University Press, New York, NY.

Keen, H. A., Nelson, O. L., Robbins, C. T., Evans, M., Shepherdson, D. J. and Newberry, R. C. (2014). Validation of a novel cognitive bias task based on difference in quantity of reinforcement for assessing environmental enrichment. *Animal Cognition*, 17, 529-541.

Kelling, A. S., Synder, R. J., Marr, M. J., Bloomsmith, M. A., Gardner, W. and Maple, T. L. (2006). Color vision in the panda *(Ailuropoda melanoleuca). Learning and Behavior*, 34, 154-161.

MacDonald, S. E. (1994). Gorillas' (*Gorilla gorilla gorilla*) spatial memory in a foraging task. *Journal of Comparative Psychology*, 108, 107-113.

MacDonald, S. E. and Agnes, M. M. (1999). Orangutan (*Pongo pygmaeus abelii*) spatial memory and behavior in a foraging task. *Journal of Comparative Psychology*, 113, 213-217.

MacDonald, S. E. and Wilkie, D. M. (1990). Yellow-nosed monkeys' (*Cercopithecus ascanius whitesidei*) spatial memory in a simulated foraging environment. *Journal of Comparative Psychology*, 104, 382-387.

MacDonald, S. E., Pang, J. and Gibeault, S. (1994). Marmoset (*Callithrix jacchus jacchus*) spatial memory in a foraging task: Win-stay versus win-shift strategies. *Journal of Comparative Psychology*, 108, 328-334.

Page, R., Merten, S. and Simers, B. (2011) Associative memory or algorithmic search: a comparative study on learning strategies of bats and shrews. *Animal Cognition*, 15, 495-504.

Perdue, B. M., Snyder, R. J., Pratte, J., Marr, M. J. and Maple, T. L. (2009). Spatial memory recall in the giant panda (*ailuropoda melanoleuca*). *Journal of Comparative Psychology*, 123, 275-279. doi:http://dx.doi.org.huaryu.kl.oakland.edu/10.1037/a0016220.

Perdue, B., Snyder, R., Zhihe, Z., Marr, J. and Maple, T. (2011) Sex differences in spatial ability: A test of the range size hypothesis in order carnivore. *Animal Behaviour*, 7, 380-383.

Tarou, L. R. (2004). An examination of the role of associative learning and spatial memory in foraging of two species of bear (family: Ursidae) (*Ailuropoda melanoleuca, Tremarctos ornatus*). *Dissertation Abstracts International: Section B: The Sciences and Engineering*, 64, 5260.

Thorpe, C. M., Hallett, D. and Wilkie, D. M. (2007). The role of spatial and temporal information in learning interval time-place tasks. *Behavioural Processes*, 75, 55-65. doi: http://dx.doi.org/10.1016/j.beproc.2007.01.002.

Vonk, J. and Beran, M. J. (2012). Bears "count" too: Quantity estimation and comparison in black bears (*Ursus Americanus*). *Animal Behaviour*, 84, 231-238.

Vonk, J., Jett, S. E. and Mosteller, K. W. (2012). Concept formation in American black bears (*Ursus americanus*). *Animal Behaviour*, 84, 953-964.

West, S., Jett, S. E., Beckman, T. and Vonk, J. (2010). The Phylogenetic roots of cognitive dissonance. *Journal of Comparative Psychology*, 124, 425-432.

Zamisch, V. and Vonk, J. (2012). Spatial memory in captive American black bears (*Ursus americanus*). *Journal of Comparative Psychology*, 12, 0735-7036. doi:10.1037/a 0028081.

In: Spatial, Long-and Short-Term Memory
Editor: Edward A. Thayer
ISBN: 978-1-63484-148-1

Chapter 4

Visuospatial Working Memory in Children with Nonverbal Learning Disabilities: Impairment in Encoding Spatial Configuration

Tadamasa Narimoto
Tokyo University of Social Welfare, Department of Psychology
Kita-ku, Tokyo, Japan

Abstract

There have been a substantial number of reports indicating the existence of children who have intact verbally based learning but not visuospatially based learning. Rourke (1995) and Semrud-Clikeman, Walkowiak, Wilkinson, & Christopher (2010) described these children as having nonverbal learning disabilities (NLD). Normally, they show a large discrepancy between high verbal and lower performance scores on IQ testing, and generally have a pattern of cognitive and emotional impairment coupled with postulated right hemisphere brain dysfunction. Cornoldi et al. (2003) indicated that children with NLD who exhibited low visuospatial intelligence but intact verbal intelligence showed deficits in visual and spatial working memory (more specifically a storage component for visuospatial coded materials in the working memory system called the visuospatial sketchpad, or VSSP). It could be argued that because children with NLD exhibit impaired visuospatial working memory, the cause could be deficits in the memory capacity of VSSP. Specifically, the storage function of VSSP is impaired; therefore, these children perform significantly lower on visuospatial working memory tests than normally developing children. However, one study indicated that impaired visuospatial working memory could not be explained solely by deficits in VSSP, if at all. Mammarella and Pazzaglia (2010) reported that children at risk of NLD show severe impairments in visuospatial working memory tests, and show impairments in perceptual tests in which memory processes are not involved. Because some studies indicate simply perceiving visual features and spatial configurations is impaired in children with NLD, there is the possibility that their impaired performance on visuospatial working memory tests is due to a problem in the encoding phase. However, there have been few studies to investigate the above problem. In this chapter, I introduce a study conducted by Narimoto, Matsuura,

Takezawa, Mitsuhashi, and Hiratani (2013) to show that difficulty encoding relational information between spatial locations presented in random positions simultaneously is responsible for impaired visuospatial working memory. Their results indicated that children with NLD indeed have difficulty in encoding relational information. Specifically, it was hard for children to encode a visual configuration formed by each spatial location. In other words, they seemed to encode each individual absolute position. It is important to understand the causal relationship between the encoding process and visuospatial working memory in order to further provide effective support to children with NLD.

Keywords: Nonverbal learning disabilities, visuospatial working memory, relational information between spatial locations, visuospatial sketchpad

INTRODUCTION

Children with Deficits in Visuospatial Processes

A substantial number of experimental studies have provided evidence indicating the existence of children who have deficits in visuospatial processes but not in verbal processes. Rourke (1989, 1995) has described these children as having "nonverbal learning disabilities" (NLD). According to Rourke and his colleagues (e.g., Harnadek & Rourke 1994; Pelletier, Ahmad & Rourke 2001), children with NLD have deficits in visual-perceptual-organizational abilities, complex psychomotor skills, tactile perception, and nonverbal problem-solving skills, with age-appropriate development of rote verbal, simple motor, and psycholinguistic skills and abilities. These children also have deficits in mathematical abilities. Rourke and his colleagues (Pelletier et al., 2001; Rourke & Del Dotto 1994) also introduced the term R-S to describe children with poor single-word reading and spelling skills (R-S children). These children show deficits in verbal processes but not in visuo-perceptual-organizational abilities. Harnadek and Rourke showed that performance of the NLD group was significantly lower than that of the R-S and control groups on tests measuring visual-perceptual-organizational abilities (e.g., visual scanning and visual-spatial short-term memory), while the NLD group's levels of performance did not significantly differ from those of the control group on the tests measuring verbal abilities (e.g., single-word reading and spelling skills). On the other hand, performance of the R-S group was significantly lower than that of the NLD and control groups on tests measuring verbal abilities, while performance on tests measuring visual-spatial-organizational abilities was intact. Similarly, Pelletier et al. showed that children in the S-R group had a mean Verbal IQ (on WISC/WISC-R) that was significantly lower than that exhibited by children in the NLD group. Children in the S-R group also had marked deficiencies on the tests measuring reading and spelling abilities.

Although Rourke and his colleagues argued that children with NLD have deficits not only in visual-spatial-organizational abilities but also in mathematical and psychosocial skills, Forrest (2004) proposed that deficits in visuospatial abilities could be the core of NLD. In her study, children who showed a low performance IQ on the WISC, low arithmetic scores on the WRAT, and slowed psychomotor speed performed significantly lower in visuospatial perceptual and memory tests than children in the control group and group with deficits in verbal processes. However, there was no significant difference in mathematical abilities among the three groups. In addition, contrary to expectation, internalized psychopathology (e.g., depression, psychosis, or withdrawal) was greater in the group with deficits in verbal processes.

Furthermore, Cornoldi, Rigoni, Tressoldi, and Vio (1999) and Cornoldi, Dalla Vecchia, and Tressoldi (1995) found that children with NLD, who exhibited low visuospatial intelligence and high verbal intelligence, showed difficulty performing "spatial" and "visual" short-term memory tests. Similarly, Lepore, Celentano, Conson, and Grossi (2008) reported a case study of a 9-year-old child who showed normal general intelligence but had a discrepancy between verbal and performance scores on the WISC-R scale, and had difficulty in performing neuropsychological tests measuring spatial short-term memory. Similar findings were also reported by Mammarella, Lucangeli, and Cornoldi (2010) and Mammarella & Pazzaglia (2010).

Visuospatially Coded Materials and Working Memory

It has been widely agreed that working memory is a cognitive system for information processing. The most popular model of working memory is a multi-component model introduced by Baddeley (1986; Baddeley and Logie 1999). In this model, working memory consists of three storage subcomponents and one controlling system. Visuospatially coded materials are considered to be temporarily stored in the visuospatial sketchpad (VSSP). There are two other storage components: the "phonological loop" responsible for retaining verbally coded material and the "episodic buffer" (Baddeley, 2000a). This latter component is assumed to be for storage of an integrated episode that is bound across domains (see also Baddeley, Allen & Hitch 2011; Respovs & Baddeley 2006). Each of these storage components is considered to have a limited pool of cognitive resources, though they are supervised by an attentional system called the central executive (Baddeley and Logie 1999). The central executive is considered to control higher cognitive processes, such as planning (Gilhooly, Wynn, Phillips, Logie & Della Sala, 2002), updating mental representations (Morris & Jones, 1990; van der Linden, Bredart & Beerten 1994), inhibition of irrelevant information (Baddeley, 1996; Salway & Logie 1995), and coordination of verbal and visuospatial storage (Loisy & Roulin 2003).

It could be argued that deficits in visuospatial processes manifested by children with NLD are attributable to a low capacity of VSSP. However, it could also be true that visuospatial deficits manifested by such children are attributable to the difficulty in encoding visuospatial information. In the latter case, it would be the functional deficiencies of the central executive system (i.e., an attentional system) and not VSSP (i.e., storage component) that causes low performance on visuospatial tasks.

Objective of Narimoto et al.'s Study (2013)

Needless to say, it is very important to understand the causal relationship between the encoding process and visuospatial memory in order to provide effective support to children with NLD. However, there have been few studies to clearly explain these mechanisms. Our study specifically investigated whether difficulty encoding a spatial configuration could be a cause for impaired spatial short-term memory. Previous studies provide evidence that spatial items presented simultaneously in random positions are encoded with relational information between them, but not encoded individually. Because children with NLD normally show impaired spatial memory, they could have difficulty encoding this relational information. For example, Woodman, Vecera, and Luck (2003) argued that "perceptually grouping" spatial positions presented simultaneously is an important cognitive process for visuospatial short-term memory. They showed evidence that targets that are grouped together tend to be stored together, and also emphasized that perceptual grouping is not a controlled process requiring attentional resources, but rather a bottom-up (i.e., automatic) process. Similarly, Jiang, Olson, and Chun (2000) conducted experiments to investigate whether spatial targets presented simultaneously in random positions are encoded with relational information between them. Their results indicated that participants encoded relational information between spatial positions, but did not encode each absolute position of the spatial configuration.

The above evidence and the experimental results reported by Mammarella and Pazzaglia (2010) together seem to indicate that impaired spatial memory shown by children with NLD is attributed to an impaired automatic process of perceptual grouping. In other words, their storage function (i.e., VSSP) is not impaired, and because Woodman et al. argued less involvement of controlled process in encoding relational information, attentional function (i.e., central executive) is also not impaired. The aim of our study was to examine whether difficulty in encoding relational information between spatial positions presented in random positions simultaneously is responsible for their impaired spatial short-term memory.

METHODS

Participants

Children with difficulty in visuospatial processes (or NLD), but not in verbal and executive processes, were selected from a larger sample of over two hundred students referred to clinical services at the Hiratani Pediatric Clinic for Disabled Children in Japan, due to their difficulties at regular elementary school. The selected children were not diagnosed as having other developmental disorders and showed no indication of having emotional impairment. In addition, the Full Scale Intelligence Quotient (FSIQ) of selected children having NLD was in the normal range. Five children with NLD (3 boys and 2 girls) who fulfilled the selection criteria were selected from the larger sample. Their mean age was 9.8 years (range 8–11 years). Each child showed a discrepancy (at least 15 points) between verbal IQ (M = 104.4, SD = 4.96) and performance IQ (M = 80.6, SD = 5.12) as measured by the WISC-III. Their FSIQ, which represents children's overall cognitive ability, was greater than or equal to 86 (M = 92.4, SD = 4.88). The children were also selected based on scores in Verbal Comprehension (VC) and Perceptual Organization (PO), as Forrest (2004) underwent these scales to specify children with NLD. Their mean scores were 106.0 (SD = 5.90) for VC and 83.2 (SD = 8.86) for PO. Because we carefully selected children with NLD who had FSIQ scores in the normal range and showed a discrepancy between verbal IQ and performance IQ, the sample size inevitably became small.

Five children without NLD (3 boys and 2 girls) were selected from the same sample as a control group. Their mean age was 10.6 years (range 9–12 years). Each child showed a discrepancy (at least 15 points) between verbal IQ ($M = 73.2$, $SD = 7.44$) and performance IQ ($M = 104.6$, $SD = 7.17$) as measured by the WISC-III. Their FSIQ was greater than or equal to 82 ($M = 87.0$, $SD = 4.43$). Their mean scores on the WISC-III for VC and PO were 73.6 ($SD = 8.09$) and 101.4 ($SD = 7.39$), respectively. This group was set up to make sure that verbal processes were not involved in the spatial memory task. Unless the spatial memory task required verbal processes, the performance level of children in this group would be similar to that of normally developing children.

Five normally developing children (4 boys and 1 girl) were also selected from regular elementary school classrooms as another control group. They showed no impairments in visuospatial or verbal processes. Their mean age was 10.6 years (range 8–12 years). Although their schoolteachers and parents reported that the children had no academic problems, by way of caution we measured their mental abilities with the Wechsler Intelligence Scale for Children (fourth edition). The FSIQ mean score was 107.0 ($SD = 8.19$). The Working Memory Index (WMI), which assesses their ability to memorize new information, hold it in short-term memory, concentrate, and manipulate, was 103.4 ($SD = 10.33$). There was no significant discrepancy between these two scores.

Each child participated in this experiment after parental consent was obtained. All participants had normal or corrected-to-normal vision and were unaware of the purpose of the experiment.

Preliminary Experiment

Each participant's memory span was first measured using visual and spatial memory tests to confirm that visuospatial memory performance of children with NLD was significantly lower than those of children without NLD.

Span Tests and Design in the Preliminary Experiment

For the visual memory test, children were presented with a series of two to eight non-sense figures and had to decide whether or not these figures (memory image) were identical to the previous ones (probe image). For instance, at the second level, two figures were presented, and at the third level, three figures were presented. Participants were tested three times at each level in ascending order. Each participant's memory span was defined as the last level at which he or she correctly performed at least two out of three trials. On each trial, two images were presented separated by a blank interval, as shown in Figure 1. The non-sense, black-colored figures (about 1.4 cm × 1.4 cm) were presented simultaneously at random locations on a white background. In the probe image, an equal number of figures were presented as in the memory image. Participants were required to decide whether the figures on the two images were the same or not the same. They were instructed to point to the figure on the probe image that they thought had not been presented on the memory image. In the spatial memory test, children were presented simultaneously with a series of two to eight black-colored squares positioned randomly on the memory and probe images. Participants were required to decide whether the locations of the squares on the two images were the same or different. They were instructed to point to the position on the probe image that had been changed from the memory image.

Participants initiated each trial by pressing the ENTER key on a portable 10-key calculator. In both tests, at the beginning of the procedure a blank screen appeared for 1000 ms, followed by another blank screen for 500 ms, then the non-sense figures (3000 ms), followed by another blank screen for 500 ms. After presentation of a fixation point for 1500 ms, either the same series of figures or a series differing in one figure was presented as a probe image. The experimenter recorded participants' responses. This preliminary experiment was programed with SuperLab 4 (Cedrus Corporation). All stimuli were presented on a 17-inch monitor with a viewing distance of 40 cm. Participants were tested individually in a room with normal lighting. This preliminary experiment was conducted at the Hiratani Pediatric Clinic for Disabled Children and took approximately thirty minutes.

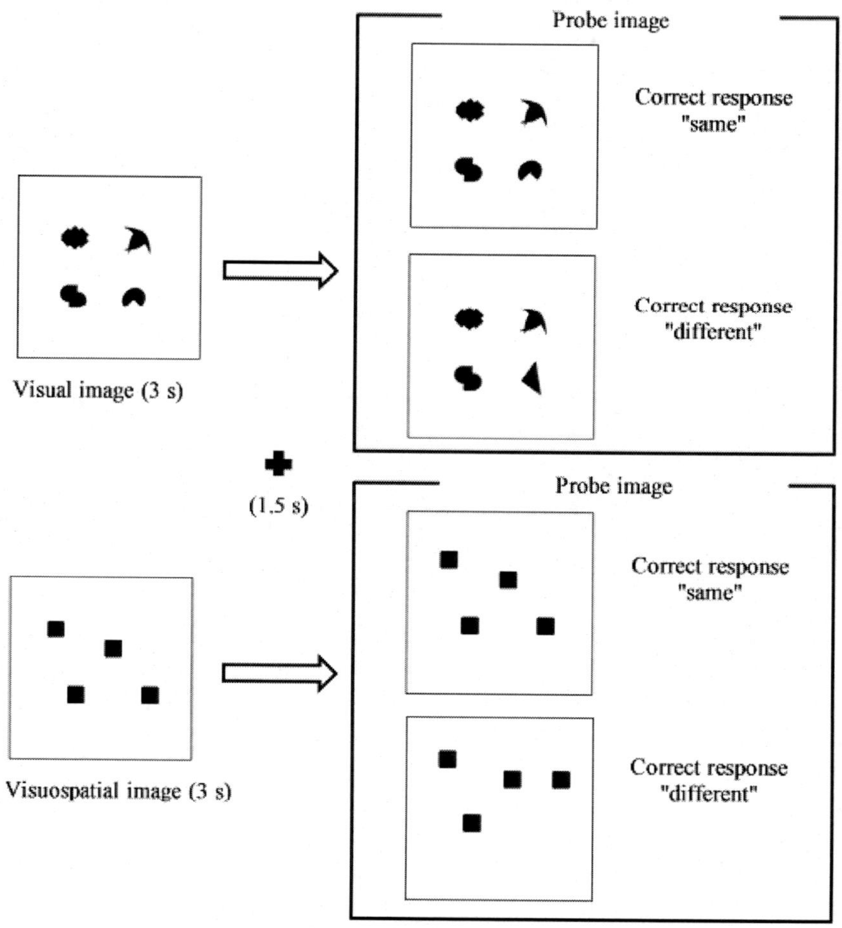

Figure 1. A schematic plot showing an example of a four-item memory set in the visual and visuospatial memory test. Originally published as Figure 1 in Narimoto et al. (2013). Spatial short-term memory in children with nonverbal learning disabilities: Impairment in encoding spatial configuration. Journal of Genetic Psychology, 174 (1), 73–87. Taylor & Francis Ltd.

Results of the Preliminary Experiment

The mean memory span scores on the visual memory test for normally developing children (control group), children without NLD (low VC group), and children with NLD (low PO group) were 5.60 ($SD = 0.49$), 5.20 ($SD = 0.75$), and 2.80 ($SD = 0.74$), respectively. The difference among the three groups was significant ($F(2, 12) = 7.88$, $p < .001$). Multiple comparison tests with Ryan's method (Ryan, 1960) showed that performance of the low PO group was significantly lower than that of both the control and low VC groups, while performance between the control and low VC groups was not statistically different. A similar pattern of results was obtained on the spatial memory test. The mean span scores for the control, low VC, and low PO groups were 7.84 ($SD = 0.66$), 7.40 ($SD = 0.80$), and 4.40 ($SD = 1.36$), respectively. The difference among the three groups was significant ($F(2, 12) = 14.18$, $p < .001$). Multiple comparison tests with Ryan's method showed that performance of the low PO group was significantly lower than that of both the control and low VC groups, while performance between the control and low VC groups was not statistically different. These results clearly show that children in the low PO group had difficulty in visuospatial processes.

Materials and Design for the Primary Experiment

On each trial, two images were presented separated by a blank interval, as shown in Figure 2. The memory image contained three, five, or seven green squares (1.2 cm × 1.2 cm) presented simultaneously at random locations on a white background. Each square was randomly positioned in an invisible 6 × 6 matrix (each cell = 1.6 cm). The second image was the probe and had two conditions. In both probe conditions an equal number of squares were presented, as in the memory image. One of the squares was outlined by a red box (1.3 cm × 1.3 cm). The other squares remained at previously presented locations (minimal location change) or were positioned randomly at previously blank locations (maximal location change). The task was to decide whether the square with a red outline box was at a new location (50% of the trials) or a previously occupied location. Participants initiated each trial by pressing the ENTER key on a portable 10-key calculator. Each trial started with a central black fixation cross (1 cm × 1 cm) lasting 1 s, followed by a blank period of 1 s. The memory image was then presented for 1 s and erased. After another blank interval of 1 s, the probe image was presented until the participant responded. Participants were instructed to press "1" on the calculator if the square with a red outline was at a previously occupied location, and to press "+" if it was at a new location.

A within-subjects design was used such that all participants performed all conditions. Each participant performed 240 experimental trials (3 memory set sizes × 2 probe types × 2 change present or absent × 20 cases). Stimulus positions were randomly chosen on each trial. Three children in each group performed the minimal location change condition first, and two children performed the maximal location change condition first. The order of set sizes was randomized. Participants performed 10 practice trials before starting experimental trials in each condition. Participants were encouraged to rest whenever they wanted. This experiment was conducted at the Hiratani Pediatric Clinic for Disabled Children and took approximately one and a half hours (including rest time).

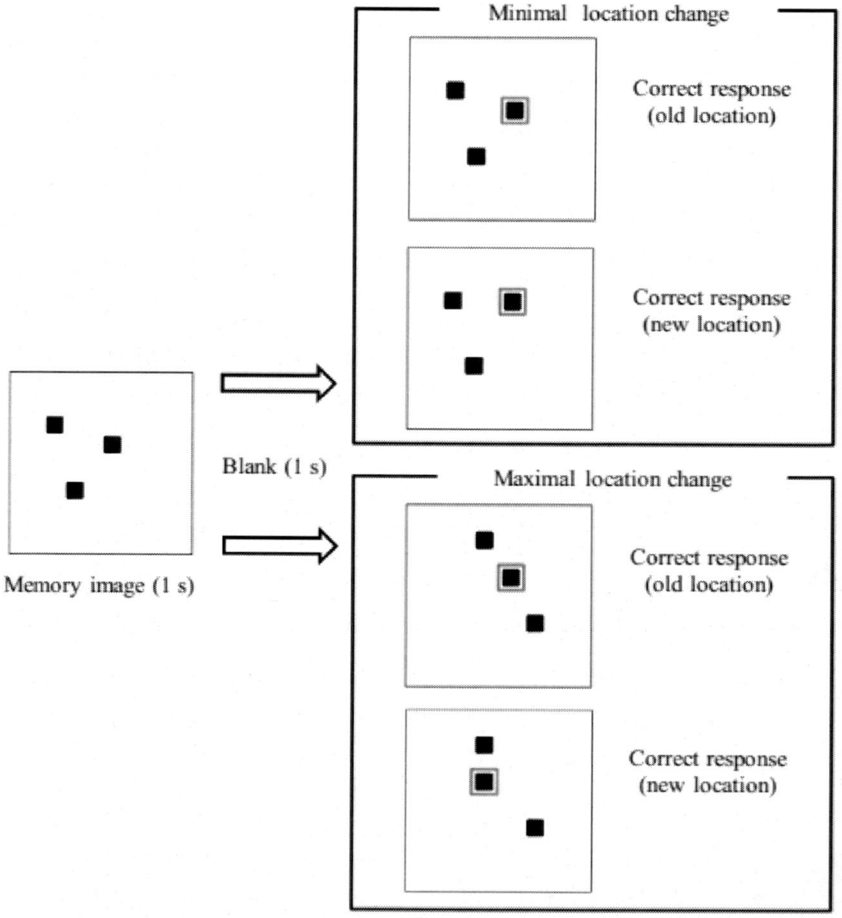

Figure 2. A schematic plot showing an example of a three-item memory set in the minimal and maximal location change conditions. Originally published as Figure 2 in Narimoto et al. (2013). Spatial short-term memory in children with nonverbal learning disabilities: Impairment in encoding spatial configuration. Journal of Genetic Psychology, 174 (1), 73–87. Taylor & Francis Ltd.

Apparatus for the Primary Experiment

The experiment was programed with SuperLab 4. All stimuli were presented on a 17-in monitor with a viewing distance of 40 cm. Participants were tested individually in a room with normal lighting.

RESULTS

A 3 × 3 ANOVA (memory set size × group) was used to test differences in the minimal and maximal location change conditions separately (see Figures 3 and 4). In the minimal location change condition, we only found a significant main effect of group ($F(2, 12) = 12.61$,

$p < .001$). Multiple comparison tests with Ryan's method showed that only the performance of the low PO group was significantly lower than the other two groups. There were no main effects of group or set size in the maximal location change condition, nor was the interaction of these two factors significant. Since there was no significant interaction of memory set size with group in either location change condition, we pooled across the set size factor and then used a group (3) × change condition (2) ANOVA. Figure 5 shows the mean percent correct on the recognition test as a function of group and change condition. We found significant main effects of group ($F(2, 12) = 8.32, p < .01$) and change condition ($F(1, 12) = 153.76, p < .001$). The interaction between group and change condition was also significant ($F(2, 12) = 13.84, p < .001$). In the minimal location condition, performance of the low PO group was significantly lower than the other two groups ($F(2, 24) = 18.67, p < .001$). In the maximal task condition, there was no significant difference in performance among the three groups. Furthermore, each group showed significantly better performance in the minimal task condition than in the maximal task condition: control group ($F(1, 12) = 103.65, p < .001$), low VC group ($F(1, 12) = 68.75, p < .001$), and low PO group ($F(1, 12) = 9.03, p < .05$).

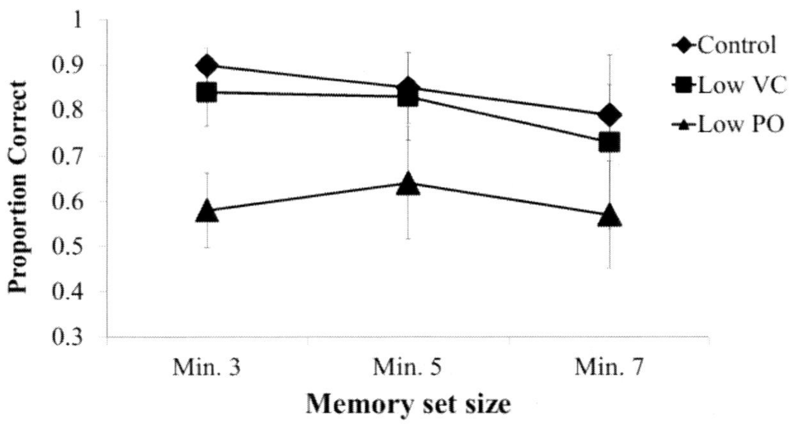

Figure 3. Mean proportion of correct responses as a function of group and memory set size in the minimal location change condition. Originally published as Figure 3 in Narimoto et al. (2013). Spatial short-term memory in children with nonverbal learning disabilities: Impairment in encoding spatial configuration. *Journal of Genetic Psychology*, *174* (*1*), 73–87. Taylor & Francis Ltd.

We also measured participants' detection sensitivity (d') and response bias in the minimal location change condition. Sensitivity was measured by determining how well an observer was able to make correct judgments and avoid incorrect ones. Response bias was measured by determining the propensity of an observer to favor a particular response over another. Since memory set size did not interact with group, we pooled across the set size factor and group when calculating false alarm rate and hit rate. The scores of d' were 2.19 ($SE = 0.11$) in the control group, 1.85 ($SE = 0.28$) in the low VC group, and 0.51 ($SE = 0.16$) in the low PO group. The sensitivity value of the low PO group was significantly lower than the other two groups ($F(2, 12) = 16.45, p < .001$). The response bias values were 2.05 ($SE = 1.04$) for the control group, 1.48 ($SE = 0.53$) for the low VC group, and 1.23 ($SE = 0.13$) for the low PO group. The differences in these values failed to reach statistical significance ($F(2, 12) = 1.51$, *n.s.*).

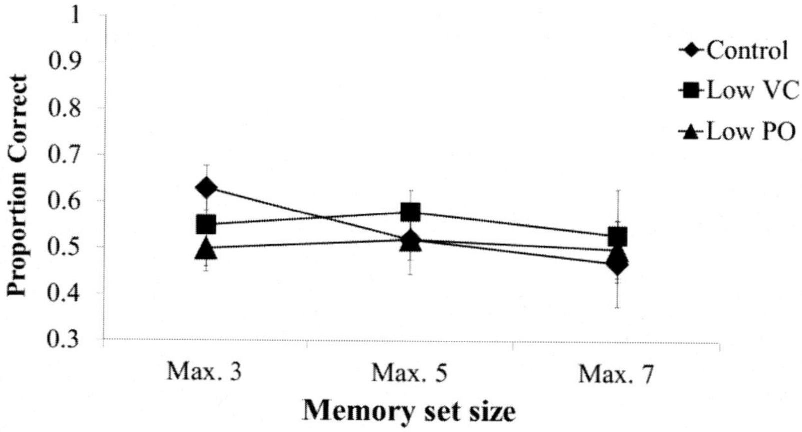

Figure 4. Mean proportion of correct responses as a function of group and memory set size in the maximal location change condition. Originally published as Figure 4 in Narimoto et al. (2013). Spatial short-term memory in children with nonverbal learning disabilities: Impairment in encoding spatial configuration. Journal of Genetic Psychology, 174 (1), 73–87. Taylor & Francis Ltd.

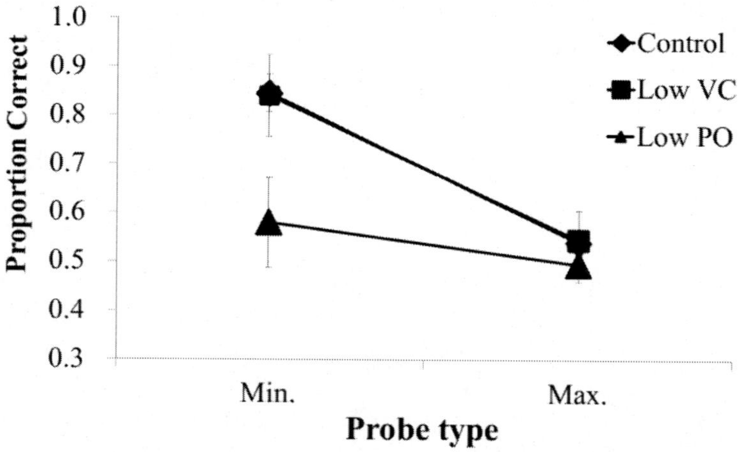

Figure 5. Mean proportion of correct responses as a function of group and probe type. Originally published as Figure 5 in Narimoto et al. (2013). Spatial short-term memory in children with nonverbal learning disabilities: Impairment in encoding spatial configuration. Journal of Genetic Psychology, 174 (1), 73–87. Taylor & Francis Ltd.

Discussion

Previous studies have provided clear evidence that children with NLD show impaired visuospatial short-term memory (e.g., Cornoldi et al., 1999; Mammarella, Cornoldi & Donadello 2003; Mammarella, Pazzaglia & Cornoldi 2008; Mammarella et al., 2010). Our study investigated specifically whether low performance in spatial location memory shown by children with NLD is attributable to the low capacity of VSSP or to the difficulty in encoding relational information among spatial locations. The results showed that children without NLD performed significantly better in the minimal location change condition than in the maximal location change condition, indicating that relational information between randomly positioned squares, not individual absolute location, is indeed encoded (e.g., Jiang et al. 2000). Performance of children with NLD was lower than that of children without NLD in the minimal location change condition, suggesting that children with NLD have difficulty encoding the relational information. Furthermore, participants' detection sensitivity and response bias in the minimal location change condition were analyzed. Sensitivity to accurate response in the minimal location change condition was significantly lower in the low PO group. More importantly, there was no significant difference in response bias values among the three groups. Therefore, the accuracy difference was not an artifact of different response criteria. These findings indicate that the cause of impaired spatial memory is not a deficit in the storage function of VSSP.

However, there is a possibility that the low performance of children with NLD, compared with children without NLD, in the minimal condition was attributable to impaired storage capacity of VSSP. Previous studies showed evidence that, in general, those children who show intact verbal and lower performance scores on IQ testing had difficulty retaining not only spatial locations but also visual features regardless of simultaneous or sequential presentations (Mammarella et al., 2010). Even though it would not be important to encode relational information for temporal retention of each visual feature, children with NLD showed lower performance in visual (feature) memory tests. This fact indicates that storage capacity of VSSP in children with NLD is impaired, as visual materials are considered to be also stored in VSSP. However, a number of studies have provided evidence that VSSP is not a single storage component for visuospatial coded materials, but may be further divided into two subcomponents for spatial locations and visual features. Actually, Klauer and Zhao (2004; also, Kessels, Postma & de Haan 1999; Smith, Jonides, Koeppe, Awh, Schumacher & Minoshima 1995; Tresch, Sinnamon & Seamon 1993) argued that VSSP is composed of a visual subcomponent for retaining visual properties of objects and a spatial subcomponent for retaining spatial locations. Following these authors' claim, it is possible to argue that the capacity for visual features may be different between children with and without NLD, whereas the capacity for spatial locations in children with NLD is not impaired. The idea that the spatial subcomponent (i.e., storage capacity of spatial locations) is intact in children with NLD was further supported by the results of our study. That is, we showed there was a significant difference between the minimal and maximal location change conditions in the performance of children with NLD. If impaired capacity of the spatial subcomponent were a cause of low performance in spatial location memory, then their performance would not have differed between the two conditions. This fact seems to indicate that impaired spatial location memory is attributed to difficulty encoding relational information.

There is another possible alternative accounting for the impaired spatial location memory shown by children with NLD. It could be attentional (or executive) functions that are damaged; therefore, their performance in the minimal location change condition was significantly lower than that of children without NLD. However, it is not unreasonable to consider that children with NLD simply had difficulty directing their attention on the memory tests, because, as mentioned earlier, response bias values of children in the low PO group were the same as those of children in other groups. This fact indicates that impaired spatial memory is not explained solely by executive dysfunction, if at all. If they had difficulty directing their attention in the present study, the response bias values of children in the low PO group would not have been similar to the other groups.

Our study required children to retain positions of spatial items for only 1 s and found that the performance of children with NLD was significantly worse on memory tests in the minimal location change condition than children in the low VC and control groups. This impaired memory performance appears to be caused by difficulty encoding relational information between item positions. Moreover, Semrud-Clikeman et al. (2010) conducted experiments to investigate whether performance on the visuospatial tasks was different among children with either NLD, Asperger syndrome (AS), or attention deficit hyperactivity disorder (ADHD). They reported that these difficulties were present only for the NLD group even when motor disability was not present, and that no difference was found among the AS, ADHD, or control groups on visual-spatial ability. The above study indicates that the lower performance shown by children with NLD in the present study is not attributable to executive dysfunction, because if a deficit in executive processes were the cause of lower spatial location memory, there would have been no difference in performance between children with NLD and children with ADHD in the Semrud-Clikeman et al. study.

However, it is also not unreasonable to suggest that difficulty encoding a spatial configuration is the only factor accounting for impaired spatial location memory in children with NLD. The results of our study do not rule out involvement of factors such as low memory capacity (e.g., Cornoldi, Rigoni, Venneri & Vecchi 2000). For instance, it might be true that because children with NLD were unable to visually relate each position of spatial items presented simultaneously, they were forced to encode individual absolute location, inevitably putting a lot of strain on their memory capacity. Therefore, they would even have difficulty retaining locations of three items if the memory capacity is indeed smaller than normally developing children.

Weakness of the Present Study

One possible weakness in our study was the small sample size, as a result of carefully selecting children with NLD (i.e., low PO group) and without NLD (i.e., low VC group) from the larger sample (more than two hundred children). Consequently, the power to detect a significant difference in performance among small groups could be low. However, our study provided clear results showing statistical differences in performance between children with and without NLD. These clear results were obtained because we cautiously selected children with NLD and without NLD and required each child to perform a large number of experimental trials (forty trials) in each condition, so as to obtain reliable and consistent data. Therefore, the results supporting the hypothesis that impaired spatial location memory in children with NLD is attributable to difficulty with encoding relational information between spatial items could not be denied because of the small sample size.

Finally, difficulty encoding the relational information, but not the storage function of VSSP, is firmly considered as an important factor for impaired spatial location memory exhibited by children with NLD. However, the experimental results supporting the above hypothesis were obtained by a single experiment that may not address all aspects of the impairment. Therefore, further research may be necessary to ascertain the hypothesis with a variety of experimental design methods and large number of experimental participants.

REFERENCES

Baddeley, A. D. (1986). *Working memory*. New York, NY: Oxford University Press.

Baddeley, A. D. (1996). Exploring the central executive. *Quarterly Journal of Experimental Psychology*, *49*, 5–28.

Baddeley, A. D. (2000a). The episodic buffer: A new component of working memory? *Trends in Cognitive Sciences*, *4*, 417–423.

Baddeley, A. D., Allen, R. J., & Hitch, G. J. (2011). Binding in visual working memory: the role of the episodic buffer. *Neuropsychologia*, *49*, 1393–1400.

Baddeley, A. D., & Logie, R. H. (1999). Working memory: The multiple-component model. In A. Miyake & P. Shah (Eds.), *Models of working memory* (pp. 28–61). Cambridge, UK: Cambridge University Press.

Cornoldi, C., Della Vecchia, R., & Tressoldi, P. E. (1995). Visuo-spatial working memory limitations in low visuo-spatial high verbal intelligence children. *Journal of Child Psychology and Psychiatry*, *36*, 1053–1064.

Cornoldi, C., Rigoni, F., Tressoldi, P. E., & Vio, C. (1999). Imagery deficits in nonverbal learning disabilities. *Journal of Learning Disabilities*, *32*, 48–57.

Cornoldi, C., Rigoni, F., Venneri, A., & Vecchi, T. (2000). Passive and active visuo-spatial memory: Double dissociation in developmental learning disabilities. *Brain and Cognition*, *43*, 117–120.

Forrest, B. (2004). The utility of math difficulties, internalized psychopathology, and visual-spatial deficits to identify children with the nonverbal learning disability syndrome: Evidence for a visualspatial disability. *Child Neuropsychology*, *10*, 129–146.

Gilhooly, K. J., Wynn, V., Phillips, L. H., Logie, R. H., & Della Sala, S. (2002). Visuo-spatial and verbal working memory in the five-disc Tower of London task: An individual differences approach. *Thinking & Reasoning*, *8*, 165–178.

Harnadek, M. C. S., & Rourke, B. P. (1994). Principal identifying features of the syndrome of nonverbal learning disabilities in children. *Journal of Learning Disabilities*, *27*, 144–154.

Jiang, Y., Olson, I. R., & Chun, M. M. (2000). Organization of visual short-term memory. *Journal of Experimental Psychology: Learning, Memory, and Cognition*, *26*, 683–702.

Kessels, R. P. C., Postma, A., & de Haan, E. H. F. (1999). Object Relocation: A program for setting up, running, and analyzing experiments on memory for object locations. *Behavior Research Methods, Instruments, & Computers*, *31*, 423–428.

Klauer, K. C., & Zhao, Z. (2004). Double dissociation in visual and spatial short-term memory. *Journal of Experimental Psychology: General*, *133*, 355–381.

Lepore, M., Celentano, K., Conson, M., & Grossi, D. (2008). On the nature of nonverbal working memory fractionation: A case of selective spatial short-term memory deficit in a child. *Child Neuropsychology*, *14*, 438–452.

Loisy, C., & Roulin, J. L. (2003). Multiple short-term storage: A task to evaluate the coordination function of the central executive. *International Journal of Psychology*, 38, 1–10.

Mammarella, I. C., Cornoldi, C., & Donadello, E. (2003). Visual but not spatial working memory deficit in children with spina bifida. *Brain and Cognition*, *53*, 311–314.

Mammarella, I. C., Lucangeli, D., & Cornoldi, C. (2010). Spatial working memory and arithmetic deficits in children with nonverbal learning difficulties. *Journal of learning disabilities*, *43*, 455–468.

Mammarella, I. C., & Pazzaglia, F. (2010). Visual perception and memory impairments in children at risk for nonverbal learning disabilities. *Child Neuropsychology*, *16*, 564–576.

Mammarella, I. C., Pazzaglia, F., & Cornoldi, C. (2008). Evidence for different components in children's visuospatial working memory. *British Journal of Developmental Psychology*, *26*, 337–355.

Morris, N., & Jones, D. M. (1990). Memory updating in working memory: The role of the central executive. *British Journal of Psychology*, *81*, 111–121.

Narimoto, T., Matsuura, N., Takezawa, T., Mitsuhashi, Y., & Hiratani, M. (2013). Spatial short-term memory in children with nonverbal learning disabilities: Impairment in encoding spatial configuration. *Journal of Genetic Psychology*, *174*, 73–87.

Pelletier, P. M., Ahmad, S. A., & Rourke, B. P. (2001). Classification rules for basic phonological processing disabilities and nonverbal learning disabilities: Formulation and external validity. *Child Neuropsychology*, 7, 84–98.

Repovs, G., & Baddeley, A. D. (2006). The multi-component model of working memory: Explorations in experimental cognitive psychology. *Neuroscience*, *139*, 5–21.

Rourke, B. P. (1989). *Nonverbal learning disabilities: The syndrome and the model*. New York: Guilford Press.

Rourke, B. P. (1995). *Syndrome of nonverbal learning disabilities: Neurodevelopmental manifestations*. New York: Guilford Press.

Rourke, B. P., & Del Dotto, J. E. (1994). *Learning disabilities: A neuropsychological perspective*. Thousand Oaks, CA: Sage.

Salway, A. F. S., & Logie, R. H. (1995). Visuospatial working memory, movement control and executive demands. *British Journal of Psychology*, *86*, 253–269.

Semrud-Clikeman, M., Walkowiak, J., Wilkinson, A., & Christopher, G. (2010). Neuropsychological differences among children with Asperger syndrome, nonverbal learning disabilities, attention deficit disorder, and controls. *Developmental Neuropsychology*, *35*, 582–600.

Smith, E. E., Jonides, J., Koeppe, R. A., Awh, E., Schumacher, E. H., & Minoshima, S. (1995). Spatial vs. object working memory: PET investigations. *Journal of Cognitive Neuroscience*, *7*, 337–356.

Tresch, M. C., Sinnamon, H. M., & Seamon, J. G. (1993). Double dissociation of spatial and object visual memory: Evidence from selective interference in intact human subjects. *Neuropsychologia*, *31*, 211–219.

van der Linden, M., Bredart, S., & Beerten, A. (1994). Age-related differences in updating working memory. *British Journal of Psychology*, *85*, 145–152.

Woodman, G. F., Vecera, S. P., & Luck, S. J. (2003). Perceptual organization influences visual working memory. *Psychonomic Bulletin & Review*, *10*, 80–87.

In: Spatial, Long-and Short-Term Memory
Editor: Edward A. Thayer

ISBN: 978-1-63484-148-1

Chapter 5

SHORT AND LONG TERM MEMORY IN PEDIATRIC IDIOPATHIC EPILEPSY: FUNCTIONS AND EFFECT OF INTERVENTIONS

***Yael Schaffer*[1] *and Prof. Ronny Geva*[2]**

[1]Department of Psychology
The Gonda Brain Research Center, Bar-Ilan University, Ramat Gan, Israel
[2]Head of Developmental Neuropsychology lab, Department of Psychology,
The Gonda Brain Research Center, Bar Ilan University, Ramat Gan, Israel

ABSTRACT

Multiple diseases affect memory, but only in a few pathological processes, memory systems are discretely affected, allowing to study short and longterm - resilience and susceptibility of memory systems, in the absence of other background cognitive deficits. Idiopathic epilepsies (IE) are considered to have relatively good prognoses and normal or near normal developmental outcomes. Nevertheless, accumulating studies demonstrate memory and executive functions deficits in this population. The aim of this chapter is to describe in details memory systems in children with IE and to present a new structured cognitive group intervention protocol in children with mild memory deficits.

The intervention program is designed to improve auditory verbal short term and long term memory using strategic abilities in a specific manner. The program is composed of 5 weekly sessions in a group format. 33 children with IE, ages 9-14 years participated in the research protocol and were compared to 27 age and education matched healthy control. Initial results demonstrate that auditory verbal short term memory skills which were frequently deficient at baseline were improved as a result of the intervention. Further analysis indicated that executive functions mediated the intervention effect. The effects were such that participants with higher EF functioning gained less from the intervention and improved their auditory memory less than participants with lower baseline EF. Results suggest that group therapy for children with mild memory impairments such as children with IE may benefit from short term intervention which is specifically tailored to limit the degree of the persistent auditory verbal memory deficits.

Based on these results, the chapter presents a theoretical model for memory intervention paths, designed for pediatric populations with mild memory deficits with emphasis on the role of executive functions in short term memory rehabilitation in these patients.

Future studies that will focus on pediatric populations with mild memory deficits and widen the knowledge on executive functions role in memory rehabilitation, utilization of retrieval strategies in memory intervention protocols and methods that help assimilate strategies learned are recommended in addition to examining long term effect and ecology of the model presented.

INTRODUCTION

Epilepsy, a group of disorders that cause disturbances in electrical signaling in the brain, is a fairly common in the general population [1]. An epileptic seizure occurs when an electric pulse surges rapidly due to abnormal, excessive or synchronous neural activity in the brain [2]. This brief electrical surge can transpire in a limited brain region, or it can affect the whole brain. Depending on the affected area, this surge can produce changes in a person's sensations or state of consciousness. It can also instigate uncontrolled movements of certain parts of the body or of the whole body [3]. There are three main types of epilepsy: idiopathic (elicited by an unknown cause), symptomatic (activated by an identifiable etiology), or cryptogenic (with an un-known cause). Idiopathic epilepsy can be partial (seizures involving only part of the brain) or generalized (seizures involving both sides of the brain) [4, 5]. Idiopathic epilepsy tends to appear during childhood or adolescence [6]. People with idiopathic epilepsy (IE) typically display normal intelligence and typical neurological and MRI results [6], yet electroencephalogram (EEG) tests, which measures electrical impulses in the brain, may show epileptic discharges affecting the entire or part of the brain [7-9]. IE was considered for many years to result in a preserved cognitive profile, as well as in preserved memory. Nevertheless, data from the recent decade indicate that memory difficulties represent the most common clinical complaints in patients with epilepsy, including those with IE type [10, 11], suggesting that the cognitive impact of epilepsy has been at times underestimated.

MECHANISMS FOR MEMORY LOSS IN EPILEPSY

Basic neurophysiological work suggests that seizures can modify, slow down, or accelerate a wide range of unique processes that take place during development and that are essential for the correct formation and function of brain circuitry and for memory [12].

According to several studies, three main factors are considered to be involved in IE patients' memory impairments. The first factor is the underlying etiology for epilepsy. For example, memory impairments resulting from childhood absence epilepsy [13] are different from impairments resulting from idiopathic generalized epilepsy or rolandic epilepsy [14-16]. The second factor has to do with the effects of seizures/epileptiform EEG discharges themselves, which insult consolidation during sleep of declarative memories [17]. In addition, memory impairments can result from the effects of chronic repetitive spikes that inhibit or disrupt activity in the same cortical area for many years [7]. The third factor concerns the effects of antiepileptic drugs (AEDs), as several AEDs, such as Topiramate and

Phenobarbital, are associated with memory problems in children [18]. Though most patients with epilepsy are successfully treated with a single antiepileptic drug (monotherapy), this sometimes does not lead to complete seizure control, and thus in at times a combination of antiepileptic medications are prescribed (polytherapy) [18, 19]. Several studies have shown polytherapy results in more pervasive cognitive deficits than monotherapy [18, 20]. With this in mind, it seems important to explore what particular memory deficits are expected in IE.

DISCRETE MEMORY DEFICITS IN IE

Memory is a multi-system construct [21] with different types of memory systems affected to varying degrees in childhood epilepsy [11, 14, 22, 23]. Most cognitive theoreticians address memory as a continuous process that involves different stages, including: encoding, storage and retrieval [21]. One common theoretical framework used to define memory differentiates between three types of time-dependent memory systems: short term memory (STM; 24, 25), long term memory (LTM; 26, 27-30); and working memory (WM; 31, 32-34).

STM in idiopathic epilepsy: Research regarding whether or not STM is affected in children with IE have yielded conflicting results. Several studies have demonstrated that processes of encoding and immediate recall are preserved in children with IE [11, 14, 23, 35, 36], while others have discovered greater risks for STM deficits in this population [15, 16, 37, 38]. Several factors may play into this discrepancy. One reason may be attributed to the fact that some studies were conducted when the participants were in remission as during remission, many patients show improved performance in a general intellectual test [15]. Other reasons may be related to differences in test sensitivity or task impurity [39].

A third explanation for these discrepancies may arise from diverse etiologies that fall under the category of idiopathic. Some idiopathic syndromes are benign, such as benign epilepsy with centrotemporal spikes [4], whereas others involve different brain substrates, such as is often the case in primary generalized epilepsy [5]. These diverse etiologies may form different memory impairments [40]. *LTM in IE*: Unlike in STM, LTM, and especially auditory verbal LTM [16] has been determined as a major area of deficit in children with IE. These deficits usually include delayed recall and recognition [14-16, 23, 35-38, 41, 42].These deficits may indicate the impairment in LTM may possibly result from deficits in storage and retrieval of information. *WM in IE*: While there may be significant individual variations, it was found that there is a high probability of relative deficits in aspects of processing speed and working memory in childhood epilepsy regardless of specific etiology [43], more specifically in children with recently diagnosed epilepsy [44], in particularly in children with idiopathic generalized epilepsy [16, 36, 38, 45, 46] and in children with benign epilepsy with centrotemporal spikes [14-16, 37, 47].

MODALITY DIFFERENCES IN IE

In recent years studies point to the role of modality in memory impairments in epilepsy, highlighting a particular sensitivity in coding and memorizing auditory verbal material as compared with nonverbal or visual stimuli [14-16, 35]. These deficits seem to also extend to other types of epilepsy, namely with benign epilepsy with centrotemporal spikes [for instance; 37, 47, 48-50] and Panayiotopoulos epilepsy [for instance 51, 52]. More specifically, whereas STM impairments are eminent in both auditory verbal and in nonverbal systems, LTM and WM deficits are mainly noted in response to auditory verbal cues. These deficits have been noted using canonical tools such as the digit span test and Rey auditory verbal test [14, 53].

Overall, it seems that children with IE tend to suffer from a pervasive auditory verbal memory impairments in STM, LTM and WM; as well as a marked susceptibility in STM, evident by deficits in holding in STM both verbal and nonverbal information. There is no consensus, however, whether STM impairments in this population are transient or chronic.

Considering Rehabilitation of Memory Deficits in IE

Deficits in global cognition [54], processing speed and memory [16, 42, 55] are associated with poorer quality of life in children with epilepsy, highlighting the need for early identification and intervention.

For this reason, designing a rehabilitation program suitable for children with IE, focusing mainly on auditory verbal impairments, while taking into account patient's preserved intelligence, seems warranted. Moreover, recent studies on memory rehabilitation among children have highlighted executive functions' role in memory rehabilitation [56] and in cognitive behavioral therapy [57, 58]. For this reason examining EF role in IE seems warranted when designing memory rehabilitation for this population.

Executive Functions May Support Short and Long Term Memory in Pediatric IE

The term "executive function" refers to a set of higher order cognitive skills that allow purposeful, goal-directed activity, such as initiation of behaviors, planning in order to complete a desired activity, and self-regulation of behavior [59-61]. The study of executive dysfunction in pediatric epilepsy is particularly important, as the development of these cognitive skills follows a protracted course paralleling functional maturity of the frontal systems [61]. In addition, executive functions play a central role in memory functions and memory rehabilitation [56, 62-65].

Executive functions deficits are frequently found to affect children with IE [22, 66-70]. Interestingly, there is a strong relation between severity of executive function deficits and epilepsy severity [69].

Considering the integrity of EF, it is important to explore the role of age and development. From school age through adolescents, executive attention and cognitive strategies go through a marked developmental spurt, with some young patients enjoying the advents of fairly mature EF networks and others having to rely on immature ones. A recent review on efficacy of memory interventions with children who suffer from childhood CNS disorders suggests that the use of memory rehabilitation techniques that rely on executive components after 7 years of age yields better outcomes [56]. In that review, we suggested that there is a possible mediating roles of executive functions and metacognitive abilities in supporting memory during in middle childhood [71, 72]. Hence it seems important to consider the mediating role of EF in understanding memory intervention effects in IE.

MEMORY INTERVENTION PROTOCOL FOR CHILDREN WITH IE

In view of the above information, we designed a group memory intervention procedure for children aged 9-14 who suffer from IE. Our approach to rehabilitation was guided by encouraging memory intervention results in other pediatric populations, such as children with CNS disorders of childhood [73-76], fetal alcohol syndrome [77] and other disorders [78, 79], all pointing to the notion that auditory verbal WM and STM may possibly improve as a result of comprehensive memory interventions [56]. The program presented in the current chapter was specifically designed for children with IE and the specific cognitive challenges children in this population face [11, 16].

The underlying mechanism that explains how intervention improves memory functions is not clear. There is a debate in the literature concerning whether memory itself can be improved as a result of practicing strategies, or whether mediating factors are actually being targeted for intervention [56]. In the current framework, we explored three possible paths (see figure 1):

a) A direct path: improvements in memory are caused directly by learning memory strategies.
b) A mediating path concerning EF: improvements in memory are moderated by improvements in executive skills [16, 65].
c) A mediating path concerning medication: improvements in memory are moderated by medication profile, with children who receive monotherapy improving more so than children who receive polytherapy [18].

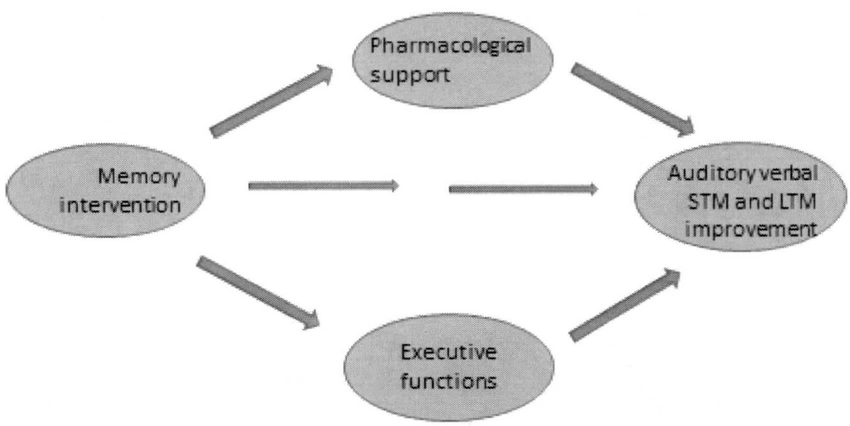

Figure 1. Direct and indirect path s for memory improvement in IE.

Memory Intervention Protocol Tailored for Children with IE

The intervention program was developed as a brief, 5 group session training program (approximately 10 child-training hours in total, two hours per group meeting) that teaches strategies designed to improve auditory verbal memory daily functioning with an emphasis on self-monitoring and self-efficacy stances. We opted for specifically targeting auditory verbal memory deficits, given its central role in IE, and hypothesized a domain specific effect, such that a tailored intervention would affect auditory verbal memory more than it would affect less directly targeted domains, namely visual memory.

The focus of the memory training module was on learning a variety of strategies and techniques to improve organizational and memory skills. The first memory training session began with an open discussion of the rehabilitation program goal, including its aims and objectives. This session was followed by interactive memory games that incorporated participant's personal characteristics (e.g., names and hobbies) while presenting auditory verbal STM memory strategies [80]. The game was followed by a discussion about the idea that forgetting can occur at different rates, for different reasons and it can affect successful encoding and retrieval (e.g., attention, fatigue, physical limitations, pain, medication, stress). At the completion of the first session, self-awareness of individual memory slips, such as forgetting to complete homework assignments or to deliver a message, was promoted by encouraging participants to maintain a "slips" log throughout the week. In addition participants were briefly asked to practice the strategy that they learned in the session.

The second training session continued the focus on external strategies. It began with a review and discussion of memory slips that participants logged throughout the week and of practicing memory strategies. The use of strategies such as smartphone© reminders was practiced and encouraged [81, 82]. For example, each child received a note with a specific hour and programed the smartphone reminder. During the session, participants were asked to press a bell placed in the middle of the room on the specific time they received. At the same time, additional auditory verbal elaborative encoding technique and strategies for enhancing remembering were practiced [83], such as connecting knowledge and background story for the information that should be remembered. Diverse objects were placed in the middle of the room and participants were asked to remember the objects by telling a story or connecting the object to past experience. The children were amazed to discover that after connecting the object to past experience they remembered better. At the conclusion of this session, participants were asked as homework to practice the strategy and to send a message to the group counselor on specific date by using a Smartphone reminder.

The primary focus of training sessions 3 to 5 was to practice a variety of internal strategies which help to encode information in a deep and meaningful way and implement using external memory aids in daily life. For these purposes, participants were introduced and practiced the following strategies: visualization, categorization, question asking and association [21] all improving auditory verbal STM. Each strategy was taught using games and materials suitable for children. For example visualization was practiced using drawings of the material learned, and categorization was practiced using daily chores of each child making the memory intervention relevant for the children's life. As for daily memory functioning, learning the importance of routines and habits was one of the memory intervention goals (placing keys or cellular phone in the same location in the house ensures being able to find them when needed) and participants were introduced to the idea and asked to practice it through the following weeks. In addition training of everyday memory compensatory aids was done by using Smartphone reminders in daily life and during the sessions. As homework between sessions 3 to 5, participants were given assignments for practicing the various strategies and planning the Smartphone reminder in order to perform several tasks during the week in their natural home/school settings. For example participants were asked to send messages for each other, to use categorization in order to plan the afternoon assignments etc. Although participants were encouraged to learn and practice all strategies, it was recognized that different strategies work for different children in different situations and that combinations of strategies are commonly used.

Intervention Efficacy: Promising Pilot Results

Participants and design: We have conducted a study with thirty-three 9-14 year olds (mean age M = 10.88, SD = 1.5; 51% female) who were diagnosed with IE, and 27 healthy control participants, aged 9-14 years (mean age M = 10.18, SD = 1.4; 52% female). All fluent in Hebrew (their native language) were enrolled in the study [84] All participants had an estimated intelligence score within normal limits based on the block design subtest from the WISC-IV [85] (Estimated intelligence quotient, ESIQ >79), and were enrolled in mainstream schooling.

For the IE group, children were enrolled through the neurology department at Sheba hospital and at the neurology department at Schneider Children's hospital at the Rabin Medical Centre, Israel. Medical history, electroencephalography, and imaging data were reviewed by the treating neurologists according to the International League against Epilepsy (ILAE) criteria for IE [4]. Inclusion criteria consisted of at least one unprovoked non-febrile seizure or status epilepticus in the past, but no current seizures (balanced condition). Further all participants were classified with idiopathic etiology: benign Rolandic epilepsy (n = 18), absence epilepsy (n = 4), and generalized epilepsy (n = 11). Exclusion criteria included temporal epilepsy, structural epilepsy, metabolic epilepsy, co-morbid neurological disorders other than ADHD [86], co-morbid chronic illness (e.g., diabetes and asthma), major depression [86], psychosis, and prescribed use of Topiramate and Phenobarbital AEDs.

The control participants were comprised of 27 children (14 females, 13 males) who were matched to the epilepsy group for age and sex. These children showed no evidence of any neurological or other disorder. Children were randomly recruited from mainstream public schools in the (central) district of Israel via word-of-mouth (snowball recruitment) and were exposed to the same educational curriculum as the epilepsy group. Their past medical history, as reported by their parents, was unremarkable. The same inclusion criteria used for the epilepsy group was also used for the control group with regard to age, intelligence, reported head injuries, schooling, psychiatric involvement, and/or medication.

Intervention efficacy was tested using two comparable pre-post intervention testing sessions that employed comparable, yet non-identical assessment items in order to limit item exposure effects (further details in [84]). The pre-assessment conducted one to two weeks before intervention provided baseline measures and the post-assessment assessed participants' performance in the two weeks following completion of the intervention. The training sessions were administered to groups of 4– 6 participants in carefully matched ages and mixed genders. Missed attendance was negligible (3% missing attendance), with make-up sessions provided to ensure that all participants received the same amount of training. Homework task completion was monitored between sessions, using parental mediation via emails, in order to maximize efficacy and to ensure comparability.

RESULTS

Direct Path: Memory Systems Analysis

In the analysis conducted to examine whether intervention will affect auditory verbal memory more than it will affect visual memory, a significant effect for mode was found such that auditory memory was lower relative to visual memory. In addition, a significant main effect for intervention was seen, such that an improvement in memory functions was evident in both modalities (auditory and visual memory) as a result of intervention. There was no interaction between mode and intervention indicating a domain general effect of intervention [84].

In the next step an investigation of the specific memory system (STM, WM and LTM) was conducted. We included verbal STM, LTM and WM scores in a repeated measures analysis, comparing memory systems pre- and post-intervention. Results showed a moderate effect for memory system and a near significant interaction between memory system and intervention effect though post-hoc examination highlighted a post-intervention improvement only in verbal STM [84].

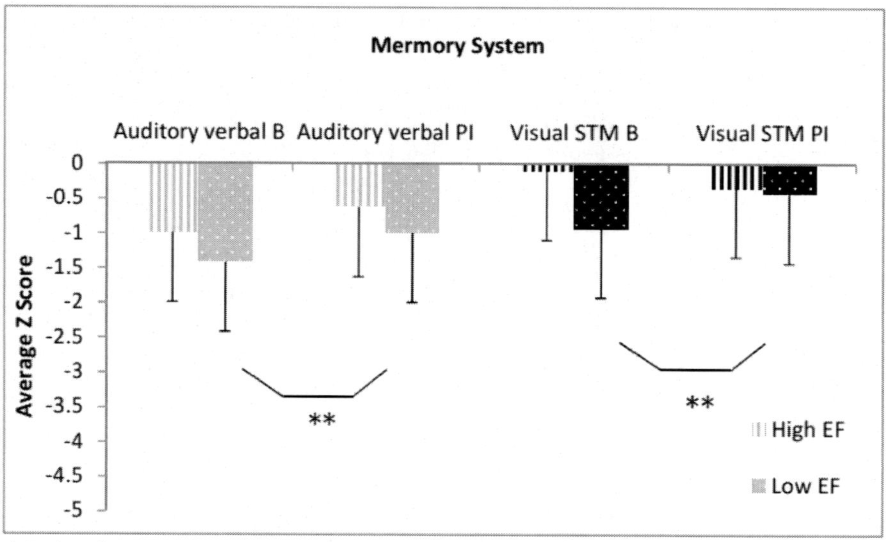

Legend: B, baseline assessment; PI, post intervention assessment.
*p < 0.05; **p < 0.01.

Figure 2. Intervention effect: Auditory memory versus visual memory as a function of executive functions.

Lastly, frequency of normalized performance as a function of intervention was performed. Results demonstrated that at baseline, participants with IE were at a higher risk for auditory verbal memory and for verbal STM more than controls.

In the post treatment analysis, the risk for auditory verbal memory and for verbal STM post intervention was markedly reduced [84].

EF moderation path: Findings showed that the children with IE have lower executive functioning than controls and that post intervention no EF improvement was seen [84]. Then, we examined the role of executive functions (EF) as measured at baseline in memory outcome comparing auditory verbal memory and visual memory before and after intervention as a function of EF (high vs low, defined by a median-split). This analysis resulted in a moderate main effect for mode ($F_{(1,26)} = 28.124$, $p < 0.0001$, $\eta^2 = 0.529$) and intervention ($F_{(1,26)} = 8.888$, $p < 0.01$, $\eta^2 = 0.262$). In addition a significant interaction between mode, intervention and EF was found ($F_{(1,25)} = 6.820$, $P < 0.05$, $\eta^2 = 0.214$), such that participants with lower functioning of EF tended to show improved auditory verbal memory relative to participants with higher EF. This suggests that auditory verbal memory improvement was moderated by EF (see Figure 2).

Moderation of pharmacological support: To explore whether the noted improvement after intervention is related to the intervention protocol alone, or rather is moderated by the participant's routine care prescribed pharmacological intervention, we conducted the same analysis with pharmacological intervention as a between subjects variable (2 levels: monotherapy versus polytherapy) . Analysis indicated that the above results were preserved; indicating that pharmacological intervention does not account for further explained variance [84].

To conclude, these results showed that auditory verbal memory and visual memory improved as a result of our intervention and that baseline EF played a role in auditory verbal improvement. In addition medication profile did not play a role in intervention outcome.

DISCUSSION

The main goal of the current chapter was to present an intervention that is specifically designed to support short- and long term auditory verbal memory deficits in children with IE. Furthermore, this research aimed to deepen the understanding of the mechanisms involved in the intervention process. To do this, we examined the roles of EF and pharmacological profile on memory outcome of this population. Data showed that a susceptible neuropsychological domain (i.e., auditory verbal memory) was improved as a result of this intervention protocol. Further, analysis showed that baseline EF played a role in these effects, such that children with low EFs profited more from the intervention than children with high EF, although both groups demonstrated improvements in memory post intervention. The implications of these findings are briefly discussed below.

The cognitive profile of children with IE is characterized by intelligence within normal range with diverse moderate memory and EF impairments [7, 15, 16, 69, 70]. This specific cognitive profile doesn't characterize children with IE only, but is eminent in other neurological disorders such as post-concussion or after minor traumatic brain injuries that may cause mild memory deficits [87, 88]. For this reason results may underscore a promising direction for other samples with mild memory deficits as current results seem to indicate efficacy for short term focused intervention programs with children with a comparable neuropsychological profile.

The intervention program results demonstrate auditory verbal memory amenability to intervention that is mediated by EF. Two points emerge from this result; the first concerns the particular sensitivity of auditory verbal memory to intervention; and the second concerns role of executive functions in memory rehabilitation.

Auditory Verbal Short and Long Term Memory in Rehabilitation for Children with IE

Results seem to demonstrate that children with IE can benefit from specifically tailored memory rehabilitation to improve their most affected memory system, auditory verbal memory [14-16]. This finding may be promising, in that auditory verbal memory is important for all ages, but specifically at school age. Children at school age face multiple challenges in dealing with auditory verbal memory tasks, especially when learning new materials. Auditory verbal memory is also important in social interactions, such as in forming autobiographical memories (i.e., recalling personally experienced events), keeping a conversation going and remembering content [89-92]. This suggests that improving short and long term auditory verbal memory in children with IE, who suffer from a deficit in this specific memory system, may help improve social functioning as well as auditory verbal memory impairments.

However, the investigation made in order to discover which memory system was most amenable to intervention discovered that short term memory improved the most as a result of intervention.

Apparently improving long term memory seems to be a complicated task [56, 93, 94] although children were taught mainly elaborative encoding strategies that theoretically improve LTM as well as STM [21]. In order to delve into this question we went back to results and deepen the examination of different memory systems in LTM. It is well known that LTM can be divided into two parts sub-systems: an explicit system whereby auditory verbal material that is retrieved explicitly using recall questions (the child tells what he or she remembers from a story) and an implicit one, whereby auditory verbal material that is retrieved implicitly using recognition questions (using multi choice questions or yes or no questions) [21]. In this view, when examining our results again we discovered that current results seem to indicate improvement in the implicit LTM network, evident by improvements occurred only when recognition questions were asked and that using an average score of LTM befogged this finding. This pattern possibly points on *retrieval difficulties* rather than un-improvement in LTM memory consolidation of system as a whole information. This notion seems to be strengthened by several studies pointing on retrieval difficulties in children with IE [36, 95] and in other CNS disorders [96, 97].

On a similar vein, anecdotal information indicates that an interesting phenomenon occurred in many participants in our study: often children could not say explicitly what they have gained from intervention and what strategy they used. Nevertheless observation during assessments discovered implicit utilization of strategies with supremacy to rehearsal techniques. What does this observation can teach us about the role of implicit memory in pediatric memory interventions?

It is known that implicit memory develops early in life and reaches to adults' level very soon [98]. Considering this and taking into account intervention outcome, children with mild memory deficits may gain from interventions even if they do not recognize it. Similar mode of intervention is evident in errorless learning method [99] in which clients learns implicitly auditory verbal material [100-103]. In this regard, our results may point to the importance of practicing memory strategies even if explicit retrieval of a learnt method is not accessible. In comparison to our sample, a study with participants with mild-moderate memory impairments showed that implicit memory strategy (using errorless learning), produced greater accuracy in name recall than did trial-and-error learning [104]. These results seem to also strengthen our observation with regard to improvements in implicit LTM and calls for future studies aiming to promote retrieval strategies in this population. Nevertheless the use of diverse memory rehabilitation strategies aiming to improve STM and LTM, seems to be effective in improving auditory verbal memory as a whole, but needs further research in order to investigate what effects explicit LTM as well. The lack of efficient retrieval strategy may be related to compromises in strategy use, deficits in retrieval and/or be related to deficits in systems supporting executive abilities (Figure 3).

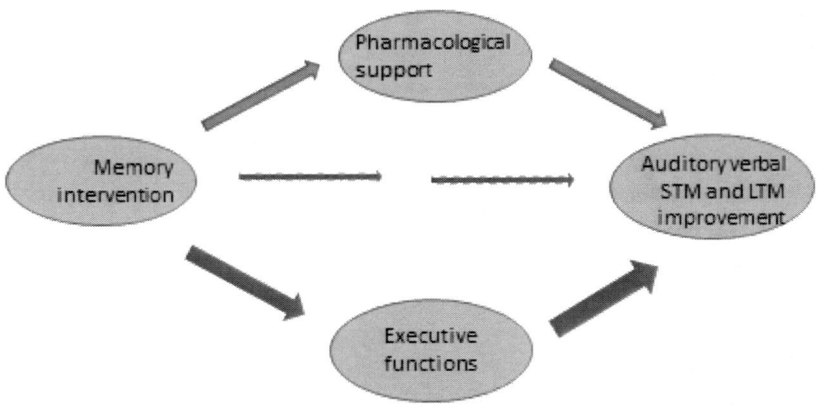

Legend: In red: significant path; In blue: nonsignificant path.

Figure 3. Outcome of intervention: direct and indirect path for memory improvement in IE.

EF Role in Memory Rehabilitation

Current results showed that the presented intervention, which highlights specific strategies to improve memory, did not improve executive functions, but rather relied on the child's baseline executive functions to improve memory functions. This finding extends a compatible finding noted with elderly people with subjective complaints of cognitive or memory decline [105] and with adults who show a variety of suspected neurological and psychiatric conditions, including head injury, dementia, vascular disorders and neoplasms [106], underscoring the role of preserved executive functions in memory rehabilitation and calls for further investigation on the mechanisms which cognitive behavioral interventions rely on. Such a notion would merit further studies with other clinical cohorts.

Clinical Implications

First, the current results point the role of EF in improving verbal memory in this population. These results call for assessing the neuropsychological profile of children with mild memory deficits, as a careful delineation of the memory deficits may be fruitful in order to plan the efficient rehabilitation intervention.

Moreover, structuring EF interventions for children in order to improve baseline EF may strengthen memory intervention efficacy in children with mild memory impairments.

Combining explicit memory strategies, specific strategies to improve retrieval and implicit memory strategies may be fruitful and enhance children profit from memory intervention.

Finally, interventions with children are recommended to address family issues, as the family often experience stress associated with their child's condition. In this regard, an interesting observation was that the parents created an unintended support group. It was noted that the parents had shared their experiences and gave and received emotional support by waiting together and letting themselves meet each other. For this reason, perhaps a more structured support group, with estimation for parental support may be highly useful.

Conclusion

The chapter presents a theoretical model for memory intervention paths, designed for pediatric populations with mild memory deficits with emphasis on the role of executive functions in short term memory rehabilitation in these patients. The model supports using short term group intervention protocol for children with IE who suffer from mild memory impairments. Results highlight that while retrieval of information from LTM is more resistant to intervention in this population. STM is amenable to intervention. Moreover, baseline EF seems to play a significant role in rehabilitation of this population pointing on the mediating roles of executive functions and metacognitive abilities in supporting memory.

This study points to the importance of intervention specifically designed to improve short and long term memory deficits in pediatric IE in particular and perhaps other neurological population with mild verbal auditory memory impairments.

References

[1] Palencia R: Prevalence and incidence of epilepsy in childhood. *Revista De Neurologia.* 2000, *30(s):*1-4.

[2] Fisher R, van Emde Boas W, Blume W, et al.: Epileptic seizures and epilepsy: definitions proposed by the International League Against Epilepsy (ILAE) and the International Bureau for Epilepsy (IBE). *Epilepsia.* 2005, *46:*470-472.

[3] Aldenkamp A, Dreifuss F, Reiner W, Suurmeijer T: *Epilpesy in children and adolescents*. Boca Raton: CRC press, 1995.

[4] Scheffer IE, Berkovic SF, Capovilla G, et al.: The organization of the epilepsies: Report of the ILAE Commission on Classification and Terminology. 2014.

[5] Panayiotopoulos C: *Idiopathic Generalised Epilepsies*: Springer, 2010.

[6] Camfield P, Camfield C: Epileptic syndromes in childhood: clinical features, outcomes, and treatment. *Epilepsia.* 2002, *43:*27-32.

[7] Nicolai J, Van Der Linden I, Arends JB, et al.: EEG characteristics related to educational impairments in children with benign childhood epilepsy with centrotemporal spikes. *Epilepsia.* 2007, *48:*2093-2100.

[8] Aldenkamp A, Weber B, Overweg-Plandsoen W, Reijs R, van Mil S: Educational underachievement in children with epilepsy: a model to predict the effects of epilepsy on educational achievement. *Journal of Child Neurology.* 2005, *20:*175-180.

[9] Kellaway P: The electroencephalographic features of benign centrotemporal (rolandic) epilepsy of childhood. *Epilepsia.* 2000, *41:*1053-1056.

[10] Kadis D, Stollstorff M, Elliott I, Lach L, Smith M: Cognitive and psychological predictors of everyday memory in children with intractable epilepsy. *Epilpesy and Behavior.* 2004, *5:*37-43.

[11] Gascoigne MB, Barton B, Webster R, et al.: Accelerated long-term forgetting in children with idiopathic generalized epilepsy. *Epilepsia.* 2012, *53:*2135-2140.

[12] Holmes G: Pathogenesis of learning disabilities in epilepsy. *Epilepsia.* 2001, *42:*13-15.

[13] Nolan M, Redoblado M, Lah S, et al.: Memory function in childhood epilepsy syndromes. *Journal of Paediatric and Child Health.* 2004, *40:*20-27.

[14] Goldberg-Stern H, Gonen O, Sadeh M, et al.: Neuropsychological aspects of benign childhood epilepsy with centrotemporal spikes. *Seizure.* 2010, *19:*12-16.

[15] Bhise VV, Burack GD, Mandelbaum DE: Baseline cognition, behavior, and motor skills in children with new-onset, idiopathic epilepsy. *Developmental Medicine and Child Neurology.* 2010, *52:*22-26.

[16] Schaffer Y, Ben Zeev B, Cohen R, Shufer A, Geva G: Auditory verbal memory and psychosocial symptoms are related in children with idiopathic epilepsy *Epilepsy & Behavior.* 2015, *ahead-of-print.*

[17] Galer S, Urbain C, De Tiège X, et al.: Impaired sleep-related consolidation of declarative memories in idiopathic focal epilepsies of childhood. *Epilpesy and Behavior.* 2015, *43:*16-23.

[18] Ijff D, Aldenkamp A: Cognitive side-effects of antiepileptic drugs in children. *Handbook of clinical neurology.* 2012, *111:*707-718.

[19] Schmidt D, L G: Monotherapy versus Polytherapy in epilepsy. *CNS Dtugs.* 1995, *3:*194-208.

[20] Andrew T, Milinis K, Baker G, Wieshmann U: Self reported adverse effects of mono and polytherapy for epilepsy. *Seizure.* 2012, *21:*610-613.

[21] Sohlberg MM, Mateer CA: *Cognitive rehabilitation: An integrative neuropsychological approach.* New York: Guilford Press, 2001.

[22] Nicolai J, Aldenkamp AP, Arends J, Weber JW, Vles JS: Cognitive and behavioral effects of nocturnal epileptiform discharges in children with benign childhood epilepsy with centrotemporal spikes. *Epilepsy & Behavior.* 2006, *8:*56-70.

[23] Giordani B, Caveney A, Laughrin D, et al.: Cognition and behavior in children with benign epilepsy with centrotemporal spikes (BECTS). *Epilepsy Research.* 2006, *70:*89-94.

[24] Geva R: Short term memory. In S. Norbert (ed), *Encyclopedia of the sciences of learning.* New York: Springer, 2012, 3058-3061.

[25] Baddeley A, Thomson N, Buchanan M: Word length and the structure of short-term memory. *Journal of Verbal Learning and Verbal Behavior.* 1975, *14:*575-589.
[26] Jonides J: Working memory and the brain. *Paper presented at the International Neuropsychology Society*. Denver, CO, 2000.
[27] Squire L: Declarative and nondeclarative memory: Multiple brain systems supporting learning and memory. *Journal of Cognitive Neuroscience.* 1992, *4:*232-243.
[28] Baddeley A, Warrington E: Amnesia and the distinction between long-and short-term memory. *J Verbal Learning Verbal Behav.* 1970, *9:*176-189.
[29] Baddeley A: The influence of acoustic and semantic similarity on long-term memory for word sequences. *Quarterly Journal of Experimental Psychology.* 1966, *18:*302-309.
[30] Wood R, Baxter P, Belpaeme T: A review of long-term memory in natural and synthetic systems. *Adaptive Behavior.* 2012, *20:*81-103.
[31] Baddeley AD, Hitch G: Working memory. *Psychology of learning and motivation.* 1974, *8:*47-89.
[32] Engle RW, Kane MJ: Executive attention, working memory capacity, and a two-factor theory of cognitive control. *Psychology of learning and motivation.* 2004, *44:*145-200.
[33] Miyake A, Friedman NP, Emerson MJ, et al.: The unity and diversity of executive functions and their contributions to complex "frontal lobe" tasks: A latent variable analysis. *Cognitive psychology.* 2000, *41:*49-100.
[34] Baddeley A: Working memory. *Science.* 1992, *255:*556-559.
[35] Croona C, Kihlgren M, Lundberg S, Eeg-Olofsson O, Eeg-Olofsson K: Neuropsychologicalfindings in childrenwith benign childhoodepilepsy with centrotemporal spikes. *Developmental Medicine & Child Neurology.* 1999, *41:*813-818.
[36] Davidson M, Dorris L, O'Regan M, Zuberi SM: Memory consolidation and accelerated forgetting in children with idiopathic generalized epilepsy. *Epilepsy & Behavior.* 2007, *11:*394-400.
[37] Baglietto MG, Battaglia FM, Nobili L, et al.: Neuropsychological disorders related to interictal epileptic discharges during sleep in benign epilepsy of childhood with centrotemporal or Rolandic spikes. *Developmental Medicine & Child Neurology.* 2001, *43:*407-412.
[38] Henkin Y, Sadeh M, Kivity S, et al.: Cognitive function in idiopathic generalized epilepsy of childhood. *Developmental Medicine and Child Neurology.* 2005, *47:*126-132.
[39] Miyake A, Friedman NP: The Nature and Organization of Individual Differences in Executive Functions: Four General Conclusions. *Current Directions in Psychological Science.* 2012, *21:*8-14.
[40] You S: Cognitive function of idiopathic childhood epilepsy. *Korean Journal of Pediatrics.* 2012, *55:*159-163.
[41] Jambaqué I, Dellatolas G, Dulac O, Ponsot G, Signoret J-L: Verbal and visual memory impairment in childrem with epilepsy. *Neuropsychologia.* 1993, *31:*1321-1337.
[42] Schouten A, Oostrom KJ, Pestman WR, et al.: Learning and memory of school children with epilepsy: a prospective controlled longitudinal study. *Developmental Medicine and Child Neurology.* 2002, *44:*803-811.
[43] Reilly C, Atkinson P, Das K, et al.: Cognition in school-aged children with "active" epilepsy: A population-based study. *Journal of Clinical and Experimental Neuropsychology.* 2015, *37:*429-438.

[44] Hermann B, Jones J, Sheth R, et al.: Children with new-onset epilepsy: Neuropsychological status and brain structure. *Brain.* 2006, *129:*2609-2619.
[45] Aldenkamp A, Arends J: Effects of epileptiform EEG discharges on cognitive function: is the concept of "transient cognitive impairment" still valid? *Epilpesy and Behavior.* 2004, *5:*S25-S34.
[46] Sonmez F, Atakli D, Sari H, Atay T, Arpaci B: Cognitive function in juvenile myoclonic epilepsy. *Epilpesy and Behavior.* 2004, *5:*329–336.
[47] Metz-Lutz MN, Kleitz C, de Saint Martin A, et al.: Cognitive development in benign focal epilepsies of childhood. *Developmental neuroscience.* 1999, *21:*182-190.
[48] Massa R, de Saint–Martin A, Carcangiu R, et al.: EEG criteria predictive of complicated evolution in idiopathic rolandic epilepsy. *Neurology.* 2001, *57:*1071-1079.
[49] Pinton F, Ducot B, Motte J, et al.: Cognitive functions in children with benign childhood epilepsy with centrotemporal spikes (BECTS). *Epileptic Disorders.* 2006, *8:*11-23.
[50] Völkl-Kernstock S, Willinger U, Feucht M: Spacial perception and spatial memory in children with benign childhood epilepsy with centro-temporal spikes (BCECTS). *Epilepsy research.* 2006, *72:*39-48.
[51] Germanò E, Gagliano A, Magazù A, et al.: Benign childhood epilepsy with occipital paroxysms: neuropsychological findings. *Epilepsy research.* 2005, *64:*137-150.
[52] Gülgönen S, Demirbilek V, Korkmaz B, Dervent A, Townes BD: Neuropsychological functions in idiopathic occipital lobe epilepsy. *Epilepsia.* 2000, *41:*405-411.
[53] Gathercole S, Hitch G, Service E, Martin A: Phonological short-term memory and new word learning in children. *Developmental Psychology.* 1997, *33:*966-979.
[54] Ferro M, Camfield C, Levin S, et al.: Trajectories of health related quality of life in children with epilepsy: A cohort study. *Epilepsia.* 2013, *54:*1889–1897.
[55] Hrabok M, Sherman E, Bello-Espinosa L, Hader W: Memory and health-related quality of life in severe paediatric epilepsy. *Pediatrics.* 2013, *131:*525–532.
[56] Schaffer Y, Geva R: Memory outcomes following cognitive interventions in children with neurological deficits: A review with a focus on under-studied populations. *Neuropsychological Rehabilitation.* 2015*:*1-32.
[57] Mischel W: Towerd an integrative model for CBT: encompassing behavior, cognition, affect and process. *Behavior and Therapy.* 2004, *35:*185-203.
[58] Grave J, Blissett J: Is cognitive behavior therapy developmentally appropriate for young children? A critical review of the evidence. *Clinical Psychological Review.* 2004, *24:*399-420.
[59] Elliott R: Executive functions and their disorders. *British Medical Bulletin.* 2003, *65:*49-59.
[60] Lezak M: *Neuropsychological assessment (4th ed.)* New York Oxford University Press, 2004.
[61] Samango-Sprouse C: *Frontal lobe development in childhood.* New York: The Guilford Press, 2007.
[62] Isaacs E, Vargha-Khadem F: Differential course of development of spatial and verbal memory span: A normative study. *British Journal of Developmental Psychology.* 2011, *7:*377-380.
[63] Gathercole S: Cognitive approaches to the development of short-term memory. *Trends in Cognitive Sciences.* 1999, *3:*410-419.

[64] Bryck R, Fisher P: Training the brain: practical applications of neural plasticity from the intersection of cognitive neuroscience, developmental psychology, and prevention science. *The American Psychologist.* 2012, *67:*87-100.
[65] Rabipour S, Raz A: Training the brain: fact and fad in cognitive and behavioral remediation. *Brain and Cognition.* 2012, *79:*159-179.
[66] Vuilleumier P, Assal F, Blanke O, Jallon P: Distinct behavioral and EEG topographic correlates of loss of consciousness in absences. *Epilepsia.* 2000, *41:*687-693.
[67] Caplan R, Levitt J, Siddarth P, et al.: Frontal and temporal volumes in childhood absence epilepsy. *Epilepsia.* 2009, *50:*2466-2472.
[68] Parrish J, Geary E, Jones J, et al.: Executive functioning in childhood epilepsy: Parent-report and cognitive assessment. *Developmental Medicine and Child Neurology.* 2007, *49:*412-416.
[69] MacAllister W, Bender H, Whitman L, et al.: Assessment of executive functioning in childhood epilepsy: the Tower of London and BRIEF. *Child Neuropsychology.* 2012, *18:*404-415.
[70] Kellermann T, Bonilha L, Lin J, Hermann B: Mapping the landscape of cognitive development in children with epilepsy. *Cortex.* 2015, *66.*
[71] Brocki K, Bohlin G: Executive functions in children aged 6 to 13: A dimensional and developmental study. *Developmental Neuropsychology.* 2004, *26:*571-593.
[72] Anderson V, Anderson P, Northam E, Jacobs R, Catroppa C: Development of executive functions through late childhood and adolescence in an Australian sample. *Developmental Neuropsychology.* 2001, *20:*385-406.
[73] van't Hooft I, Andersson K, Sejersen T, Bartfai A, von Wendt L: Attention and memory training in children with acquired brain injuries. *Acta pediatrica.* 2003, *92:*935-940.
[74] van't Hooft I, Andersson K, Bergman B, et al.: Beneficial effect from a cognitive training programme on children with acquired brain injuries demonstrated in a controlled study. *Brain injury.* 2005, *19:*511-518.
[75] van't Hooft I, Andersson K, Bergman B, et al.: Sustained favorable effects of cognitive training in children with acquired brain injuries. *Neurorehabilitation.* 2007, *22:*109-116.
[76] Patel SK, Katz ER, Richardson R, Rimmer M, Kilian S: Cognitive and Problem Solving Training in Children with Cancer: A Pilot Project. *Journal of pediatric hematology and oncology.* 2009, *9:*670-677.
[77] Loomes C, Rasmussen C, Pei J, Manji S, Andrew G: The effect of rehearsal training on working memory span of children with fetal alcohol spectrum disorder. *Research In Developmental Disabilities.* 2008, *29:*113-124.
[78] Conners FA, Rosenquist CJ, Arnett L, Moore MS, Hume LE: Improving memory span in children with Down syndrome. *Journal of Intellectual Disability Research.* 2008, *52:*244-255.
[79] King AA, White DA, McKinstry M, Noetzel M, DeBaun MR: A pilot randomized education rehabilitation trial is feasible in sickle cell and strokes. *Neurology.* 2007, *68:*2008-2011.
[80] Wilson B, Moffat N: *Clinical managment of memory problems.* London: Chapman and Hall, 1992.

[81] DePompei R, Gillette Y, Goetz E, et al.: Practical applications for use of PDAs and smartphones with children and adolescents who have traumatic brain injury. *Neurorehabilitation.* 2008, *23:*487-499.
[82] Wilson B, Emslie H, Evans J, et al.: The NeuroPage system for children and adolescents with neurological deficits. *Developmental Neurorehabilitation.* 2009, *12:*421-426.
[83] Brown S, Craik F: Encoding and retrieval of information. In E. Tulving and F. Craik (eds), *The Oxford handbook of memory.* New York: Oxford University Press, 2000, 93-107.
[84] Schaffer Y, Geva R: Cognitive rehabilitation intervention in children with idiopathic epilepsy: uncovering factors supporting intervention efficacy on memory and psychosocial characteristics. *European Archives of Psychiatry and Clinical Neurosciene.* submitted.
[85] Wechsler D: *Wechsler Intelligence Scale for Children—4th Edition (WISCIV).* San Antonio, TX: Harcourt Assessment, 2003.
[86] American Psychiatric Association: *The diagnostic and statistical manual of mental disorders: DSM 5*: bookpointUS, 2013.
[87] Dean P, Sterr A: Long-term effects of mild traumatic brain injury on cognitive performance. *Fronties in Human Neuroscience.* 2013, *12:*30.
[88] Smits M, Dippel D, Houston G, et al.: Postconcussion syndrome after minor head injury: brain activation of working memory and attention. *Human Brain Mapping.* 2009, *30:*2789-2803.
[89] Buckner RL, Carroll DC: Self-projection and the brain. *Trends Cogn Sci.* 2007, *11:*49-57.
[90] Spreng RN, Grady CL: Patterns of brain activity supporting autobiographical memory, prospection, and theory of mind, and their relationship to the default mode network. *Journal of Cognitive Neuroscience.* 2010, *22:*1112-1123.
[91] Spreng RN, Mar RA: I remember you: a role for memory in social cognition and the functional neuroanatomy of their interaction. *Brain research.* 2012, *1428:*43-50.
[92] Rabin JS, Rosenbaum RS: Familiarity modulates the functional relationship between theory of mind and autobiographical memory. *Neuroimage.* 2012, *62:*520-529.
[93] Limond J, Leeke R: Practitioner Review: Cognitive rehabilitation for children with acquired brain injury. *Journal of Child Psychology and Psychiatry.* 2005, *46:*339-352.
[94] Oberg L, Turkstra L: Use of elaborative encoding to facilitate verbal learning after adolescent traumatic brain injury. *Journal of Head Trauma Rehabilitation.* 1998, *13:*44-62.
[95] Vago C, Bulgheroni S, Franceschetti S, Usilla A, Riva D: Memory performance on the California Verbal Learning Test of children with benign childhood epilepsy with centrotemporal spikes. *Epilepsy and Behavior.* 2008, *13:*600-606.
[96] Bassett S, Slater E: Neuropsychological function in adolescents sustainig mild closed brain injury. *Journal of Pediatric Psychology.* 1990, *15:*225-236.
[97] Kizony R, Tau S, Bar O, Engel Yeger B: Comparing memory and meta-memory abilities between children with acquired brain injury and healthy peers. *Research In Developmental Disabilities.* 2014, *35:*1666-1673.
[98] de Hann M, Johnson M: *The cognitive neuroscience of development.* New York: Psychology Press, 2003.

[99] Wilson B, Baddeley A, Evans J, Shiel A: Errorless learning in the rehabilitation of memory impaired people. *Neuropsychological Rehabilitation.* 1994, *4:*307-326.

[100] Haslam C, Bazen-Peters C, Wright I: Errorless learning improves memory performance in children with acquired brain injury: a controlled comparison of standard and self-generation techniques. *Neuropsychological Rehabiltation.* 2012, *22:*697-715.

[101] Guillery-Girard B, Martins S, Parisot-Carbuccia D, Eustache F: Semantic acquisition in childhood amnesic syndrome: a prospective study. *Neuroreport.* 2004, *15:*377-381.

[102] Martins S, Guillery-Girard B, Jambaqué I, Dulac O, Eustache F: How children suffering severe amnesic syndrome acquire new concepts? *Neuropsychologia.* 2006, *44:*2792-2805.

[103] Kessels R, De Haan E: Implicit learning in memory rehabilitation: a meta-analysis on errorless learning and vanishing cues methods. *Journal of Clinical and Experimental Neuropsychology.* 2003, *23.*

[104] Haslam C, Hodder K, Yates P: Errorless learning and spaced retrieval: how do these methods fare in healthy and clinical populations? *Journal of Clinical and Experimental Neuropsychology.* 2011, *33:*432-447.

[105] Craik F, Winocur G, Palmer H, et al.: Cognitive rehabilitation in the elderly: effects on memory. *Journal of International Neuropsychological Society.* 2007, *13:*132-142.

[106] Duff K, Schoenberg M, Scott J, Adams R: The relationship between executive functioning and verbal and visual learning and memory. *Archives of Clinical Neuropsychology.* 2005, *20:*111-122.

In: Spatial, Long-and Short-Term Memory
Editor: Edward A. Thayer

ISBN: 978-1-63484-148-1

Chapter 6

EMERGENCE OF THE SELF-REFERENCE EFFECT IN EPISODIC MEMORY DURING EARLY CHILDHOOD

Michele D. Dunbar, Glenda Andrews and Karen Murphy
Menzies Health Institute Queensland and School of Applied Psychology, Griffith University, Gold Coast, Queensland, Australia

ABSTRACT

The self-reference effect in memory refers to the finding that performance on tests of episodic memory is better when information is encoded in relation to the self than when it is encoded in relation to another person. There have been many demonstrations of the self-reference effect in adults' memory, but its emergence in children's memory in less well understood. In this chapter we report three experiments in which we employed a self-reference paradigm to examine episodic memory in 4- to 6-year-old children. In the encoding phases of the three experiments, the items to be remembered were pictures of familiar objects which were presented along with a photo of the child's own face (self-reference condition) or a photo of another child's face (other-reference condition). In the test phase, memory for the items was assessed using free recall in Experiments 1 and 3, and recognition in Experiment 2. Memory for the encoding context (self versus other) was also assessed in the test phases of the three experiments using a 2-alternative forced choice task. Memory for the encoding context was tested for correctly recalled items in Experiment 1, and for correctly recognised items in Experiment 2. In Experiment 3, it was assessed for all items presented at encoding, irrespective of whether they were correctly recalled. The findings revealed significant self-reference effects on memory for the encoding context in all three experiments. That is, children were more accurate in identifying the encoding contexts in which photos of themselves rather than another child had been presented. The self-reference effect on memory for encoding context did not vary with age, indicating that 4-year-olds benefited as much from self-referent encoding as 5- and 6-year-olds did. The self-reference effect on item memory was not significant in any experiment. That is, children's recall and recognition of items did not differ when the items were encoded in relation to themselves as compared to another child. These findings extend our understanding of memory for encoding context and the role of the self in the development of episodic memory.

INTRODUCTION

Episodic memory includes item and contextual information (Yim, Dennis, and Sloutsky 2013). Memory for context is one property of episodic memory that differentiates it from semantic memory (Wheeler, Stuss and Tulving 1997). Context has been operationalised in various ways including the gender or identity of the person who presented the study items (Lindsay, Johnson and Kwon 1991), the source of the to-be-recalled information (Drummey and Newcombe 2002), and other features present at encoding such as the frequency or recency with which the items were presented (Chalmers and Grogan 2006). Episodic memory underpins many cognitive functions including the acquisition of language and knowledge (Roberts 2000), and has implications for areas such as eyewitness memory and suggestibility within forensic settings (Quas, Schaaf, Alexander and Goodman 2000). Not surprisingly, its development during childhood is of interest to researchers.

The self-reference effect (SRE) in memory, whereby information encoded in relation to the self is recalled or recognised more accurately than information encoded in relation to another person (Symons and Johnson 1997), can be interpreted in terms of context. In adults, the SRE in episodic memory is robust and is thought to occur because self-referent encoding promotes elaboration and/or organisation of the information at encoding (e.g., Symons and Johnson 1997). Self-reference advantages have been observed using various measures of memory including recall, recognition (Turk, Cunningham and Macrae 2008), and recency discrimination (e.g., Andrews, Murphy, Dunbar and Boyce 2012); and stimulus types including nouns and trait adjectives (Symons and Johnson 1997). Episodic memory necessarily involves the self as rememberer (Wheeler et al., 1997). While the *self-other* distinction appears to emerge earlier in episodic memory development than other distinctions (e.g., *thoughts-actions*; Foley, Johnson and Raye 1983), the age at which children can utilise self and other as cues in episodic memory tasks is not well researched. The present study examined this question using variations of a SRE procedure developed by Sui and Zhu (2005). The overall aim was to better understand the role of the self in the early development of episodic memory.

Fuzzy trace theory (Brainerd and Reyna 2002b) and the source monitoring framework (Johnson, Hashtroudi and Lindsay 1993) have provided explanations for the mechanisms underlying memory for contextual information, referred to in the present research as *context memory*. Fuzzy-trace theory proposes that memory comprises two types of representations, verbatim and gist, which operate independently. Whereas verbatim traces reflect episodically instantiated representations of the surface forms of recently experienced items, gist traces reflect episodic interpretations of the concepts that underpin the items' surface forms (Brainerd and Reyna 2002a). Accurate memory performance involves retrieving both verbatim and gist traces. The SRE in episodic memory might therefore reflect clearer verbatim traces (e.g., "I have *a distinct picture* of me [not my friend] telling that story.") and/or more robust gist traces (e.g., "I have *a strong sense* that I [not my friend] told that story because I remember thinking at the time that something similar happened last year.") produced through self-referent relative to other-referent encoding.

Source monitoring theory (Johnson et al., 1993) proposes that memory for contextual information involves a decision process whereby the qualitative characteristics of activated memories are evaluated. It includes the binding of particular combinations of event characteristics that can reflect perceptual (e.g., sound), contextual (e.g., spatial), affective (e.g., emotional reactions), semantic, or cognitive (e.g., elaborated) information (Johnson et al., 1993). Factors such as existing knowledge can also play a role in the decision process. For example, knowledge that *experienced* events are usually accompanied by clearer and more detailed memories than *imagined* events might increase the likelihood that less clear and less detailed memories will be rejected as having been experienced. Accordingly, the SRE in memory from this perspective might reflect more robust and richly detailed memories produced through encoding information in relation to the self compared to another person.

Relative to adults and children older than about 6 years, younger children's memory for contextual information tends to be poor, particularly when the contexts to be discriminated are highly similar (Lindsay 2008). However, when the contexts to be discriminated are highly distinctive (Lindsay 2008) or salient (Yim et al., 2013), young children's performance can be quite good. The self-other distinction is likely to be both highly discriminable and salient. Given the significance of the self in episodic memory (Wheeler et al., 1997), SREs in context memory might be expected during the same period that significant improvements in context memory are observed, the preschool years (Drummey and Newcombe 2002; Sluzenski, Newcombe and Ottinger 2004; Welch-Ross 1995). Interestingly, however, whilst some source memory research suggests that self-referential processing can enhance item memory (Crawley, Newcombe and Bingman 2010; Kovacs and Newcombe 2006; Sui and Zhu 2005), SREs in context memory have rarely been reported in children younger than 6 years.

Kovacs and Newcombe (2006) presented 4- and 5-year-old children with statements (e.g., "I like going to the circus to see the clowns"; p. 42) spoken by a male and female speaker (Exps. 1 and 3) or two female speakers (Exp. 2). At encoding, children in the self-focus condition reported whether they felt the same way (e.g., happy, scared) as the speaker; children in the other-focus condition judged how the speaker felt about what she or he was saying. Children then judged whether old and new statements had been previously presented (item memory test), and if so, who had spoken the sentence (source memory test). For item memory, overall performance was higher in the self-focus than other-focus condition (Exps. 1 and 2). For source memory, accuracy was higher in the other-focus than self-focus condition for 4-year-olds (Exp. 3) and 5-year-olds (Exps. 1 and 2). Kovacs and Newcombe (2006) explained these results as a reflection of the children being better able to use rich perceptual and emotional information and clear differences between sources to assist their memory.

Crawley et al. (2010), presented 4- and 6-year-olds with video clips depicting one of two women making statements that varied in emotional content (e.g., "My Dad gave me a present today."; "I had to eat broccoli today."; p. 284). In Experiment 1, children responded to one of five questions: (a) "How do you feel about that?" (emotional self-focus condition); (b) "How does she feel about that?" (emotional other-focus condition); (c) "What colour is your shirt?" (perceptual self-focus condition); (d) "What colour is her hair?" (perceptual other-focus condition); and (e) "Is the sound loud enough for you to hear?" (control condition). In Experiment 2, children responded to one of three questions: (a) "Have you ever done that?" (semantic-self condition); (b) "Can she really do that?" (semantic-other condition); and (c) "Is the sound loud enough for you to hear?" (control condition). For item memory, recognition was higher in the self-focus than other-focus condition for emotional questions, but not for perceptual (Exp. 1) or semantic (Exp. 2) questions. For source memory, overall accuracy was higher in the other-focus emotional than self-focus emotional condition and higher in the other-focus perceptual than self-focus perceptual condition (Exp. 1), but there was no effect of self-other focus with semantic encoding (Exp. 2). This was taken as evidence of the specialised processing of emotional information resulting in superior encoding compared to the perceptual and semantic encoding conditions. Thus, Kovacs and Newcombe's (2006) and Crawley et al.'s research demonstrates that focusing on the self-other distinction during encoding can affect children's memory for statements and the speaker of those statements.

Sui and Zhu (2005) presented 4-, 5-, and 10-year-old children with item-context stimulus displays. Each display comprised a picture of a common object (e.g., ball) paired with a photograph of the participant child (self condition) or another child (other condition) pointing to the object. During the encoding phase, children reported who (self or other) was pointing to each object. Item memory was assessed with a free recall test of the objects. Memory for context was assessed for recalled objects, whereby children reported who (self or other) had pointed to each correctly remembered object. Consistent with other research (Crawley et al., 2010; Kovacs and Newcombe, 2006), Sui and Zhu found overall item memory was facilitated by self-referent encoding for 5-year-olds (Exps. 1 and 2) and 10-year-olds when the task demands were increased (Exp. 2). In contrast, there was no effect of self-other encoding on context memory at any age in either experiment. Sui and Zhu interpreted these outcomes as the result of self-face recognition activating the self-network which faciltated better memory retreival.

Similar to Sui and Zhu (2005), Cunningham, Brebner, Quinn, and Turk (2014) presented children (aged 4-, 5-, and 6-years) with pictures of common objects paired with a photograph of the participant child or another child. During the encoding phase, children made evaluative judgments about each object ("Would you [or other child] really really like this object, or would you [or other child] not be very fussed about it?"; Exps. 1 and 2) or judgments about the location (left or right) of each object (Exp. 3). In Experiment 1, item memory only was assessed with a standard old-new recognition task. In Experiments 2 and 3, item and source memory were assessed simultaneously with an old-new recognition task whereby children judged whether each object was new (Exps. 2 and 3), shown previously with self or other at encoding (Exp. 2), or located to the left or right of the photograph at encoding (Exp. 3). Across experiments, Cunningham et al.'s results indicated a self-referent advantage for item and source memory, which they attributed as being due to automatic responses in relation to self-cues.

The SRE studies reviewed suggest that even very young children can utilise the self-other distinction in episodic memory. They also suggest that the distinction can impact item and context memory differentially. Whilst self-referent encoding produced superior item memory in each study, just one study reported SREs on context memory in children younger than age 6 (Cunningham et al., 2014). This is curious, particularly considering that contextual information and the self are intrinsic to episodic memory (Wheeler et al., 1997). In the present research, we modified Sui and Zhu's (2005) procedure to further investigate the significance of the self-other distinction in the early development of episodic memory. In three experiments we examined (a) the extent of age-related improvement in item and context memory between the ages of 4- and 6-years; (b) the extent to which self-referent encoding facilitates item and context memory in 4-, 5-, and 6-year-old children, and if so; (c) the ages at which this occurs.

EXPERIMENT 1

In the encoding phase of their first experiment, Sui and Zhu (2005) administered 12 trials: six in the self-encoding and six in the other-encoding condition. Item recall was assessed. Memory for encoding-context was tested on an average of 4.44 items for the 4-year-olds, 6.24 items for the 5-year-olds, and 7.44 for the 10-year-olds. Thus, the absence of self-other encoding effects on context memory might have resulted from there being too few items to discriminate between the conditions.

We increased the number of trials in the encoding phase in Experiment 1 in order to enlarge the item pool for the test of context memory. Another modification involved presenting picture cards of the objects and face cards of the two possible encoding contexts (self or other) during the context memory test phase. We reasoned that presenting pictures of items alongside the possible encoding contexts might reinstate the item-context bindings if these were established at encoding (Johnson and Chalfonte 1994). Based on Sui and Zhu's (2005) findings and other SRE studies (Crawley et al., 2010; Kovacs and Newcombe 2006), we expected to observe a SRE on item memory. We also assessed whether a SRE on context memory would occur with the modified procedure.

Method

Participants. Participants were 72 children from three age groups with equal numbers of girls and boys in each age group: 24, 4-year-olds (M = 53.58 months, SD = 3.92, range: 48–59); 24, 5-year-olds (M = 65.79 months, SD = 3.32, range: 60–70); and 24, 6-year-olds (M = 76.38 months, SD = 3.45, range: 72–83). Children were recruited from day-care centres and Catholic Education primary schools in middle-class suburbs of the city of Gold Coast, Queensland, Australia. Socioeconomic status (SES) was calculated (Hollingshead 1975). This measure yields scores that range from 8 to 61 with higher scores indicating higher SES. The mean SES scores according to age group in Experiments 1, 2, and 3 are presented in Table 1. For each experiment, a one-way ANOVA showed that mean SES scores did not differ across age groups.

Generation of the stimulus displays. Four picture sets each comprising 18 object line drawings were drawn from *The International Picture-Naming Project* (Szekely et al., 2004). In a pilot test, a separate sample of 14, 4-year-old children (8 girls; M = 53.93 months, SD = 3.58, range: 48–59) were shown a larger set of 138 drawings (Boyce 2005; Szekely et al., 2004) and asked to provide a label for each. Only object drawings for which the majority ($\geq$ 85%) of children had a suitable label were retained in the final four picture sets. Suitable labels were those referred to as dominant labels (e.g., tree) in the database or reasonable alternatives (e.g., plant). Chi-square analyses showed no significant associations between set (1, 2, 3, and 4) and age of acquisition (1-, 2-, and 3-years), or set and number of syllables (one and two). A one-way ANOVA revealed no significant effect of set on either frequency in the language or visual complexity. Independent-samples t-tests showed no significant effect of sex (girl, boy) on the total accuracy score for any object set.

Table 1. Socioeconomic status for the families of children who participated in experiments 1, 2, and 3

Age	Mean (*SD*)	Range
Experiment 1		
4-years	42.39 (9.99)	17.00–56.00
5-years	43.15 (8.67)	24.50–58.00
6-years	44.59 (8.86)	25.50–56.00
Experiment 2		
4-years	41.00 (9.42)	22.00–58.00
5-years	43.25 (8.46)	24.50–56.00
6-years	42.73 (8.71)	22.00–58.00
Experiment 3		
4-years	43.19 (9.96)	21.00–56.00
5-years	40.95 (5.98)	30.00–53.00
6-years	40.91 (9.16)	22.00–56.00

The drawings from Picture Sets 1 and 2 were presented in the encoding phase of Experiments 1, 2, and 3. The drawings from Picture Sets 3 and 4 were used as distracters in Experiment 2. A copy of each drawing from Picture Sets 1 and 2 was printed and laminated (9 × 9 cm), and used in the context memory test phase.

Photographs of 12 children: 2 girls and 2 boys at each of three ages (4-, 5-, and 6-years) were used in the *other* encoding-context condition. These individuals were children of undergraduate psychology students from Griffith University who received course credit for their child's participation, or children of colleagues known to the first author. These children attended day-care centres and schools different to those of participant children and were not known to the participant children. A black-and-white digital photograph was taken of each participant child's face and of each other child's face. Children representing the other encoding-context condition were matched to participant children according to sex, age, and hair colour (fair, dark). Digital images of the faces, a black-and-white line drawing of an androgynous body representation, and object line drawings from Picture Sets 1 and 2 were used in the stimulus displays presented during the encoding phase (see Figure 1). For the self encoding-context condition, a photograph of the participant child's own face was linked to the body representation (self face-body image). For the other encoding-context condition, the photograph of a matched child's face was linked to the body representation (other face-body image).

The pairing of face-body images with object line drawings was counterbalanced: 50% of the children in each age group received drawings from Picture Set 1 paired with their own face-body image and drawings from Picture Set 2 paired with the other face-body image (Presentation A). The remaining children received the opposite assignment of drawings to self and other encoding-context conditions (Presentation B). The dimensions of the face-body images and object line drawings were each 9 × 7.5 cm. A copy of the face-body image of each participant and matched child was also printed and laminated (9 × 9 cm) for use in the context memory test.

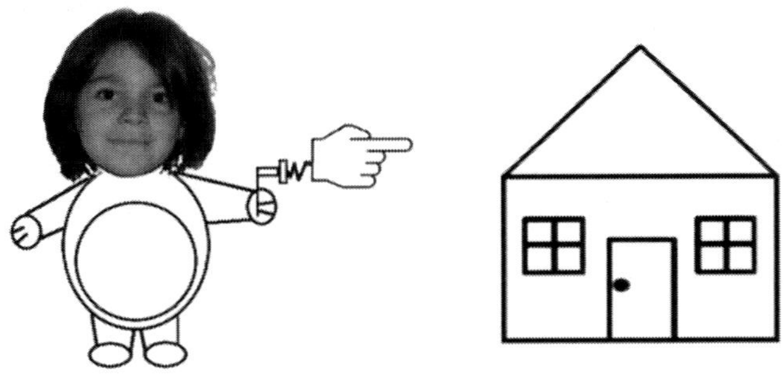

Figure 1. An example item-context stimulus display used during the encoding phase.

Procedure and apparatus. The tasks were programmed using DMDX software (Forster and Forster 2003) and run on an HP Compaq nc6400 laptop computer (2.00 GHz, 1.99 RAM) set to 1024 × 768 bit depth resolution. Prior to the day of testing, the researcher visited the day-care centre or school for the purpose of photographing each participant child's face. Photographs were taken against a white wall background. A digital camera which was attached to a tri-pod was positioned approximately 100cm from the child. Digital images of the participant child and other child were incorporated into the program. Children were tested individually in a quiet room of their day-care centre or school during normal attendance hours. The 20 min experiment comprised three phases: encoding, item memory test, and context memory test.

Encoding phase. The experimenter first read aloud the task instructions: "For this task, I'm going to show you pictures of different things. Pointing to each thing will be a picture of either you or a picture of another girl [boy]. What I'd like you to do is to say the name of the thing when it appears on the screen, and to also say who is pointing to the thing. So for example, if the thing is a picture of a house and you're pointing to it, then you would say 'I'm pointing to the house'. But if the other girl [boy] is pointing to it, then you would say 'The other girl [boy] is pointing to the house'. Let's practise so you understand what I mean."

Children were presented with two practice item-context displays (one self-condition, one other-condition) followed by 36 (18 self-condition, 18 other-condition) test item-context displays presented in random order. A 1,000 ms blank screen preceded the presentation of the item-context display. While the item-context display remained on the screen the experimenter asked: "Who is pointing to the [e.g., house]?" Children were encouraged to indicate who (self or other) was pointing to the object and to include the name of the object in their response. To ensure accurate encoding, in the event the child responded incorrectly, the experimenter pointed out the error and asked her/him to state the correct response.

Item memory test. The encoding phase was followed immediately by an incidental free recall test of the objects. Children gave spoken responses, which were noted by the researcher on a sheet containing a list of the study items. No time limit was imposed.

The item memory measure was the proportion of correctly recalled items based on 18 items in each of the self and other encoding-context conditions. Children then completed a 2-min filler task that involved drawing a picture of themselves. This was followed immediately by the context memory test.

Context memory test. Cards corresponding to the correctly recalled items were presented one at a time in a different order than during the encoding phase. Children were asked: "When you saw this [e.g., house] before during the game, who was pointing to it, was it you or was it the other girl [boy]?" The two face cards (self and other) were presented and children could respond verbally (saying "me" or "other girl [boy]") and/or point to one of the face cards. Context memory was measured as the proportion of correct judgments made for correctly recalled items.

Results and Discussion

Preliminary analyses indicated the presentation (A or B) children received during the encoding phase had no significant effect on any dependent measure in this or subsequent experiments. Data were therefore collapsed across this variable.

Item memory and context memory scores were examined separately using mixed factorial 2 (sex: girl, boy) × 3 (age: 4-, 5-, and 6-years) × 2 (encoding-context: self, other) ANOVAs, with sex and age as between-subjects variables and encoding-context as a within-subjects variable. Scheffe post-hoc tests were conducted where appropriate.

Item memory. The mean proportions of correctly recalled items are presented in Table 2. The ANOVA yielded only an effect of age, $F(2, 66) = 4.92$, $p = .01$, $\eta_p^2 = .13$. Six-year-olds ($M = .26$, $SE = .02$) recalled significantly more items than 4-year-olds ($M = .18$, $SE = .02$; $p = .017$), and marginally more items than 5-year-olds ($M = .20$, $SE = .02$; $p = .073$). Item recall for the 4- and 5-year-olds did not differ significantly.

Context memory. Single-sample *t*-tests showed the mean accuracy for self- and other-encoded items was significantly above chance level (.50) for each age group (see Table 2). The ANOVA yielded only an effect of encoding-context, $F(1, 66) = 6.13$, $p = .016$, $\eta_p^2 = .09$. Accuracy was higher for self-encoded ($M = .79$, $SE = .03$) than other-encoded items ($M = .68$, $SE = .03$). It is plausible that this SRE on context memory might reflect a response bias toward selecting the "self" photograph. Such a bias would produce a high number of self responses and a low number of other responses, resulting in a negative correlation between context memory scores for self-encoded items and other-encoded items. Pearson correlation analyses, however, revealed no evidence of this. Context memory scores for self- and other-encoded items were not significantly negatively correlated either for the entire sample, $r = .09$, $p = .46$, or for any age group, largest $r = .49$, $p = .014$ (5-year-olds).

Thus, consistent with Sui and Zhu (2005), a significant SRE on episodic memory was observed in Experiment 1. However, whereas Sui and Zhu observed a SRE on item memory but not context memory, the opposite pattern occurred in the current study. Self-referent encoding enhanced children's context memory, but not item memory.

The absence of a SRE on item memory might reflect the effortful nature of the free recall test. However, this cannot be a complete explanation because Sui and Zhu tested item memory using free recall and observed a SRE on item memory. Another possibility is that the larger number of items increased memory load which might have meant children could not benefit from any additional processing that's self-referenced items may have received (Kobasigawa 1974).

Table 2. Mean proportions of correctly recalled items and correct encoding-context judgments within each age group in experiment 1 (N = 72)

	Encoding-context	
Memory Test	Self	Other
Item		
4-years	19 (.03)	17 (.02)
5-years	18 (.02)	21 (.01)
6-years	27 (.02)	25 (.03)
Context		
4-years	76 (.07)*	65 (.06)*
5-years	82 (.06)*	72 (.04)*
6-years	79 (.05)*	67 (.06)*

Note. Standard errors are in parentheses. $n = 24$ in each age group. *Age group's mean context memory score was significantly higher than chance (.50) as assessed by a single-sample t-test.

EXPERIMENT 2

In Experiment 2, we attempted to circumvent the above issues. The free recall test of item memory was replaced with an old-new recognition test of the items. It could be argued that old-new recognition is a more age-appropriate technique for assessing item memory because it does not require strategic retrieval to the same extent that free recall does (Bjorklund and Douglas 1997). If so, it might better differentiate between self-referent and other-referent encoding in item memory for young children, while also providing a larger number of items for which context memory can be assessed (i.e., greater power to detect self-other effect). That SREs on item memory have been observed in young children using recognition tests (Crawley et al., 2010; Cunningham et al., 2014; Kovacs and Newcombe 2006) supports this proposal.

The use of old-new recognition for the item memory test in Experiment 2 addressed a second procedural issue identified within the episodic memory literature: the use of different types of tests to assess item memory and context memory, namely, free recall and a two-alternative forced-choice task, respectively. These tests are not comparable in terms of their retrieval demands and reliance on strategic processes (Brown 1975; Craik and McDowd 1987; Flavell 1970; Whiting and Smith 1997). Thus, observed differences in item and context memory might reflect the difficulty differences of the type of test used rather than differences in the type of memory. Taking into account previous research (Crawley et al., 2010; Kovacs and Newcombe 2006; Sui and Zhu 2005), the outcomes of Experiment 1, and the use of comparable item and context memory tests (old-new recognition tests), we expected self-referent encoding to facilitate item and context memory in Experiment 2.

Method

Participants. Participants were 72 children from three age groups with equal numbers of girls and boys in each age group: 24, 4-year-olds (M = 55.38 months, SD = 3.20, range:

48–59); 24, 5-year-olds (M = 65.79 months, SD = 3.22, range: 60–71); and 24, 6-year-olds (M = 78.08 months, SD = 2.92, range: 73–83).

Procedure. The encoding phase was identical to Experiment 1. Item memory was assessed using an old-new recognition test. The 36 items presented during the encoding phase, along with 36 novel distracter items (18 drawn from each of Picture Sets 3 and 4), were displayed on the computer screen in two randomised blocks each of 36 trials. Each block contained 18 old and 18 novel object drawings. Objects were displayed one at a time and remained on the screen for a maximum of 4,000 ms. The experimenter asked children: "Did you see this [e.g., house] before during the game?" After the item memory test, children completed the filler drawing task as in Experiment 1. This was followed immediately by the context memory test. Memory for encoding-context of correctly recognised items was assessed as in Experiment 1.

Results and Discussion

Except where noted, data were analysed as in Experiment 1.

Item memory. Item memory responses were expressed as hits and false alarms. Hit rates reflected the proportion of old items presented at encoding that were correctly recognised. False alarm rates reflected the proportion of new items incorrectly recognised as old. The effect of self versus other encoding-context was assessed on hit rates, but not false alarm rates. New items were those that had not been presented at encoding, thus it is not possible to examine the impact of encoding-context on false alarms.

Single-sample t-tests compared the mean hit rates for each age group and each encoding-context condition to chance level (.50; see Table 3). For self and other encoding-context conditions, the mean hit rate for each age group was significantly better than chance.

A mixed factorial ANOVA revealed a main effect of encoding-context, $F(1, 66) = 3.95$, $p = .046$, $\eta_p^2 = .06$, such that children recognised more self-encoded (M = .86, SE = .02) than other-encoded (M = .83, SE = .02) items.

Table 3. Mean item hit and false alarm rates and proportions of correct judgments for encoding-context within each age group in experiment 2 (N = 72)

	Encoding-context		
Age group[a]	Self	Other	
	Item Memory		
	Hits		False Alarms
4-years	.88 (.02)*	.87 (.02)*	.14 (.05)
5-years	.86 (.03)*	.81 (.04)*	.23 (.07)
6-years	.85 (.04)*	.81 (.05)*	.03 (.01)
	Memory for Encoding-context		
4-years	.83 (.03)*	.58 (.04)*	
5-years	.79 (.03)*	.61 (.04)*	
6-years	.78 (.05)*	.61 (.05)*	

Note. Standard errors are in parentheses. *Age group's mean item hit rate or memory for encoding-context performance was significantly higher than chance (.50) as assessed by a single-sample t-test. [a]n = 24 in each age group.

This small overall SRE on hits is different to Experiment 1, but consistent with Sui and Zhu (2005) and other research using old-new recognition to assess item memory (Crawley et al., 2010; Cunningham et al., 20014; Kovacs and Newcombe 2006). Hence, recognition might be a more sensitive measure of this aspect of episodic memory in young children when longer study lists are employed.

The main effect of sex, $F(1, 66) = 9.82$, $p = .003$, $\eta_p^2 = .13$, showed that girls ($M = .90$, $SE = .02$) recognised more items than boys ($M = .80$, $SE = .02$). This differs to Experiment 1 where girls' and boys' item recall was comparable.

Analysis of false alarm rates using a 2 (sex) × 3 (age) ANOVA (see Table 2 for relevant descriptive statistics) showed a marginally significant effect of sex, $F(2, 66) = 3.82$, $p = .055$, $\eta^2 = .06$, whereby girls ($M = .08$, $SE = .04$) tended to make fewer false alarms than boys ($M = .19$, $SE = .04$). Thus, boys incorrectly judged new items as old more frequently than girls. Girls' higher hit rates in item recognition did not come at the cost of a higher false alarm rate relative to boys.

Neither Sui and Zhu (2005) nor Cunningham et al. (2014) reported sex effects on item memory; presumably there were none. Crawley et al. (2010) found no effect of sex on item memory for their 4- to 6-year-olds. Sex differences in item memory have not been frequently discussed in the SRE literature. It is therefore unclear whether girls and boys perform differently on the different types of tests (i.e., item recall versus item recognition), or whether free recall is insufficiently sensitive to detect sex differences. More data are needed to provide a clearer picture about whether girls' and boys' item memory develops differentially during the preschool period.

The main effect of age on false alarms was significant, $F(2, 66) = 4.39$, $p = .016$, $\eta^2 = .12$. Scheffe post-hoc tests showed that 6-year-olds made fewer false alarms than 5-year-olds ($p = .016$), but not 4-year-olds ($p = .292$). The difference between 4- and 5-year-olds was not significant. We questioned whether the differential false alarm rates could account for the null effect of age on hits. Consequently, we examined the possibility that the two youngest age groups were prone to a "yes" response bias, which would inflate their item recognition performance (hit rates). If younger children are prone to a "yes" response bias, then hit and false alarm rates would be expected to be significantly positively correlated. This was checked for the entire sample and each subgroup. However, the interpretation was not supported as the only significant finding was a negative correlation between the two scores for 5-year-old girls ($r = -.66$, $p = .020$), indicating that as the hit rate for this subgroup increased, the false alarm rate decreased.

Context memory. Context memory was expressed as the mean proportion of correct encoding-context judgments made for correctly recognised items. Single-sample *t*-tests, showed that accuracy was significantly higher than chance for self-encoded and other-encoded items for each age group (see Table 3).

A mixed factorial ANOVA revealed significant main effects of encoding-context, $F(1, 66) = 76.26$, $p < .001$, $\eta_p^2 = .54$, and sex, $F(1, 66) = 6.54$, $p = .013$, $\eta_p^2 = .09$, and a significant Sex × Encoding-context interaction, $F(1, 66) = 4.02$, $p = .049$, $\eta_p^2 = .06$ (see Figure 2). Simple effects analysis revealed more accurate context memory for self-encoded than other-encoded items for girls, $F(1, 35) = 29.26$, $p < .001$, $\eta_p^2 = .46$, and boys, $F(1, 35) = 47.80$, $p < .001$, $\eta_p^2 = .58$, with a larger SRE for boys than girls. The larger SRE for boys occurred because girls' accuracy was higher than boys' for other-encoded items, $F(1, 70) =$

10.01, $p = .002$, $\eta_p^2 = .13$, but there was no difference between girls and boys for self-encoded items.

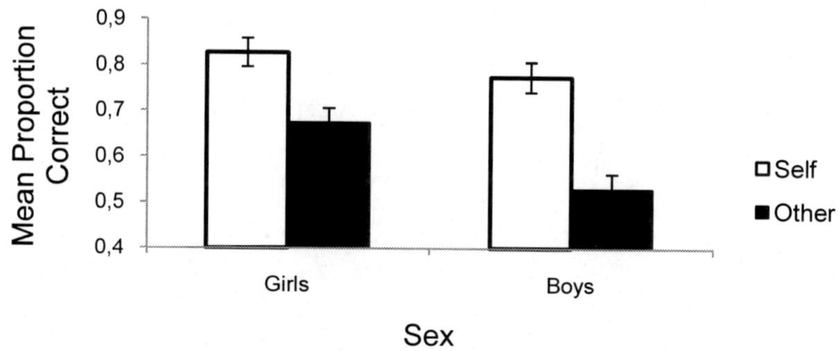

Figure 2. Mean proportions of correct encoding-context judgments according to sex and encoding-context in Experiment 2 ($N = 72$). Error bars denote standard errors.

The overall SRE on context memory is consistent with Experiment 1. The robustness of this finding is supported by the large effect size, with encoding-context accounting for around 54% of the variance in accuracy here compared to 9% in Experiment 1. This suggests that the advantage produced through self-referent encoding is amplified when more items are available for the context memory test.

In contrast to Experiment 1, the SRE on context memory was larger for boys than girls due to boys' poorer accuracy for other-encoded items. Correlation analyses further ruled out a response bias on the part of the boys as context memory accuracy for self-encoded and other-encoded items were not negatively correlated either for the entire sample, $r = .49$, $p < .001$, for girls only, $r = .50$, $p = .001$, for boys only, $r = .43$, $p = .009$, or any age group, largest $r = .72$, $p < .001$ (6-year-old girls).

As reported above, boys also had poorer item recognition (hits and false alarms). Thus, boys' item and context memory benefited more from self-referent encoding than girls' memory did. Consistent with Experiment 1 and Sui and Zhu (2005), there was no evidence of developmental improvement in children's memory for encoding-context. Whilst this differs from other research showing improvements in children's ability to discriminate contextual information between 4 and 6 years-of-age (Cunningham et al., 2014; Drummey and Newcombe 2002; Foley, Harris and Hermann 1994; Lindsay et al., 1991; Sluzenski et al., 2004; Sussman 2001; Welch-Ross 1995), differences between the current paradigm and others likely account for the disparity and are discussed in Experiment 3.

EXPERIMENT 3

In most experiments, context memory is tested for correctly remembered items only. Hence, the context memory test is not independent of the item memory test. This procedure assumes there is no memory for the context of items that are not reported at test. However, the encoding of isolated item and context features is potentially a separate process from the encoding of these features when bound together (Sluzenski, Newcombe and Kovacs 2006). Some adult research supports this idea showing that specification of an item's context is possible in the absence of memory for the item itself (Cook, Marsh and Hicks 2006; Kurilla and Westerman 2010; Starns, Hicks, Brown and Martin 2008).

It appears no child research has considered the above possibility, therefore in Experiment 3 we tested context memory for all items presented at encoding, irrespective of whether item memory was demonstrated. We were interested in whether the SRE on context memory still occurs, and if so, whether its magnitude varies when context memory is based on all items presented at encoding rather than the usual practice of testing it based on correctly recalled items only. Additionally, we examined the extent to which 4- to 6-year-old children can access contextual information without demonstrating item recall. As in Experiment 1, item memory was assessed using free recall. This enabled the differential effects of self-referent and other-referent encoding on item memory to be further investigated using the procedure with which Sui and Zhu (2005) observed SREs in 5-year-olds. However, assessing context memory for all items ensured sufficient items were available for this test to evaluate sex, age, and encoding-context effects. Where appropriate, we compared outcomes between the relevant experiments. For item memory, the effects of sex, age, and encoding-context on item recall were examined further by including data from Experiments 1 and 3 in the same analysis. Given the similar procedures, no significant effect of experiment and no interaction involving experiment were anticipated.

Method

Participants. Participants were 72 children from three age groups with equal numbers of girls and boys in each age group: 24, 4-year-olds ($M = 55.29$ months, $SD = 3.39$, range: 48–59); 24, 5-year-olds ($M = 64.58$ months, $SD = 3.79$, range: 56–71); and 24, 6-year-olds ($M = 77.33$ months, $SD = 3.71$, range: 72–83).

Procedure. The encoding phase, item memory test, and filler drawing task were identical to Experiment 1. Context memory was assessed as in Experiment 1 with one exception: Context memory was assessed for all items, irrespective of whether they were correctly recalled.

Results and Discussion

Except where indicated, data were analysed as in Experiment 1.

Item memory. Item memory was measured as the mean proportion of correctly recalled items. A mixed factorial ANOVA showed only a main effect of age, $F(2, 66) = 4.81$, $p = .011$, $\eta_p^2 = .13$. Six-year-olds ($M = .22$, $SE = .02$) recalled more items than 4-year-olds ($M = .15$, $SE = .02$; $p = .016$), but not 5-year-olds ($M = .20$, $SE = .02$); 5-year-olds recalled marginally more items than 4-year-olds ($p = .087$). Thus, consistent with Experiment 1, there was no SRE on item memory. We discuss potential reasons for the disparity between the present finding and Sui and Zhu's (2005) in the section below where item memory across experiments is compared.

Context memory. The context memory test was based on (1) all items, whereby accuracy was measured as the mean proportion of correct encoding-context judgments made for all items presented at encoding; and (2) items for which item memory was demonstrated.

Table 4. Mean proportions of correct encoding-context judgments for recalled items and all items within each age group in experiment 3 (N = 72)

	Encoding-context	
Memory test	Self	Other
Recalled Items[a]		
4-years	.90 (.06)*	.62 (.08)
5-years	.84 (.05)*	.69 (.07)*
6-years	.83 (.05)*	.62 (.07)
All Items[a]		
4-years	.80 (.03)*	.70 (.03)*
5-years	.83 (.03)*	.76 (.03)*
6-years	.83 (.02)*	.77 (.03)*

Note. Standard errors are in parentheses. *Age group's mean context memory score for recalled items or all items was significantly higher than chance (.50) as assessed by a single-sample *t*-test. [a]$n = 24$ for each age group.

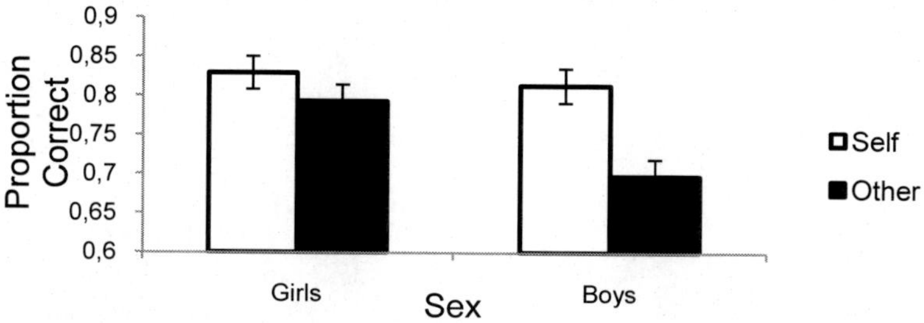

Figure 3. Mean proportions of correct encoding-context judgments for all items according to sex and encoding-context in Experiment 3 ($N = 72$). Error bars denote standard errors.

Context memory based on all items presented at encoding. The results of single-sample *t*-tests and descriptive statistics for accuracy based on all items are presented in the lower section of Table 4. In each condition and age group, mean context memory accuracy was higher than chance (.50).

A mixed factorial ANOVA revealed main effects of encoding-context, $F(1, 66) = 15.49$, $p < .001$, $\eta_p^2 = .19$, and sex, $F(1, 66) = 5.56$, $p = .021$, $\eta_p^2 = .08$, and a significant Sex × Encoding-context interaction, $F(1, 66) = 4.36$, $p = .041$, $\eta_p^2 = .06$ (see Figure 3).

Simple effects analyses showed that the SRE on context memory was significant for boys $F(1, 35) = 14.21$, $p < .001$, $\eta_p^2 = .29$, but not for girls, $F(1, 35) = 2.62$, $p = .115$, $\eta_p^2 = .07$. The SRE for boys was due to their poorer accuracy for other-encoded items compared to girls. Girls' context memory was more accurate than boys' for other-encoded items, $F(1, 70) = 9.68$, $p = .003$, $\eta_p^2 = .12$, but not self-encoded items, $F(1, 70) = 0.27$, $p = .606$, $\eta_p^2 = .004$.

The SRE on context memory was not due to a self response bias as the self-encoded and other-encoded context memory scores were not significantly negatively correlated either for the entire sample, $r = .23$, $p = .052$, any age group, largest $r = .47$, $p = .019$ (4-year-olds), or sex group, boys, $r = .16$, $p = .366$, girls, $r = .34$, $p = .051$.

Context memory based on correctly recalled items. The single-sample *t*-test results and descriptive statistics for accuracy based on recalled items are presented in the upper section of Table 4. For self-encoded items, accuracy in each age group was higher than chance. For other-encoded items, accuracy was higher than chance for 5-year-olds, but did not differ from chance for 4- and 6-year-olds.

A mixed factorial ANOVA revealed a main effect of encoding-context, $F(1, 66) = 15.60$, $p < .001$, $\eta_p^2 = .19$, whereby context memory was more accurate for self-encoded ($M = .86$, $SE = .03$) than other-encoded items ($M = .64$, $SE = .04$). The SRE was not due to a self response bias as the scores for self-encoded and other-encoded items were not negatively correlated for the entire sample, $r = -.02$, $p = .852$, or any age group, largest $r = -.11$, $p = .600$ (6-year-olds).

In summary, the SRE on context memory was observed irrespective of whether context memory was based on all items or correctly recalled items only. When assessed for recalled items only, girls and boys performed similarly, however, when assessed for all items, boys' context memory accuracy was poorer than girls' for other-encoded items. Thus, a SRE was evident for boys but not girls, which was not from a self response bias on the part of boys. This represented the principal difference between the two methods and is considered in the cross-experiment comparisons below.

Between Experiment Comparisons

A 3 (age) × 3 (experiment) factorial ANOVA showed SES did not vary significantly according to age or experiment and there was no significant Age × Experiment interaction.

Item memory. Item memory was assessed in the same way in Experiments 1 and 3, so the two experiments were compared. A 2 (sex) × 2 (experiment) × 3 (age) × 2 (encoding-context) mixed factorial ANOVA revealed there was no SRE on item memory. The absence of a SRE on item recall relative to Sui and Zhu (2005) likely reflects some task modifications (e.g., stimulus display presentation time), which are considered in the general discussion.

There was a significant main effect of age, $F(2, 132) = 8.82$, $p < .001$, $\eta_p^2 = .118$. Six-year-olds ($M = .24$, $SE = .01$) recalled significantly more items than 4-year-olds ($M = .16$, $SE = .01$; $p < .001$), and marginally more items than 5-year-olds ($M = .20$, $SE = .01$; $p = .089$); the difference between 4- and 5-year-olds was not significant. These developmental improvements replicate those observed by Sui and Zhu (2005), and more generally, reflect strategic processing developments during the preschool years (Bjorklund and Douglas, 1997). Taken together, the experiments yielded similar findings, as indicated by the nonsignificant effect of experiment and the absence of any significant interactions involving experiment.

Context memory. Context memory in the three experiments was compared. In the first analysis, context memory scores for Experiment 3 were based on correctly recalled items only. A 2 (sex) × 3 (experiment) × 3 (age) × 2 (encoding-context) mixed factorial ANOVA yielded a main effect of encoding-context, $F(1, 198) = 49.71$, $p < .001$, $\eta_p^2 = .201$, indicating more accurate context memory for self-encoded ($M = .82$, $SE = .02$) than other-encoded ($M = .64$, $SE = .02$) items. The three experiments yielded similar findings, as indicated by the nonsignificant effect of experiment and the absence of any significant interactions involving experiment. Furthermore, the significant SREs on context memory that were observed in all three experiments did not differ significantly in magnitude.

In the second analysis, context memory scores for Experiment 3 were based on all items presented during encoding. A 2 (sex) × 3 (experiment) × 3 (age) × 2 (encoding-context) mixed factorial ANOVA revealed main effects of encoding-context, $F(1, 198) = 50.29$, $p < .001$, $\eta_p^2 = .203$, experiment, $F(2, 198) = 4.40$, $p = .013$, $\eta_p^2 = .043$, and sex, $F(1, 198) = 4.96$, $p = .027$, $\eta_p^2 = .024$, and a significant Encoding-context × Experiment interaction, $F(2, 198) = 3.99$, $p = .020$, $\eta_p^2 = .039$ (see Figure 4). The main effect of sex showed that girls' ($M = .77$, $SE = .02$) accuracy was higher than boys' ($M = .71$, $SE = .02$).

The simple effect of encoding-context was significant in Experiment 1, $F(1, 71) = 6.32$, $p = .014$, $\eta_p^2 = .08$, Experiment 2, $F(1, 71) = 73.86$, $p < .001$, $\eta_p^2 = .51$, and Experiment 3, $F(1, 71) = 15.32$, $p < .001$, $\eta_p^2 = .18$, such that a SRE was evident in each experiment. The effect sizes and the means in Figure 4 suggest that the SRE was largest in Experiment 2, and comparable in Experiments 1 and 3. Simple effects analyses revealed that the smaller SRE in Experiment 3 was due to the other encoding condition, $F(2, 213) = 7.82$, $p = .001$. Context memory in the other encoding condition when assessed for all items (Exp. 3) was higher than when assessed for correctly recognised items only (Exp. 2; $p = .001$). Context memory in the other encoding condition when assessed for correctly recalled items (Exp. 1) was at an intermediate level that did not differ significantly to context memory based on all (Exp. 3) or correctly recognised (Exp. 2) items. The effect of experiment on context memory was not significant in the self encoding condition.

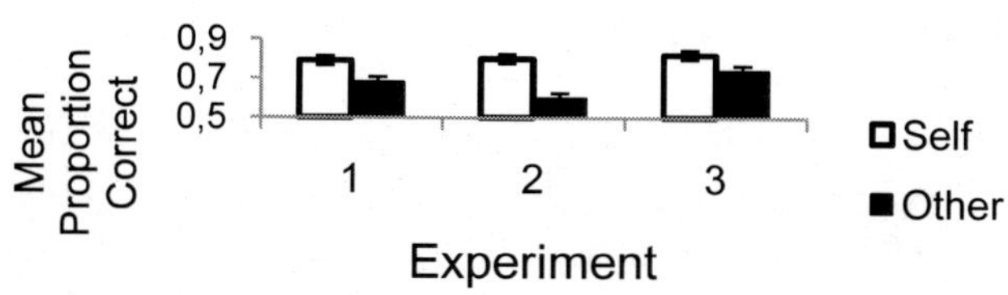

Figure 4. Mean proportions of correct encoding-context judgments according to experiment and encoding-context for combined data of Experiments 1, 2, and 3 (N = 216). Context memory was based on recalled items (Exp. 1), recognised items (Exp. 2), and all items (Exp. 3). Error bars denote standard errors.

General Discussion

In three experiments, the SRE was examined on two types of item memory tasks: item recall (Exps. 1 and 3) and item recognition (Exp. 2). The SRE was also examined on memory for the context of correctly recalled items (Exps. 1 and 3), correctly recognised items (Exp. 2), and for all items presented during the encoding phase (Exp. 3).

Consistent with other studies that used a recognition test of items (Crawley et al., 2010; Cunningham et al., 2014; Kovacs and Newcombe, 2006), self-referent encoding produced superior item memory than other-referent encoding did (Exp. 2). In contrast, however, self-referent encoding did not facilitate item recall (Exps. 1 and 3). This second outcome is inconsistent with Sui and Zhu (2005) who observed SREs on item recall for 5-year-olds. In all experiments, self-referent encoding produced superior context memory than other-referent encoding did and the SRE did not vary across age groups. Furthermore, the SRE on context memory could not be accounted for by differences in SES. Thus, consistent with Cunningham et al. (2014), these findings extend Sui and Zhu's (2005) to show that children's context memory prior to 6 years-of-age can benefit from self-referent encoding.

The two main differences in outcomes between the current research and Sui and Zhu's (2005) were that (1) self-referent encoding did not produce better item recall than other-referent encoding did, whereas in Sui and Zhu's study it did; and (2) self-referent encoding facilitated more accurate context memory than other-referent encoding did in the present research, whereas in Sui and Zhu's study it did not. Self-referent encoding exerts its advantage by facilitating elaboration and organisation in memory (Symons and Johnson, 1997). However, factors including the duration of item presentation at encoding and the retention interval between the encoding and test phases can moderate the magnitude of the SRE in episodic memory (Symons and Johnson 1997). These factors might explain the discrepancies between our findings and Sui and Zhu's.

First, the magnitude of the SRE can diminish with extended item exposure, possibly because it promotes greater processing of other-encoded information (Symons and Johnson 1997). In turn, this additional processing of other items might counteract the more rapid and automatic benefits of self-referential processing (Symons and Johnson 1997). In the present study, the item-context stimulus presentation time for each encoding trial was longer (no time limit imposed) than it was in Sui and Zhu's (2005; 4 sec). Thus, extended exposure might have neutralised the potential advantage of self-referent encoding on item recall. That item recall for other-referent items in our research was higher than it was in Sui and Zhu's (2005) study supports this account. Whereas we found that children recalled an average of 2.72 and 3.43 other-referent items (4- and 5-year-olds, respectively; Exps. 1 and 3 combined), the same-aged children in Sui and Zhu's study recalled an average of 2.29 and 2.60 (4- and 5-year-olds, respectively; Exp. 1). Additionally, Sui and Zhu (2005) found 10-year-olds did not demonstrate a SRE on item memory when the stimulus presentation time was longer (Exp. 1) relative to when it was shorter (Exp. 2).

Second, longer retention intervals between encoding and retrieval are associated with larger SREs in episodic memory, possibly because other-referent encoding involves less effective strategies (e.g., rehearsal) than self-referent encoding (Symons and Johnson 1997). The longer stimulus presentation time at encoding in the present research also meant our participants had to retain information longer than Sui and Zhu's (2005). Thus, the observed SRE on context memory but not item recall might reflect the modified procedure, whereby additional processing in the other encoding condition during encoding facilitated memory for items but not context. The item-context bindings in the other encoding condition might have decayed at a faster rate over the retention interval than item-context bindings in the self encoding condition.

We investigated whether the SRE still occurs when context memory is based on all items presented at encoding rather than the usual practice whereby context memory is based on items that were recalled or recognised only. Our findings showed that the SRE is still observed but its magnitude is reduced, apparently because context memory based on all items selectively benefits accuracy for other-referent items. To some degree, this outcome supports adult research showing that memory for context information is possible in the absence of item recall or recognition (Cook et al., 2006; Kurilla and Westerman 2010; Starns et al., 2008).

Two possible explanations for the selective enhancement of context memory for other-referent items are as follows.

Fuzzy trace theory asserts that experienced items serve as good retrieval cues for verbatim traces (Brainerd and Reyna 2002). Thus, in the absence of demonstrated item memory, re-presentation of the original item might facilitate access to the verbatim trace for context where the trace is sufficiently strong. However, because self-referent encoding automatically engages strategic processing, which generates multiple retrieval cues (Symons and Johnson 1997), no additional advantage is gained. Conversely, because other-referent encoding engages less strategic processing, fewer retrieval cues are generated (Symons and Johnson 1997), therefore re-presentation of the original item serves as a cue to the verbatim trace for context, thereby enhancing context memory for other-referent items.

Alternatively, from a source monitoring perspective (Johnson et al., 1993), children might engage a decision process which results in the encoding context being attributed to the other child when their memory lacks the clarity of detail normally expected for events involving self. This decision process can be explained as follows. The nature of the two-alternative forced-choice context memory task is such that for any given item, either *self* or *other* must be selected as context. In instances when the item-context representation is weak and children are uncertain about an item's context, they might reason that if they had pointed to the item, then they would remember it more clearly, therefore the other child must have pointed to it. The consequence of this form of reasoning would be to increase the accuracy of context judgments for other-encoded items, but not for self-encoded items when certainty is low. Of course, whether young children are able to utilise meta-memory rules such as this, is in itself open to question (Foley et al., 1983; Roberts 2000). Further clarification on the issue is required.

Another finding indicates that the magnitude of the SRE on context judgments is not dependent on the number of items available for the context memory test. Fuzzy trace theory (Brainerd and Reyna 2002a) asserts that verbatim representations are relied on heavily for retrieving contextual information, but that these representations decay with time. Fuzzy trace theory might account for the observed SRE on context memory in terms of different decay rates. That is, contextual information may decay faster in the other-referent encoding condition than self-referent encoding condition. The present findings might therefore reflect context degradation that is in line with the durational differences between the encoding phase and context memory test phase across the experiments. The duration was longest when context memory was based on correctly recognised items (Exp. 2), followed by all items (Exp. 3) and correctly recalled items (Exp. 1), respectively. It is therefore reasonable to suppose that context degradation would follow this pattern. The outcomes obtained fit reasonably well with this supposition in that the magnitude of the SRE was greatest in Experiment 2 and smaller in Experiments 1 and 3.

Unfortunately, the above assertion highlights a limitation of the current paradigm and its use of separate, successive tests of item and context memory. Due to the possibility that differential context degradation occurred between the experiments, the extent to which the SRE on context memory is enhanced by the availability of more items for the memory for context test is not clear. Future research could address this by incorporating a recognition test that assesses children's item and context memory simultaneously. Given our findings showing poorer episodic memory for boys than girls and that boys benefited more than girls from self-referent encoding, future research should also consider sex differences in the early development of the SRE in episodic memory.

Conclusion

From a theoretical perspective, the current research contributes to a better understanding of how episodic memory develops during childhood. Episodic memory involves memory for content as well as contextual information and it necessarily involves the self as rememberer (Wheeler et al., 1997). The nature of the self's involvement in this type of memory therefore represents a central aspect in understanding its development. The present findings have implications for this understanding because they provide evidence that the self-other distinction emerges early in development, being present in 4-year-olds and that this distinction facilitates relational links between item and contextual information. Second, they suggest that involvement of self, in the form of self-referential encoding, produces more robust item-context representations, which aid retrieval of context. Furthermore, the present findings indicate that even by 4 years-of-age, the self represents a cognitive structure around which information can be organised to promote episodic memory.

Acknowledgment

The authors thank Dr. Ruth Ford, Department of Psychology, Anglia Ruskin University, Cambridge UK for her insightful feedback on this manuscript.

References

Andrews, G., Murphy, K., Dunbar, M., & Boyce, J. (2012). Self-referent encoding facilitates recency discrimination and recognition in episodic memory. In G. Andrews & D. L. Neumann (Eds.), Beyond the Lab: Applications of Cognitive Research in Memory and Learning (pp. 43-55). Hauppauge, NY: Nova Science Publishers.

Bjorklund, D. F., & Douglas, R. N. (1997). The development of memory strategies. In N. Cowan & C. Hulme (Eds.), The development of memory in childhood (pp. 201-246). East Sussex, United Kingdom: Psychology Press.

Brainerd, C. J., & Reyna, V. F. (2002a). Fuzzy-trace theory and false memory. *Current Directions in Psychological Science,* 11, 164-169. doi: 10.1111/1467-8721.00192.

Brainerd, C. J., & Reyna, V. F. (2002b). Fuzzy-trace theory: Dual processes in memory, reasoning, and cognitive neuroscience. *Advances in Child Development and Behavior,* 28, 41-100.

Brown, A. L. (1975). Recognition, reconstruction, and recall of narrative sequences by preoperational children. *Child Development, 46,* 156-166. Retrieved from http://www.jstor.org/stable/1128844.

Chalmers, K. A., & Grogan, M. J. (2006). Developmental differences in judgments of recency and frequency: Quantitative or qualitative? *Cognitive Development,* 21, 72-79. doi: http://dx.doi.org/10.1016/j. cogdev.2005.11.001.

Cook, G. I., Marsh, R. L., & Hicks, J. L. (2006). Source memory in the absence of successful cued recall. *Journal of Experimental Psychology: Learning, Memory and Cognition,* 32, 828-835. doi: 10.1037/0278-7393.32.4.828.

Courage, M. L., Edison, S. C., & Howe, M. L. (2004). Variability in the early development of visual self-recognition. *Infant Behavior and Development,* 27, 509-532. doi: 10.1016/j.infbeh.2004.06.001.

Craik, F. I. M., & McDowd, J. M. (1987). Age differences in recall and recognition. *Journal of Experimental Psychology: Learning, Memory, and Cognition,* 13, 474-479. doi: 10.1037/0278-7393.13.3.474.

Crawley, S. L., Newcombe, N. S., & Bingman, H. (2010). How focus at encoding affects children's source monitoring. *Journal of Experimental Child Psychology,* 105, 273-285. doi: 10.1016/j.jecp.2009.12.003.

Cunningham, S. J., Brebner, J. L., Quinn, R., & Turk, D. (2014). The self-reference effect on memory in early childhood. *Child Development, 85*, 808-823. doi: 10.1111/cdev.12144.

Drummey, A. B., & Newcombe, N. S. (2002). Developmental changes in source memory. *Developmental Science,* 5, 502-513. doi: 10.1111/1467-7687.00243.

Flavell, J. H. (1970). Developmental studies of mediated memory. In H. W. Reese & L. P. Lipsitt (Eds.), *Advances in child development and behavior* (Vol. 5, pp. 181-211). New York, NY: Academic Press.

Foley, M. A., Harris, J. F., & Hermann, S. (1994). Developmental comparisons of the ability to discriminate between memories for symbolic play enactments. *Developmental Psychology,* 30, 206-217. doi: 10.1037/0012-1649.30.2.206.

Foley, M. A., Johnson, M. K., & Raye, C. L. (1983). Age-related changes in confusion between memories for thoughts and memories for speech. *Child Development,* 54, 51-60. Retrieved from http://www.jstor.org/stable /1129860.

Forster, K. I., & Forster, J. C. (2003). DMDX (Version 3). Tucson, AZ: University of Arizona.

Glisky, E. L., Rubin, S. R., & Davidson, S. R. (2001). Source memory in older adults: An encoding or retrieval problem? *Journal of Experimental Psychology: Learning, Memory, and Cognition,* 27, 1131-1146. doi: 10.1037//0278-7393.27.5.1131.

Hashtroudi, S., Johnson, M. K., Vnek, N., & Ferguson, S. A. (1994). Aging and the effects of affective and factual focus on source monitoring and recall. *Psychology and Aging,* 9, 160-170. doi: 10.1037/0882-7974.9.1.160.

Hollingshead, A. B. (1975). Four Factor Index of Social Status. Unpublished manuscript. Yale University, New Haven, CT.

Johnson, M. K., & Chalfonte, B. L. (1994). Binding complex memories: The role of activation and the hippocampus. In D. L. Schacter & E. Tulving (Eds.), Memory systems (pp. 311-350). Cambridge, MA: MIT Press.

Johnson, M. K., Hashtroudi, S., & Lindsay, D. S. (1993). Source monitoring. *Psychological Bulletin,* 114, 3-28. doi: 10.1037/0033-2909.114.1.3.

Kee, D. W., & Bell, T. S. (1981). The development of organizational strategies in the storage and retrieval of categorical items in free-recall learning. *Child Development,* 52, 1163-1171. Retrieved from http://www.jstor.org /stable/1129502.

Keenan, J. P., Wheeler, M. A., Gallup, G. G., & Pascual-Leone, A. (2000). Self-recognition and the right prefrontal cortex. *Trends in Cognitive Sciences,* 4, 338-344. doi: 10.1016/S1364-6613(00)01521-7.

Kobasigawa, A. (1974). Utilization of retrieval cues by children in recall. *Child Development,* 45, 127-134. Retrieved from http://www.jstor.org /stable/1127758.

Kovacs, S. L., & Newcombe, N. S. (2006). Developments in source monitoring: The role of thinking of others. *Journal of Experimental Child Psychology,* 93, 25-44. doi: 10.1016/j.jecp.2005.06.006.

Kurilla, B. P., & Westerman, D. L. (2010). Source memory for unidentified stimuli. *Journal of Experimental Psychology: Learning, Memory, and Cognition,* 36, 398-410. doi: 10.1037/a0018279.

Lindsay, D. S. (2008). Source monitoring. In H. L. Roediger (Ed.), Learning and memory: A comprehensive reference (Vol. 2, pp. 325-348). Oxford, United Kingdom: Academic Press.

Lindsay, D. S., Johnson, M. K., & Kwon, P. (1991). Developmental changes in memory source monitoring. *Journal of Experimental Child Psychology,* 52, 297-318. doi: 10.1016/0022-0965(91)90065-Z.

Quas, J. A., Schaaf, J. M., Alexander, K. W., & Goodman, G. S. (2000). Do you really remember it happening or do you only remember being asked about it happening? Children's source monitoring in forensic contexts. In K. P. Roberts & M. Blades (Eds.), *Children's source monitoring* (pp. 197-226). Mahwah, NJ: Lawrence Erlbaum Associates.

Roberts, K. P. (2000). An overview of theory and research on children's source monitoring. In K. P. Roberts & M. Blades (Eds.), *Children's source monitoring* (pp. 11–57). Mahwah, NJ: Lawrence Erlbaum Associates.

Sluzenski, J., Newcombe, N. S., & Kovacs, S. L. (2006). Binding, relational memory, and recall of naturalistic events: A developmental perspective. *Journal of Experimental Psychology: Learning, Memory, and Cognition,* 32, 89-100. doi: 10.1037/0278-7393.32.1.89.

Sluzenski, J., Newcombe, N. S., & Ottinger, W. (2004). Changes in reality monitoring and episodic memory in early childhood. *Developmental Science,* 7, 225-245. doi: 10.1111/j.1467-7687.2004.00341.x.

Starns, J. J., Hicks, J. L., Brown, N. L., & Martin, B. A. (2008). Source memory for unrecognized items: Predictions from multivariate signal detection theory. *Memory & Cognition,* 36, 1. doi: 10.3758/MC.36.1.1.

Sui, J., & Zhu, Y. (2005). Five-year-olds can show the self-reference advantage. *International Journal of Behavioral Development,* 29, 382-387. doi: 10.1177/01650250500172673.

Sussman, A. L. (2001). Reality monitoring of performed and imagined interactive events: Developmental and contextual effects. *Journal of Experimental Child Psychology,* 79, 115-138. doi: 10.1006/jecp.2000. 2575.

Symons, C. S., & Johnson, B. T. (1997). The self-reference effect in memory: A meta-analysis. *Psychological Bulletin,* 121, 371-394. doi: 10.1037 /0033-2909.121.3.371.

Szekely, A., Jacobsen, T., D' Amico, S., Devescovi, A., Andonova, E., Herron, D., Mehotcheva, T. (2004). The international picture-naming projectRetrieved 3rd July, 2006, from http://crl.ucsd.edu/~aszekely/ipnp

Turk, D. J., Cunningham, S. J., & Macrae, C. N. (2008). Self-memory biases in explicit and incidental encoding of trait adjectives. *Consciousness and Cognition,* 17, 1040-1045.

Welch-Ross, M. K. (1995). Developmental changes in preschoolers' ability to distinguish memories of performed, pretended, and imagined actions. *Cognitive Development,* 10, 421-441. doi: 10.1016/0885-2014(95)90005-5.

Wheeler, M. A., Stuss, D. T., & Tulving, E. (1997). Toward a theory of episodic memory: The frontal lobes and autonoetic consciousness. *Psychological Bulletin,* 121, 331-354. doi: 10.1037/0033-2909.121.3.331.

Whiting, W. L., & Smith, A. D. (1997). Differential age-related processing limitations in recall and recognition tasks. *Psychology and Aging,* 12, 216-224. doi: 10.1037/0882-7974.12.2.216.

Williams, K. G., & Goulet, L. R. (1975). The effects of cueing and constraint instructions on children's free recall performance. *Journal of Experimental Child Psychology,* 19, 464-475. doi: 10.1016/0022-0965(75)90076-4.

Yim, H, Dennis, S. J, & Sloutsky, V. M. (2013). The development of episodic memory: Items, contexts, and relations. *Psychological Science,* 24, 2163-2172. doi: 10.1177/0956797613487385.

In: Spatial, Long-and Short-Term Memory
Editor: Edward A. Thayer

ISBN: 978-1-63484-148-1

Chapter 7

OPTICAL MEMORY MODEL OF THE HUMAN BRAIN

Tetsuya Hoshino[1,*], Toyohiko Yatagai[2] and Masahide Itoh[1]

[1]Institute of Applied Physics, University of Tsukuba, Tsukuba, Ibaraki, Japan

[2]Center for Optical Research and Education, Utsunomiya University,Utsunomiya, Tochigi, Japan

ABSTRACT

We developed models that can explain the working of the human brain. It is important to identify the source of memory. For example, it could be the distance, size, shape, or absorption capability of the neuron. Moreover, it may be multiple values or a single value memory.

Considering the low density of neurons, the type of memory should be a multiple value memory. In our study, we employ a multiple value memory, whose source of information is distance. The distance information is defined as the distance between the neurons.

Further, it is necessary to know how the brain processes the information stored in memory for thinking functions. We classify optical memory as temporary and long-term. We assigned long-term memory with the multiple value memory of distance. Fourier transforms are used to convert long-term memory into temporary memory.

The information stored in long-term memory is Fourier transformed into a hologram so that the brain can think associatively. Here, the hologram is a temporary image. The hologram has merit to explain easily the working of associative memory in the human brain. It is shown that the human brain is superior to a semiconductor computer especially in the field of associative memory. Further, a hologram is suitable for associative memory because it can easily recall total information from partial information. Finally, we explain the characteristics of the human brain by this model. A neuron can be representative of an image such as that of a grandmother and is therefore

* E-mail:hoshino@gabor.bk.tsukuba.ac.jp.

called a grandmother neuron. If one neuron represents an image, injury to the brain should destroy the memory of the image; however, it actually does not. The neuron is merely a tentative center to represent the image.

The mechanism is as follows. The information is represented as the distance from the tentative center neuron to the other neurons. The memory consists of one center and other columns of redundant information. The center may stay at any position, as long as it is outside the corresponding neurons. If the tentative center is destroyed, another center takes over as an alternative center.

1. Introduction: Human Brain and Computer's IC Chip

A robot is controlled by a computer whose brain is an IC chip (Figure 1). The pitch of wires of an IC chip is several tens of nanometers in size. On the other hand, the thickness of a neuron of the human brain is on the order of several tens of micrometers [1]. Although the pitch of the IC chip is one thousand times finer than the neuron, humans can process tasks that are more complex compared with a robot. Humans have five senses and they can integrate the information received from these senses smoothly. For example, a human can sweep a room, babysit a child, and cook various dishes; performing these tasks much better than a computer [2]. The type of human memory and the treatment of the information may have the key to handling these complex tasks well. Therefore, we research the key.

A worldwide top-level super computer has 10^9 transistors per IC chip [3-5] and 10^5 chips per computer [6]. Thus, the total number of transistors is 10^5 billion (10^{14}). On the contrary, the number of neurons that make up the human brain is between 50 and 100 billion [7, 8], of which 10 billion belong to the cerebral cortex [9, 10]. The human brain records memories by trial and error and another person cannot arrange the stack of memory. Furthermore, memories are said to be delocalized; therefore, if a part of it is lost, the memory does not vanish completely [11-14]. These things demand considerable degeneracy of the human memory and the same memory may be recorded in several parts of the brain [15, 16].

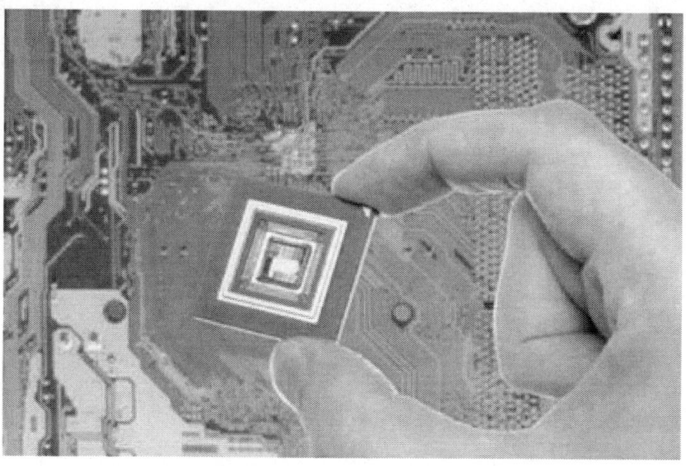

Figure 1. IC chip and its wiring pattern.

The computer has a large number of memory units, which are arranged well; however, this arrangement is inferior to the human brain. Therefore, the number of the neurons is too small a parameter to explain the brain's high-performance capacity, if each individual neuron is assumed to correspond to a transistor.

1.1. Importance of Modeling the Brain

Although identifying the working mechanism of the brain is indeed a promising field of study, there is often insufficient theory to explain its operation. For example, researches in this field still cannot define an engram, which is the source of memory. In the beginning of the study, it is important to present a well-mannered assumption. If there is no model, it is like going through a maze without markings.

To research this unknown mechanism, researchers have developed a tentative model of the mechanism and have performed simulations to examine it [17-19]. We should find the key mechanism because even though the brain is very complex, the process may be reasonably simpler and effective.

1.2. Importance of Optical Memory Model for Association

A human is superior to a computer especially in terms of associative ability. For example, a human can easily infer the emotion of another person from facial expressions; however, a computer is unable to do so without a complex program. For a regulated problem such as a game of chess, the computer is often superior to a human; however, for an associative problem, a human is superior to the computer. Holography for the neuron system has been studied as one of the associative memories [20, 21]. Holographic memory is delocalized memory. Associative memory can also be explained by a computational neural network, which covers the human body from brain to hand, eye, and ear [17, 22-24]. This neural network works in the field of electrical computers and needs another concrete method. On the other hand, a hologram is an optical memory that can be examined in a concrete system [25].

Neurons transmit information through electric signals, which consists of pulse trains [8]. On the other hand, information in an optical memory is transmitted as light. The electric signal and light travel based on different laws. One possibility to explain the difference is that the pulse train of an electric signal corresponds to the periodic amplitude modulation of light. The pulse train of a neuron has several periodicities and can be analyzed by Fourier transformation [26]. If two pulse trains from different neurons interfere at the screen, they make a modulated pattern owing to the distance between the sources of the pulses [27, 28]. In the holographic memory, this modulation helps us determine the distance [29].

2. Source of Memory

We developed models that can explain the working of the human brain. It is important to identify the source of memory. For example, it could be the distance, size, shape, or absorption capability of the neuron. Moreover, it may be a multiple or single value memory. Considering that the brain has a small number of neurons and high capacity, the type of memory should be a multiple value memory. Multiple value memory can store a considerable amount of information in the limited density of neurons as compared to single value memory [30, 31]. Some researchers have reported that quantum memory is the solution [32, 33]. This memory can solve many problems simultaneously and has high-density capacity. However, since the lifetime of this memory is very short, its possibility to contribute to enhance the memory capacity of the brain is low [34]. Thus, classical multivalued memory is the remaining candidate to enhance the memory capacity.

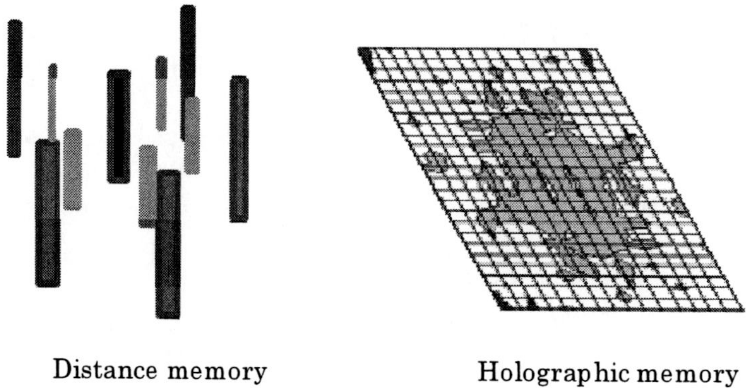

Figure 2. Types of optical memory.

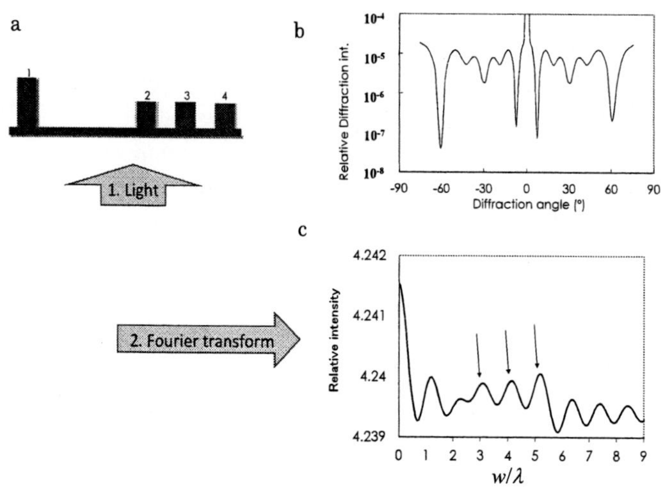

Figure 3. Characteristics of distance memory: (a) Shape of the scatterers, (b) diffraction pattern of the scatterers, and (c) Fourier transformed pattern of the diffraction pattern. w is the distance from the scatterer 1 to the scatterer 2, 3 or 4, λ is the wavelength, and the arrows indicate each distance.

We used two types of memories as shown in Figure 2. The first type of memory that we employed is the multiple value memory of distance. The distance information is given by the distance between the neurons. We represent the neuron as a column and the information is the distance from the specific column to the others (Figure 3). Incident light is scattered by an array of scatterers. The diffraction pattern is plotted against the diffraction angle (Figure 3(b)). When the specific column has a strong scattering intensity, the Fourier transformed data of the diffraction pattern gives the distance from the other column to the specific column [28]. This type of memory is supported by the following facts: (i) single neurons can store complex information [35], and (ii) subtle changes in neurons underlie the process of memorization [36].

We employed the hologram as the second type of memory. The information is spread, and it cannot be seen in itself (Figure 4). The information is picked up by the image that resembles the information. It is seen that when a stimulus is applied to the holographic memory, the rest of the information is drawn from the memory [37]. The data of the brain signal is converted into another format that is not invariant [38]. An example of this type of memory is shown in the cat striate cortex (V1), which is represented by a sinusoidal wave and is useful for signal processing [35]. The hologram has been a major candidate for optical memory [20, 39, 40]. It has been a candidate for associative memory [41], which is a characteristic memory of the brain [11, 20, 21, 42]. The hologram provides a concrete memory system [43, 44]. The optical system is composed of lenses, mirrors, and photosensitive materials [45, 46], and it can be realized as a concrete system.

A hologram is a data set that can be Fourier transformed into the original image, for example, the pigeon as shown in Figure 4.

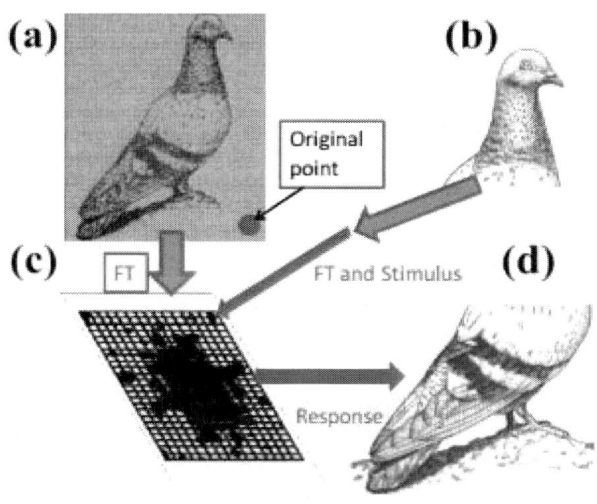

Figure 4. Function of holographic memory: (a) Memory of original image, (b) image of stimulus, (c) Fourier transformed data of original image (hologram), and (d) retrieved image for the stimulus.

Inversely, the image of the pigeon can be Fourier transformed into the hologram. If the head of the pigeon is Fourier transformed and projected onto the original hologram, the whole image is regenerated [37]. Normally, phase information is needed for saving the data set of a hologram. Phase is time dependent and is not stored as a normal two-dimensional photograph [27]. The original image is not restored fully without phase information. However, even if phase information is not used for the holographic optical memory, the original image can be restored for a "certain" hologram. We use one strong scatterer at the original point and an image of the pigeon as shown in Figure 4. We memorize the intensity distribution of the

Fourier transformed image. The regenerated information is the distance from the strong scatterer to the other scatterers [28].

The hologram has the merit of easy parallel calculations [45]. To recognize the image, considerable information is processed simultaneously. The projection of the image on to holographic memory is accompanied by considerable information processing. Furthermore, holography enables us to perform successive calculations. In Figure 5, there are several layers of holograms, through which the holographic data of the pigeon's head passes. If one of the holograms is that of a pigeon, light is scattered by the hologram [20], else if there are no holograms of a pigeon, the light is not scattered.

Using holograms and light, one can also perform numerical calculations [46-48]. These are also performed as parallel information processing [25]. We used both holographic and distance memories to explain the mechanism of the brain. Though the hologram is famous as associative memory, distance memory has its own merits.

The first advantage is that the distance memory can have high density. Tanaka et al. suggested that a hologram is not necessarily a high-density memory [49]. Table 1 shows that the memory density of the distance memory is higher than that of the holographic memory as long as the resolution and precision are the same [50]. The ON/OFF type information in the table is provided by conventional memories such as DVD or Blu ray. They read 0 or 1 signal from the pit on the disk [51].

Table 1. Comparison of the densities of memory types

Memory unit	Information type	Resolution (λ)	Precision (λ)	Number of points (1/bit)	Bit density ($1/\lambda^2$)
1 bit	ON/OFF	1	0.01	1	1
Multiple bit	Columns	1	0.01	0.26	3.8
	Hologram	1	0.01	0.89	1.1

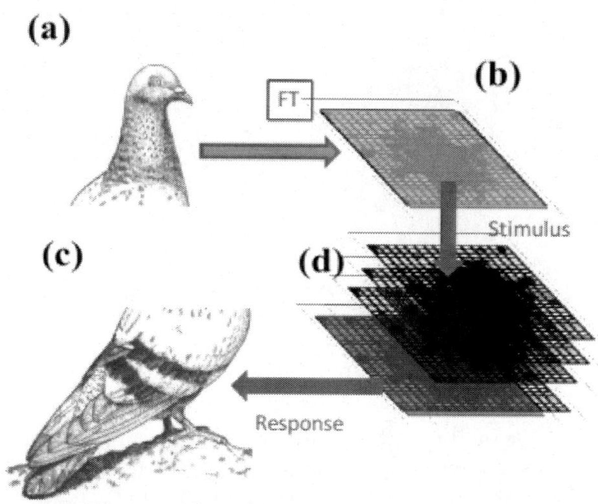

Figure 5. Example of association by holographic memory: (a) Image of the stimulus, (b) Fourier transformed data of stimulus image, (c) retrieved image for the stimulus, and (d) an array of a variety of holograms including the original image of a pigeon.

The second merit is that it is suitable for the model of the "grandmother cell" [52, 53]. The grandmother cell represents the face of the grandmother. Here, "grandmother" is used as example since the face of the grandmother is too complex to be represented by a single neuron. This can be explained by distance memory. If the strong scatterer of the distance memory depicts the grandmother cell, the face of grandmother can be expressed not only by the grandmother cell but also by a combination of the grandmother cell and many other cells that are the hidden weak scatterers.

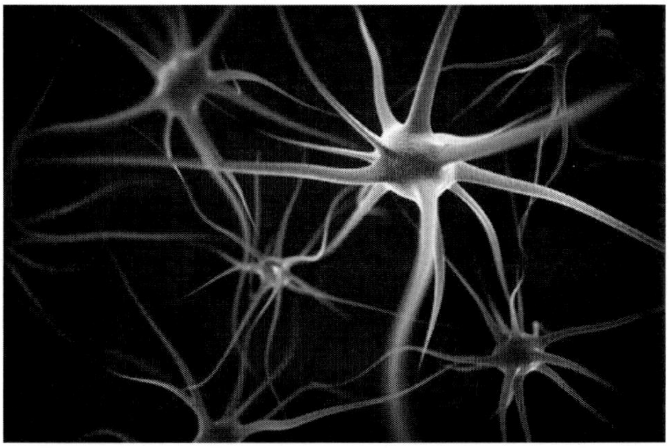

Figure 6. Grandmother cell.

Table 1 shows that distance memory has the highest density capacity; however, we think that it is insufficient, because if the number of transistors in the computer is 10 times more than the neurons in the brain, multiplicity of the memory may be more than 10 times. There exist other mechanisms such as absorption, or shape that can enhance the capacity.

Both the shape and absorption of the scatterer can provide information for the distance memory. When information of the shape and the absorption of the scatterer are added to the distance memory, memory density can be enhanced. The shape of the scatterer changes the diffraction pattern, which provides additional information. The isosceles triangle and the scalene triangle in Figure 7 have different diffraction patterns as shown in Figure 8.

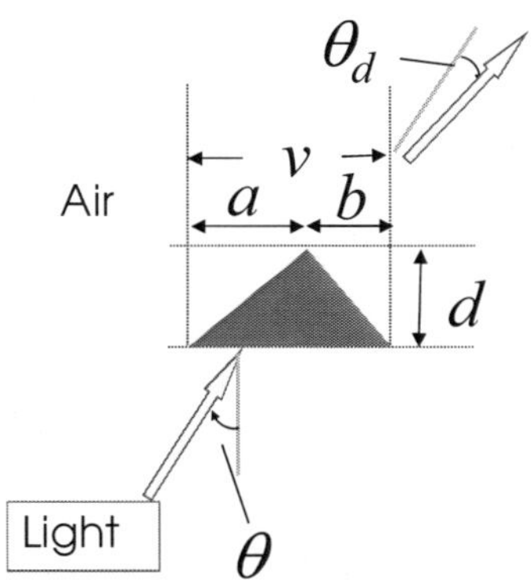

Figure 7. Scheme of incidence angle and shape of the scatterer in the air.

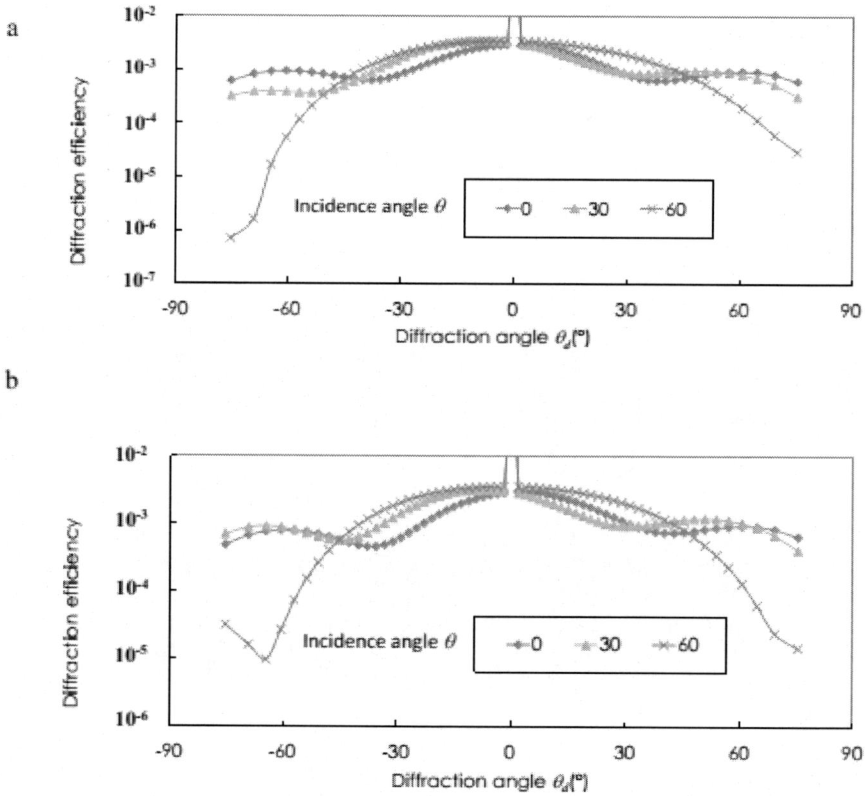

Figure 8. Diffraction pattern of the scatterer: (a) Isosceles triangle with $v = 3$, $d = 1$, and refractive index $n = 1.5$. (b) Scalene triangle with $a = 1.8$, $b = 1.2$, $d = 1$, and refractive index $n = 1.5$.

The difference is clear if we focus on the relative intensity of different incidence angles at the diffraction angles of ±60°. Thus, it is seen that shape changes the diffraction pattern. Therefore, the distance memory can be a candidate for the high-density memory of the brain.

Another source of memory is absorption. The total transmissive diffraction intensity of refractive index $n + ik$ is given by $f(k)$ and it does not include the non-diffracted light. The peak of non-diffracted light is at 0° as shown in Figures 7 and 8.

The scatterer is an isosceles triangle that has a size of $v = 3$ and $d = 1$. Its refractive index is $n + 4i(1+\sin(\pi\lambda/\mu m))$, where λ is the wavelength. The scattering intensity of a sphere particle is said to be proportional to $(1/\lambda)^4$ [54]. We find that the absorption of the triangle is proportional to $(1/\lambda)^2$, when the shape is two-dimensional. In Figure 9, $f_0(k)$ is multiplied by λ^2, to negate the effect of the size of the triangle as mentioned above.

The $f_0(k)\bullet\lambda^2$ changes in proportion to the extinction coefficient *k,* where *k* defines the absorption. Therefore, absorption can be used to represent a memory value, when the level of the absorption corresponds to information. We assume that there are three types of engrams of memory, which are distance between scatterer, the shape and size of scatterer, and absorption. We assume that there are three types of engrams of memory, which are distance between scatterer, the shape and size of scatterer, and absorption.

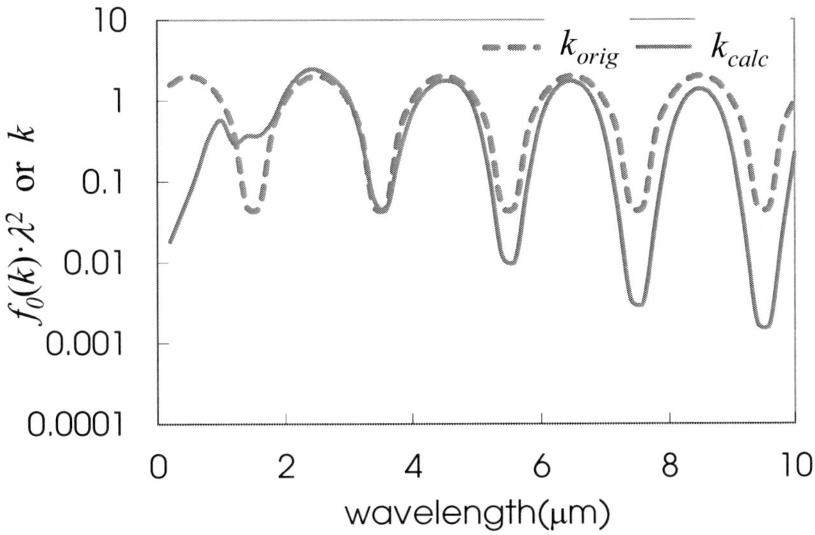

Figure 9. Absorption spectrum of the scatterer. k_{orig} is k and k_{calc} is $f_0(k_{\text{orig}})\bullet\lambda^2$.

$$f_0(k) = f(k) / f(0) \tag{1}$$

Information of the distance can give four times more density than that of an ON/OFF type memory. If information of color is three: red, green and blue, and each color has 4 levels of absorption, the total color information is $4 \times 4 \times 4$, which is equal to 2^6. In Figure 7, if information of triangular shape is the ratio a:b and a changes from 0 to 2.1 by step distance 0.3; it provides an information of 11. Thus, the total information is $2^4 \times 2^6 \times 8$, which can be written as 2^{13}. It suggests that the information density can be enhanced 13 times. This enhancement is useful for improving the memory density.

As mentioned above, the distance memory is superior to holographic memory in terms of capacity of the memory its and similarities with the brain. We think that the long-term memory comprises distance memory, and associative memory comprises holographic memory.

3. Model of the Memory: Examination of the Model Using Recent Experimental Results

3.1. Mouse Memory

Genome engineering gives direct information in relation to the role of the protein or the enzyme in the brain. This technique can remove specific material in the brain at the level of genome. With regard to the mouse, genome engineering is very popular and the behavior of the mouse has been researched by this method. NMDA (N-methyl-D-aspartate) receptors play an important role in memorization [55]. Using the NMDA receptor in the mouse, Hasan et al. showed that associative memory is in the cerebral cortex and not in the hippocampus [56, 57].

NMDA receptors bind the neurotransmitter glutamate to the synapses and become active when several signals feed into one synapse simultaneously. In the behavior test of eyeblink conditioning, a mouse had to learn to link a tone with subsequent electrical stimulus. Without NMDA receptors in the primary motor cerebral cortex, the genetically modified mice could not remember the connection between the tone and electrical stimulus, and therefore, they kept their eyes open despite the tone. On the other hand, mice without NMDA receptors in the hippocampus are still quite capable of learning the relationship between the tone and electrical stimulus [57]. It suggests that association is performed in the primary motor cerebral cortex.

Redondo et al. used a mouse to study whether a part of the brain connected to the memory could be rewritten or not [58]. The strength of combination of the memory and brain is called valence. The brain of a mouse is given the some valence to feel "fear" or "happiness." For a mouse, the dorsal dentate gyrus (DG) of the hippocampus has temporal memory and the basolateral complex of the amygdala has long-term memory [58].

The part of the brain that stores memory is the hippocampus or the amygdale [59]. The outer information flows from the hippocampus to the amygdale. The valence associated with the hippocampal memory engram can be rewritten. In contrast, the amygdale engram cannot be rewritten [58]. It suggests that the long-term memory is stored in the amygdale. On the other hand, Hayashi et al. showed that the synapse change occurred in the spine of the neuron in the primary motor cortex and it was the memory source of motor learning [60].

3.2. Monkey Memory

It is known that an array of the neural column in the brain of a monkey contributes to visual image processing [61]. Therefore, the study on monkeys may have the key to the memory system.

The amygdale is an inferior part of the brain as shown in Figure 12 [62]. From the lesion of the monkey's amygdale, it is known that the amygdale is involved in learning associations between neutral stimulus and primary reinforces [22].

Hirabayashi et al. studied the cynomolgus monkey as shown Figure 10 [63]. The perirhinal cortex is a cortical region in the medial temporal lobe. They paid attention to the perirhinal cortex, where the visual associative memory works [64]. The primate perirhinal cortex receives information from the ventral visual pathway and participates in the storage and retrieval of the long-term memory [63]. The researchers of these studies state that there are two types of neurons in the perirhinal cortex. One is a "cue-holding" neuron, which encodes the presented object, and the other is a "pair-recall" neuron, which recalls the target. They showed that the information flows from the "cue-holding" neuron to the "pair-recall" neuron 1. Furthermore, the information flows from "pair-recall" neuron 1 to "pair-recall" neuron 2. Finally, they showed the mechanism of recalling long-term memory. The "cue-holding" and "pair-recall" neurons are located in the limbic area and neocortical area, respectively [65].

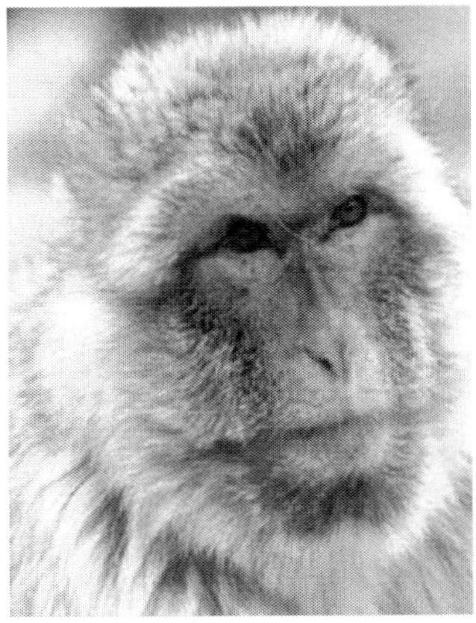

Figure 10. Species of monkey used in the study.

3.3. Human Memory

The primary brain has a folding structure. The convex surface is the cerebral gyrus and the groove is the cerebral sulcus. The cortex is divided into four parts: frontal lobe, parietal lobe, temporal lobe, and occipital lobe.

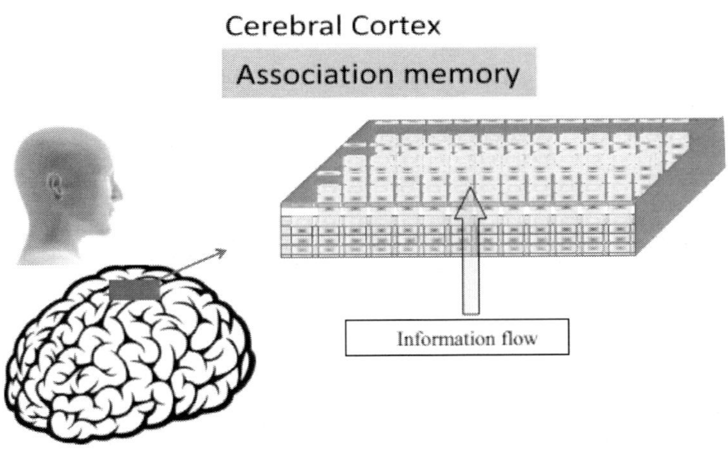

Figure 11. Human brain and the information flow in the cerebral cortex.

At the microlevel, the cerebral neocortex is made of six layers' columns and electric signal flows in the column through the layers [66]. Information flows along the longitudinal column. It enables the simultaneous treatment of information at each layer [67]. Most of the brain's surface has this layer.

The columns in the six layers are arranged such that they are roughly equidistant as shown in Figure 11 [67, 68]. It is suitable for holographic type memory whose information is not the distance between columns but the intensity of the signal in each column. This coincides with the model shown in Figures 4 and 5.

3.4. Schematic of the Mechanism of Association

Finally, we explain the schematic characteristics of the brain memory by the model of combination of holographic memory and distance memory that are described in section 2.

One of the sources of the long-term memory is in the hippocampus as shown by Redondo et al. [58]. They showed a direct proof of the presence of long-term memory in this part of the brain.

On the other hand, the cerebral cortex is important for associative memory [56, 58]. Further, the NMDA receptor is indispensable to memory. When the NMDA receptor is genetically removed from the cerebral cortex, the association function is stopped. On the contrary, when NMDA receptor is removed from the hippocampus, the association function is maintained [56]. Thus, we can infer that the hippocampus stores distance memory and the cerebral cortex stores holographic memory (Figures 12 and 13).

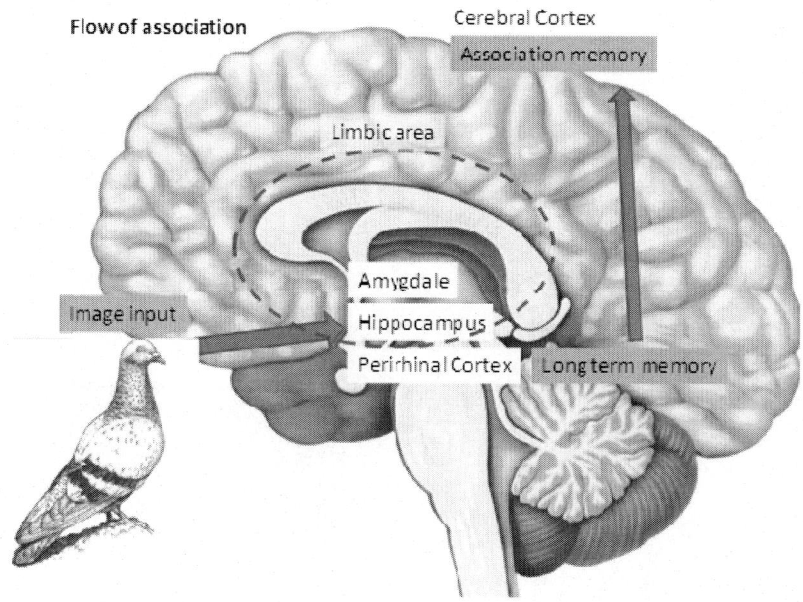

Figure 12. Scheme of the human brain and the memory function.

Hippocampal neurons are said to be related to short-term memory [12]. Image information from the eye goes through the optic nerve to the peripheral cortex, where the long-term memory is recorded. The information of the peripheral cortex is called back and projected onto the cerebral cortex when an association is performed. The information is stored in the peripheral cortex as a distance memory. When it is projected onto the cerebral cortex, it is Fourier transformed and becomes holographic memory in the cerebral cortex. The cerebral cortex has temporal memory and performs the association. The holographic memory is associative memory. When it is given a part of the image, the full image regenerates. Stimulus of the image comes from the eye and candidates of the full image come from long-term memory. Only the corresponding image out of the candidates reacts to the stimulus of the image as seen in Figure 5.

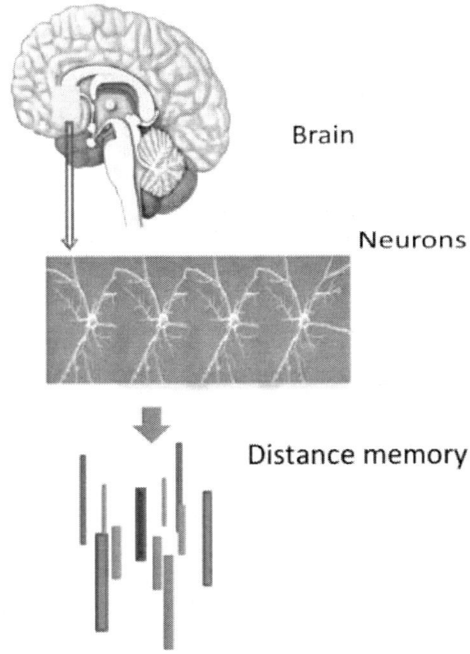

Figure 13. Human brain and the distance memory.

4. MECHANISM OF MEMORY

We redraw the working mechanism of the brain considering optical memory in this section.

The image from the eye goes through the hippocampus and a certain part of it goes to the perirhinal cortex, while the other part goes to the cerebral cortex. The long-term memory is stored in perirhinal cortex. To recollect a memory, information is transmitted from the cue-holding neuron to the pair-recall neuron [63] and the information in the pair-recall neuron is passed to another pair-recall neuron. According to this phenomenon, a variety of information from the long-term memory is projected onto the cerebral cortex, and the outer image is also projected onto the cerebral cortex as stimulus. The stimulus image goes through a variety of long-term memory and when it coincides with an old memory, the memory is amplified.

In the concrete model, the shape change of a neuron is an important factor. Brain memory has the following two structural characteristics.

(1) The sizes and shapes of neurons are categorized into four types only [1, 36].
(2) The shape changes induced by memorization are subtle [36].

Moreover, the signal from long distance neurons is amplified [36]. These characteristics help periodic signals to interfere at the screen that is away from the neurons.

Besides the shape, another important point is how to process the memory for thinking. We think the temporary memory and long-term memory. We assigned the long-term memory with the multiple value memory of distance. The long-term memory is Fourier transformed into temporary memory.

The information is Fourier transformed into a hologram so that the brain can make an association. It is a temporary image. A hologram has merit to explain the working of the human brain. It is said that the human brain is superior to a semiconductor computer especially in the field of associative memory. A hologram is suitable for associative memory, because it can recall total information from the partial information. The real field of the holographic memory is cerebral neocortex. Another type of memory is the distance memory, which may be located in the limbic area or temporal lobe [12, 69]. The memory's information is distance from a specific neuron to the other. The specific neuron has a strong signal. The information from the outer part of the brain is Fourier transformed when it changes from the distance memory to holographic memory. The holographic signal travels from one holographic memory to another to find out the best matching holographic memory.

5. Damage to Memory

It is shown that damage to the brain never erases the memory; however, the memory fades out a little by little in accordance with the damage [11]. The memory that may be the pigeon's head, tail, leg, or wing is dispersed in the brain. When these memories are connected to a specific neuron, they are recalled and projected onto the screen. The screen here refers to the holographic memory. In this model, the damage to the memory may erase a part of the information, but not all of it.

A neuron can be representative of the complex image such as that of the grandmother. Therefore, it is called the grandmother neuron. If one neuron represents an image, injury to the brain should destroy the memory of the image, but in fact, it does not. The neuron is merely the tentative center to represent the image. The mechanism is as follows. The information is represented as the distance from the tentative center to the other columns. The memory consists of one center and other columns of redundant information. The center may stay at any position, as long as it is outside the corresponding columns. If the tentative center is destroyed, the other center acts as an alternative center.

Conclusion

It has been shown that that memory does not vanish completely if any part of the brain is removed as long as it is limited to a specific part. It suggests that the memory is delocalized in the brain. It seems to contradict the model of the grandmother cell, but if the cell is not immobilized, it is possible. In the distance memory model, the role of grandmother cell is not to give information itself, but it acts as the pivot to draw information from other cells, which memorize the entire information. The distance memory is Fourier transformed into holographic memory in the cerebral cortex. The holographic memory works as an associative memory. The long-term memories and an image from the eye are projected onto the holographic memory area and the image goes through a variety of the long-term memory. Finally, the related memory is extracted from the considerable amount of information.

REFERENCES

[1] Zhang H, Hubbard PL, Parker GJM, Alexander DC. Axon diameter mapping in the presence of orientation dispersion with diffusion MRI. *NeuroImage*. 2011;56:1301–1315.

[2] Moravec H. When will computer hardware match the human brain? *Journal of Evolution and Technology*. 1998;1(1):1–10.

[3] Rabaey JM, Chandrakasan AP, Nikolic B. Digital integrated circuits. vol. 2. Prentice hall Englewood Cliffs; 2002.

[4] Kameyama M. Lithography and ITRS. Institute of Innovation Research Hitotsubashi University; 2010. 10-06. IIR Working Paper.

[5] Wikipedia. Transistor count; 2015. https://en.wikipedia.org/wiki/TransistorcountMicro processors:

[6] TOP500.org; 2015. http://top500.org/lists/2015/06/.

[7] Bloom FE, Lazerson A, Hofstadter L. Brain, mind, and behavior. New York: W.H. Freeman; 1985.

[8] Azevedo FAC, Carvalho LRB, Grinberg LT, Farfel JM, Ferretti REL, Leite REP, et al. Equal numbers of neuronal and nonneuronal cells make the human brain an isometrically scaled-up primate brain. *J. Comp. Neurol.* 2009;513:532–541.

[9] Shepherd GM. The Synaptic Organization of the Brain. 5th ed. New York: Oxford University Press; 2003.

[10] Nunez PL, Srinivasan R. Electric Fields of the Brain: The Neurophysics of EEG. New York: Oxford University Press; 2005.

[11] Lashley KS. Brain mechanisms and intelligence: A quantitative study of injuries to the brain. New York: Hafner Pub. Co.; 1964.

[12] Bloom FE, Lazerson A, Hofstadter L. 7. In: Brain, mind, and behavior. New York: W.H. Freeman; 1985. p. 177–204.

[13] Squire LR, Wixted JT, Clark RE. Recognition memory and the medial temporal lobe: a new perspective. *Nature Rev Neurosci.* 2007;8(11):872–883.

[14] Cabeza R, Ciaramelli E, Olson IR, Moscovitch M. The parietal cortex and episodic memory: an attentional account. *Nature Rev Neurosci.* 2008;9(8):613–625.

[15] Barlow HB. Single units and sensation: a neuron doctrine for perceptual psychology? *Perception.* 2009;(38):795–798.

[16] Leibold C, Kempter R. Sparseness Constrains the Prolongation of Memory Lifetime via Synaptic Metaplasticity. *Cereb Cortex.* 2008;18(1):67–77.

[17] Hopfield JJ. Neural networks and physical systems with emergent collective computational abilities. *Proc. NatL. Acad. Sci.* 1982;79:2554–2558.

[18] Abbott LF, Kepler TB. Model neurons: From hodgkin-huxley to hopfield. *Lect Notes Phys*. 1990;368:5–18.

[19] Pasemann F. A Simple Chaotic Neuron. *Physica D.* 1997;104(2):205–211.

[20] Gabor D. Associative Holographic Memories. *IBM J. Res. Dev.* 1969;13(2):156–159.

[21] Westlake PR. The possibilities of neural holographic processes within the brain. *Biological Cybernetics*. 1970;7(4):129–153.

[22] Rolls ET, Treves A. 7. In: Neural Networks and Brain function. New York: Oxford University Press; 1998. p. 136–164.

[23] Thivierge JP, Dandurand F, Cousineau D. A Multi-state Model of Cortical Memory. In: Proceedings of International Joint Conference on Neural Networks. San Jose, California, USA: IEEE; 2011. p. 133–138.

[24] Kuroyanagi S, Iwata A. Auditory Pulse Neural Network Model to Extract the Inter-Aural Time and Level Difference for Sound Localization. *IEICE T. Inf. Syst.* 1994;E77-D(4):466–474.

[25] Psaltis D, Brady D, Gu XG, Lin S. Holography in artificial neural networks. *Nature.* 1990;343:325–330.

[26] Nunez PL, Srinivasan R. 9. In: Electric fields of the brain: the neurophysics of EEG. 2nd ed. New York: Oxford university press; 2006. p. 353–431.

[27] Goodman JW. Introduction to Fourier optics. 3rd ed. Greenwood Village USA: Roberts and Company Publishers; 2005.

[28] Hoshino T, Yatagai T, Itoh M. Precise and rapid distance measurements by scatterometry. *Opt. Express.* 2012;20:3954–3966.

[29] Born M, Wolf E. 8.5. In: Principles of Optics: Electromagnetic Theory of Propagation, Interference and Diffraction of Light. 7th ed. Cambridge: Cambridge University Press; 1999. p. 436–446.

[30] Fusi S, Abbott LF. Limits on the memory storage capacity of bounded synapses. *Nat. Neurosci.* 2007;10:485–493.

[31] Zijlstra P, Chon JWM, Gu M. Five-dimensional optical recording mediated by surface plasmons in gold nanorods. *Nature.* 2009;459:410–413.

[32] Koch C, Hepp K. Quantum mechanics in the brain. *Nature.* 2006;440:611–612.

[33] Artur BDE, Anton Z. The physics of quantum information: quantum cryptography, quantum teleportation, quantum computation. Oxford: Springer Publishing Company; 2000.

[34] Tegmark M. Importance of quantum decoherence in brain processes. *Phys. Rev. E.* 2000;61(4):4194–4206.

[35] Sasaki KS, Tabuchi Y, Ohzawa I. Complex Cells in the Cat Striate Cortex Have Multiple Disparity Detectors in the Three-Dimensional Binocular Receptive Fields. *The Journal of Neuroscience.* 2010;30:(41):13826–13837.

[36] Kubota Y, Karube F, Nomura M, Gulledge AT, Mochizuki A, Schertel A, et al. Conserved properties of dendritic trees in four cortical interneuron subtypes. *Scientific Reports.* 2011;1(89):1–13.

[37] Soffer BH, Dunning GJ, Owechko Y., Marom E. Associative holographic memory with feedback using phase-conjugate mirrors. *Opt. Lett.* 1986;11:118–120.

[38] Heil P, Neubauer H, Irvine DRF, Brown M. Spontaneous Activity of Auditory-Nerve Fibers: Insights into Stochastic Processes at Ribbon Synapses. *J. Neurosci.* 1994;27(31):8457–8474.

[39] Gabor D. Holographic Model of Temporal Recall. *Nature.* 1968;217:584.

[40] Gabor D. Improved Holographic Model of Temporal Recall. *Nature.* 1968;217:1288–1289.

[41] Wess O, R¨oder U. A holographic model for associative memory chains. *Biological cybernetics.* 1977;27(2):89–98.

[42] Pribram KH. Introduction to Fourier optics. Hillsdale, N.J.: Lawrence Erlbaum Associates; 1991.

[43] Hill B. Some Aspects of a Large Capacity Holographic Memory. *Appl Opt.* 1972;11:182–191.
[44] Longuet-Higgins HC. Holographic model of temporal recall. *Nature.* 1968;217:104.
[45] ABU-MOSTAFA Y, Psaltis D. Optical neural computers. *Scientific American.* 1987;256(3):88–95.
[46] Ebersole JF. Optical image subtraction. *Optical Engineering.* 1975;14:436–447.
[47] Gabor D, Stroke GW, Restrick R, Funkhouser A, Brumm D. Optical image synthesis (complex amplitude addition and subtraction) by hollographic fourier transformation. *Physics Letters.* 1965;18(2):116–118.
[48] Lee SH, Yao SK, Milnes AG. Optical Image Synthesis (Complex Amplitude Addition and Subtraction) in Real Time by a Diffraction-Grating Interferometric Method. *J. Opt. Soc. Am.* 1970;60:1037–1041.
[49] Tanaka K, Hara M, Tokuyama K, Hirooka K, Ishioka K, Fukumoto A, et al. Improved performance in coaxial holographic data recording. *Opt. Express.* 2007;15(24):16196–16209.
[50] Hoshino T, Yatagai T, Itoh M. A Columnar Model Explaining Long-Term Memory. *Optical Memory and Neural Networks* (Information Optics). 2012;21(4):209–218.
[51] Gu M, Li X. The Road to Bit-by-Bit Optical Data Storage. *OPN Optics and Photonics News.* 2010;21(7):28–33.
[52] Gross CG. Genealogy of the Grandmother Cell. *Neuroscientist.* 2002;8(5):512–518.
[53] Quiroga R, Reddy L, Kreiman G, Koch C. Invariant visual representation by single neurons in the human brain. *Nature.* 2005;435:1102–1107.
[54] Born M, Wolf E. Principles of Optics: Electromagnetic Theory of Propagation, Interference and Diffraction of Light. 7th ed. Cambridge: Cambridge University Press; 1999.
[55] Sakimura K, Kutsuwada T, Ito I, Manabe T, Takayama C, Kushiya E, et al. Reduced hippocampal LTP and spatial learning in mice lacking NMDA receptor "1 subunit. *Nature.* 1995;(373):151–155.
[56] Hasan MT, Hernandez-Gonzalez S, Dogbevia G, Trevino M, Bertocchi I, Gruart A, et al. Role of motor cortex NMDA receptors in learning-dependent synaptic plasticity of behaving mice. *Nature communications.* 2013;4:2258.
[57] Max-Planck-Gesellschaft. Long-term memory stored in the cortex; 2013. http://www.sciencedaily.com/releases/2013/08/130827091629.htm.
[58] Redondo RL, Kim AJ, Ramirez AL, Liu XS, Tonegawa S. Bidirectional switch of the valence associated with a hippocampal contextual memory engram. *Nature.* 2014;513:426–430.
[59] Bird CM, Burgess N. The hippocampus and memory: insights from spatial processing. *Nature Rev. Neurosci.* 2008;9(3):182–194.
[60] Hayashi-Takagi A, Yagishita S, Nakamura M, Shirai F, Wu YI, Loshbaugh AL, et al. Labelling and optical erasure of synaptic memory traces in the motor cortex. Nature. 2015.
[61] Fujita I, Tanaka K, Ito M, Cheng K. Columns for visual features of objects in monkey inferotemporal cortex. *Nature.* 1992;360(6402):343–346.
[62] Nunez PL, Srinivasan R. 2. In: Cognitive Neuroscience–The Biology of the Brain. New York: W.W. Norton & Company, Inc; 1998. p. 23–68.

[63] Hirabayashi T, Takeuchi D, Tamura K, Miyashita Y. Functional microcircuit recruited during retrieval of object association memory in monkey perirhinal cortex. *Nature*. 2013;77:192–203.

[64] Miyashita Y. Cognitive memory: cellular and network machineries and their topdown control. *Science*. 2004;306:435–440.

[65] Naya Y, Yoshida M, Takeda M, Fujimichi R, Miyashita Y. Delay-period activities in two subdivisions of monkey inferotemporal cortex during pair association memory task. *European Journal of Neuroscience*. 2003;18(10):2915–2918.

[66] Bloom FE, Lazerson A, Hofstadter L. 3. In: Brain, mind, and behavior. New York: W.H. Freeman; 1985. p. 53–88.

[67] Nakada T. Neuroscience of water molecules: a salute to professor Linus Carl Pauling. *Cytotechnology*. 2009;59(3):145–152.

[68] Bloom FE, Lazerson A, Hofstadter L. 8. In: Brain, mind, and behavior. New York: W.H. Freeman; 1985. p. 205–234.

[69] Takeuchi D, Hirabayashi T, Tamura K, Miyashita Y. Reversal of interlaminar signal between sensory and memory processing in monkey temporal cortex. *Science*.2011;331:1443–1447.

In: Spatial, Long-and Short-Term Memory
Editor: Edward A. Thayer
ISBN: 978-1-63484-148-1

Chapter 8

'Spotlight on the Survival Processing Advantage': An fNIRS Study on Adaptive Memory

Patrick Bonin[1,2,*], Laura Ferreri[2], Margaux Gelin[2], Christophe Fitamen[2], Patrick Bard[2] and Aurélia Bugaiska[2]

[1]Institut universitaire de France, Paris, France
[2]Univ. Bourgogne- Franche Comté
LEAD-CNRS, Dijon, France

Abstract

In the present study, participants had to rate words for their relevance in an ancestral survival scenario (e.g., is *bottle* relevant in the fictious scenario of being stranded in the grasslands of a foreign land without basic supplies) and for their pleasantness (e.g., is *bottle* a pleasant word?). A distractor task lasting a few minutes followed and the participants were then tested on their recall of the words. We used fNIRS to bilaterally monitor the dorsolateral-prefrontal cortex (DLPFC, known to be involved in strategic encoding) during the processing of verbal material in these two deep encoding situations. At the behavioral level, we replicated the survival processing advantage in recall rates, with the result that words processed for their survival value were better remembered than words processed for their pleasantness value.

Importantly, at the neural level, we observed a lesser activation of the DLPFC during verbal encoding in the pleasantness condition compared to the survival condition, thus supporting the hypothesis that the survival processing advantage is underpinned by effortful processes, and more specifically relational processing.

Keywords: Survival processing advantage, adaptive memory, NIRS, prefrontal cortex

* Corresponding author: Patrick Bonin. LEAD-CNRS (UMR 5022), University of Bourgogne, Pôle AAFE - Esplanade Erasme, BP 26513, 21065 Dijon Cedex, France. E-mail: Patrick.Bonin@u-bourgogne.fr.

INTRODUCTION

According to the adaptive view of human memory championed by Nairne (2010, 2013; Nairne and Pandeirada 2008a), our memory systems are the product of the evolutionary pressures our species has confronted and adapted to. This view of human memory, which focuses on both ultimate and proximate explanations, is relatively recent in the literature but it has been attracting increasing interest in recent years. Evidence that supports this view of episodic memory has come mainly from the survival processing advantage (Nairne, Thompson and Pandeirada 2007, Nairne and Pandeirada 2008b, Nairne, Pandeirada and Thompson 2008). Indeed, numerous studies have shown that when items (words or pictures) are processed according to a fictional survival scenario (i.e., participants have to rate the relevance of unrelated words [e.g., *bottle*] in a survival situation [e.g., being stranded in the grasslands of a foreign land without basic supplies]), the items are better remembered than in deep control situations which are not survival-related, such as rating words for their pleasantness. Indeed, the pleasantness condition has been widely used as a benchmark to evaluate the survival processing advantage (e.g., Aslan and Baüm 2012, Bugaiska, Mermillod and Bonin 2015, Nairne et al. 2007, Nairne and Pandeirada 2008b, Nairne et al. 2008, Nairne, Pandeirada, VanArsdall and Blunt 2015; Weinstein, Bugg and Roediger III 2008). Pleasantness has been claimed to be a quintessential form of "deep processing" (Nairne et al. 2015) and, as the findings from Packman and Battig's (1978) study suggest, pleasantness is one of most powerful types of deep encoding leading to long-term retention. Several proposals have been put foreword in the literature to account for the survival processing advantage in memory (Erdfelder and Kroneisen 2013, Nairne 2013).

Likewise, different proximate mechanisms have been proposed as potential mechanisms underpinning this memory effect. These include: self-encoding (Cunningham, Brady-Van den Bos, Gill and Turk 2013), elaboration (Nouchi 2012, 2013), richness-of-encoding (Kroneisen and Erdfelder 2011), as well as both item-specific and relational processing (Burns, Burns and Hwang 2011). Broadly speaking, all these accounts assume that items are actively processed during encoding in a survival context, and that this processing is stronger than in other well-known deep encoding situations known for their high potential to boost memory performance (i.e., pleasantness, self-reference, imagery). By strong active processing, we mean that survival processing involves some form of relational processing and the building of item-specific associations (Burns et al. 2011). Moreover and importantly for the current study, virtually all accounts of the survival processing advantage share the core assumption that the mechanisms underpinning this effect are strategic, and therefore depend on cognitive resources, i.e., they are resource-dependent mechanisms. The behavioral evidence relating to the survival processing advantage therefore strongly suggests that, at the neural level, the memory processes involved in survival effects are underpinned by a brain network that has previously been identified in the memory literature as being involved in strategic and resource-demanding processes. This is a very important issue that we address in the present study. In an electrophysiological study, Fellner, Bäuml and Hanslmayr (2013) compared the encoding of related brain oscillatory activity elicited by a deep semantic judgment task (i.e., animacy) and the survival encoding condition. At the behavioral level, survival processing led to better recognition performance than the control semantic processing. Successful encoding in the semantic control condition was reflected by a considerable decrease in alpha and beta power, whereas successful encoding in the survival condition was related to increased alpha and beta long-range phase synchrony. Since phase synchronization has generally been considered to be a mechanism facilitating communication between distant cortical areas (e.g., Varela et al. 2001), the authors interpretated this increase in the cortical communication indexes as reflecting the concurrent processing of the items on several dimensions that lead to the encoding of a contextually rich episodic memory and consequently improve the probability of subsequent successful retrieval (Craik and Tulving 1975).

Interestingly, this is in line with previous behavioral studies claiming that the advantage of survival processing, as compared to other forms of semantic processing, is due to the involvement of relational and associative mechanisms rather than simple item-specific encoding processes (Burns et al. 2011).

However, to the very best of our knowledge, there has, to date, only been one neuroscientific study on the survival processing advantage and no studies have specifically investigated the hypothesis that associative and relational neural mechanisms play a crucial role in the survival encoding condition. In the present study, we used functional Near-InfraRed Spectroscopy (fNIRS) to test the involvement of the dorsolateral-prefrontal cortex (DLPFC - BA 9 and 46) in the survival processing advantage in free recall. Below, we will first review the few studies on the identified neural substrates of episodic memory and, in particular, the role of the DLPFC cortex. We then briefly describe the fNIRS used in our study to test the hypothesis that the DLPFC cortex plays an important role in the survival processing advantage in episodic memory.

Memory encoding and retrieval processes are supported by a widespread brain network involving medio-temporal and posterior parietal areas, the hippocampus and the prefrontal cortex (PFC), the latter of which is particularly important for episodic memory (Manenti, Cotelli, Robertson and Miniussi 2012; Spaniol, Davidson, Kim, Han, Moscovitch and Grady 2009). Different sub-regions of the PFC are recruited by different mnemonic processes. According to the Hemispheric Encoding/Retrieval Asymmetry (HERA) model (Tulving, Kapur, Craik, Moscovitch and Houle 1994), left PFC activation is greater during encoding than during retrieval whereas right PFC activation is greater during retrieval than during encoding. Although the PFC sub-region most constantly associated with memory in neuroimaging studies is the ventrolateral-prefrontal cortex (VLPFC - BA 44-45-47), the dorsolateral-prefrontal cortex (DLPFC - BA 9 and 46) has recently been the object of attention for the specific investigation of memory encoding processes. More particularly, it has been shown that the DLPFC, and in particular the left hemisphere, plays a crucial role in organizational, associative (Ranganath 2010; Murray and Ranganath 2007) and semantic (Innocenti, Giovannelli, Cincotta, Feurra, Polizzotto, Bianco et al. 2010) memory encoding. As discussed by Blumenfeld and Ranganath (2007), DLPFC activation seems to be more specifically sensitive to demands for organizational processing and it may support long-term memory by building associations among items that are active in memory. These are all processes that, as reviewed above, are assumed to be involved in the survival processing advantage. In effect, and most importantly, a recent fMRI study by Blumenfeld, Parks, Yonelinas and Ranganath (2010) found that DLPFC activity specifically promoted memory for relational information but not for item-specific information during encoding. Since the survival effect is assumed to be underpinned by several proximate mechanims, including relational processing (Burns et al. 2011), the implication is that the DLPFC should be involved when encoding items for their survival value.

fNIRS is an optical neuroimaging technique that can monitor cortical tissue oxygenation (oxygenated-O_2Hb and deoxygenated-HHb hemoglobin concentration changes) during cognitive, motor and sensory stimulation (Ferrari and Quaresima 2012; Jobsis 1977). Since it is portable, non-invasive and has good motion tolerance, fNIRS has been shown to be a suitable tool for psychologically-based research (Ferreri, Bigand, Perrey and Bugaiska 2014). In the field of memory research, fNIRS studies have mostly shown an increase in PFC oxygenation patterns (i.e., an increase in O_2Hb with a concomitantly smaller decrease in HHb) during working memory and attentional tasks in healthy and clinical populations (see Cutini, Basso Moro and Bisconti 2012 for a review). Some recent studies on music and memory have tested the feasibility of using NIRS in episodic memory tasks in young (Ferreri, Aucouturier, Muthalib, Bigand and Bugaiska 2013) and older adults (Ferreri, Bigand, Perrey, Muthalib, Bard and Bugaiska 2014), and the results suggest that this technique is suitable for episodic memory investigations.

In sum, the purpose of the present study was to assess whether processing words for their relevance in a survival scenario during encoding results in different memory-specific cortical patterns of activations than processing words for their pleasantness value. To this end, we used fNIRS to bilaterally monitor the DLPFC during the encoding of verbal material in these two deep encoding situations. A greater activation of the DLPFC during verbal encoding in the survival condition compared to the pleasantness condition would support the general idea that the survival processing advantage is underpinned by effortful processes. More precisely, it would support Burns et al.'s (2011) hypothesis that some form of relational processing, which has been assumed to recruit the DLPFC (e.g., Blumenfeld et al. 2010; Murray and Ranganath 2007), is involved in the survival processing advantage.

METHOD

Participants. 19 young, healthy, right-handed volunteers (14 female, mean age 21 ± 2.35 years) at the University of Bourgogne took part in the experiment in exchange for course credits. The participants were native French speakers and reported having normal or corrected-to-normal vision. None were taking medication known to affect the central nervous system. Informed written consent was obtained from all participants prior to taking part in the experiment. The study was anonymous and fully adhered to the Helsinki Declaration, Convention of the Council of Europe on Human Rights and Biomedicine.

Materials. The words consisted of 42 taxonomically unrelated concrete nouns selected from Snodgrass and Vanderwart's (1980) and Bonin, Peereman, Malardier, Méot and Chalard's (2003) databases. They were randomly divided into six lists (7 words per list, 21 words for each encoding condition) matched for number of letters and lexical frequency (New et al. 2004). Procedure. The participants were seated in a chair in front of a computer in a quiet dimmed room. Each participant then performed a memory encoding and a retrieval task while their DLPFC activation was monitored using fNIRS neuroimaging. After the 8 fNIRS probe-set was adjusted on the forehead scalp overlying the DLPFC (see fNIRS section below for a description), the participants were informed that they were about to be presented with different lists of words within two different encoding contexts: pleasantness vs. survival. They were explicitly instructed to memorize words for a test to be administrated afterwards.

In the survival situation, they were given the following instructions: "In this task, we would like you to imagine that you are stranded in the grasslands of a foreign land, without any survival equipment. In the coming months, you will have to find stable supplies of food and water and protect yourself from predators.

We will present you with a list of words and want you to rate the relevance of each word in the survival situation. Some of the words may be relevant and others not, it's up to you to decide. You must use a rating scale of 1 (totally irrelevant) to 5 (extremely relevant)." In the Pleasantness condition, the participants were given the following instructions: "In this task, you will be presented with a list of words and we would like to you rate the pleasantness of each word. Some of them may be pleasant and others not, it's up to you to decide. You must use a rating scale of 1 (extremely unpleasant) to 5 (extremely pleasant)."

The encoding phase consisted of three blocks of "survival encoding" and three blocks of "pleasantness encoding," separated by 30 second rest periods. In each block, seven words were displayed successively. The words in each block were presented at a rate of 5 s per word (35 s for the sequential presentation of 7 words).

The order of survival/pleasantness blocks was counterbalanced, as were the order of the word lists and the order of words in the lists. During the rest periods, the participants were instructed to try to relax and not to think about the task any longer. The entire encoding phase, together with fNIRS recording, took about 15 min.

The test phase was administered after a 5-minute retention interval. During this interval, the participants performed two interference tasks: an "X-O" letter-comparison task (Salthouse et al. 1997) and a "plus-minus" task (Jersild 1927, Spector and Biederman 1976). At recall, the participants were told that they had 5 minutes to write down the previously presented words in any order they liked.

fNIRS Measurements

The procedure was the same as that used in previous studies on episodic memory and music (Ferreri et al. 2013, 2014). An 8-channel fNIRS system (Oxymon MkIII, Artinis Medical Systems B.V., The Netherlands) was used to measure changes in the concentration of O_2Hb and HHb (expressed in μM) using an age-dependent constant differential path-length factor given by 4.99 + 0.0067* (age ^ 0.814) (Duncan et al. 1996).

Data was acquired at a sampling frequency of 10 Hz. The eight fNIRS optodes (4 emitters and 4 detectors) were placed symmetrically over the dorsal part of the PFC (Brodmann Areas 46 and 9, EEG electrodes AF7/8, F5/6, F3/4 and AF3/4 of the international 10/10 system) (Jurcak et al. 2007; Okamoto et al. 2004), and the distance between each emitter and detector was fixed at 3.5 cm.

To optimize signal-to-noise ratio during the fNIRS recording, the eight optodes were masked from ambient light by a black plastic cap that was kept in contact with the scalp with elastic straps, and all cables were suspended from the ceiling to minimize movement artifacts (Cui et al. 2011). During data collection, O_2Hb and HHb concentration changes were displayed in real time, and signal quality and absence of movement artifacts were verified.

Results

Behavioral Data

A t-test was performed on the number of correctly recalled words, with Encoding condition (pleasantness vs. survival) as a factor. More words were correctly recalled in the survival encoding condition (m = 8.47, sd = 2.34) than in the pleasantness condition (m = 6.11, sd = 2.77), yielding a reliable main effect of Encoding condition, $t(18) = 2.89$, $p < .005$.

fNIRS Data

For each of the eight fNIRS measurement points, the O_2Hb and HHb signals were first low-pass filtered to eliminate task-irrelevant systemic physiological oscillations (5th order digital Butterworth filter with cutoff frequency 0.1 Hz). In order to determine the amount of activation during the encoding phase for the two conditions, the data for each of the six experimental blocks was baseline corrected using the mean of the O_2Hb and HHb signals for the 5 seconds preceding the start of word encoding for each block.

In order to ascertain the level of DLPFC activation during the entire block of survival/ pleasantness encoding conditions, we ran a complete time–series analysis in which we averaged O_2Hb and HHb concentrations over 5-second windows (i.e., one average point for each 5-second period) across the entire block encoding.

This yielded 10 successive measures of concentrations (from 5 seconds preceding presentation of the first word through to the end of the words in the block, and including the first 10 seconds of the rest phase). Considering O_2Hb increases and small HHb decreases as patterns of cortical activations (Jobsis 1977), DLPFC activations were assessed by separately analyzing the baseline-corrected O_2Hb and HHb concentration changes on the averaged survival and pleasantness blocks for each participant.

Figure 1 shows the grand-average time-course series for O_2Hb (in black) and HHb (in gray) concentration changes, respectively, in the "pleasantness" (dotted line) and "survival" (solid line) conditions for the left and right DLPFC throughout the encoding block. Time-series graphic clearly indicates a substantial difference between the two conditions, with the "survival" encoding resulting in a higher pattern of activation, in the form of an increase of O_2Hb together with a decrease of HHb, compared to the "pleasantness" encoding condition.

A 2 (laterality: right vs. left) × 2 (encoding conditions: pleasantness vs. survival) x times points (10) repeated measures analysis of variance (ANOVA) was performed on O_2Hb values and HHb values. The ANOVA on O_2Hb values confirmed a main effect of the condition, $F(1, 18) = 5.19$, $p = .03$, revealing a significantly greater bilateral O_2Hb increase in the survival than in the pleasantness condition.

Moreover, the results indicated an interaction between condition and time, $F(9, 162) = 2.35$, $p = .016$. As shown in Figure 1, the O_2Hb increase and HHb decrease occurred during the encoding phase and then slowly returned to the baseline level at the end of the encoding block. Post-hoc t-test comparisons between first baseline point and following time points throughout the encoding (see Figure 1, for comparisons) revealed that the higher DLPFC activation for "survival" was mostly due to left hemisphere. Moreover, this left-lateralization was borne out by a repeated measures ANOVA on HHb values, which revealed a marginally significant main effect of laterality, $F(1, 18) = 3.56, p = .076$.

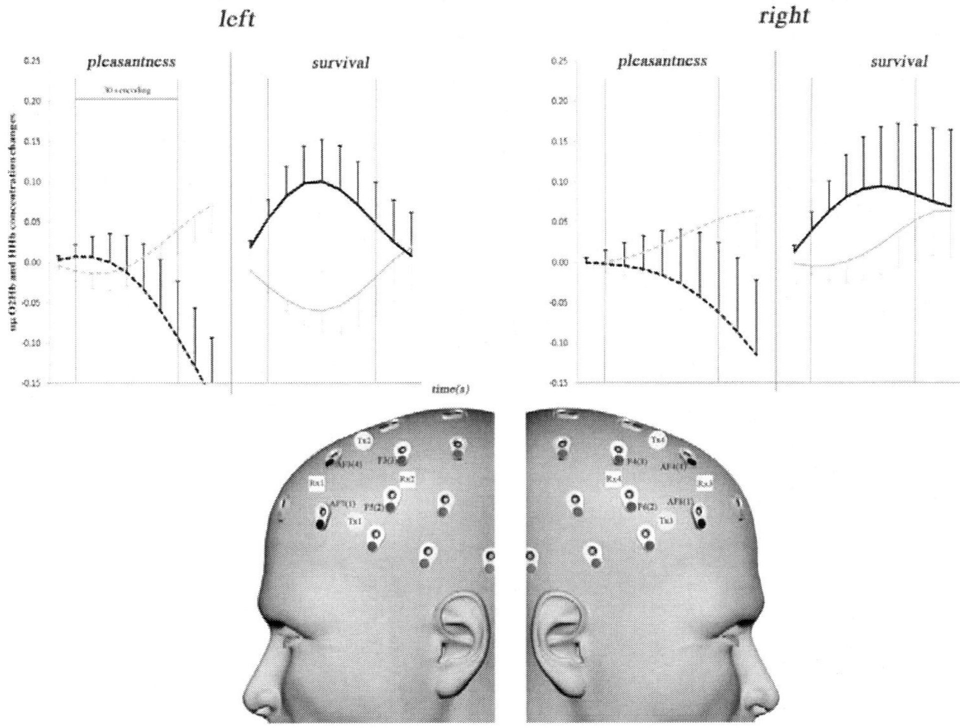

Figure 1. Grand-average time-course series for O_2Hb (in black) and HHb (in gray) concentration changes in the "pleasantness" (dotted line) and "survival" (solid line) conditions for the left and right DLPFC throughout encoding block.

DISCUSSION

In the present study, we used fNIRS to monitor the DLPFC bilaterally during the encoding of words in order to assess whether processing words for their relevance in a survival scenario results in different memory-specific cortical patterns of activation than processing words for their pleasantness value.

As reviewed in the introduction, the survival processing advantage has been clearly established at a behavioral level (Nairne et al. 2007; Nairne et al. 2008a, 2008b, see Bonin and Bugaiska 2014, Kazanas and Altarriba 2015, for reviews), but thus far the neural substrates that underlie this memory effect have been all but ignored. At the more general level, there have been a limited number of fNIRS studies (Ferreri et al. 2013, 2014; Kubota et al. 2006; Matsui et al. 2007; Okamoto et al. 2011) that have investigated encoding-retrieval processes and tested the feasibility of using fNIRS for the study of long-term memory processes.

The findings of our study are clear-cut. At the behavioral level, as observed many times in previous studies (Nairne et al. 2007; Nairne et al. 2008b), we replicated the survival processing advantage, with the result that unrelated words processed for their survival value were better remembered than words processed for their pleasantness value[1]. More importantly, at the neural level, we found a substantial difference between the two encoding conditions, with the survival encoding condition resulting in a higher pattern of activation, namely an increase in O_2Hb together with a decrease in HHb, than the pleasantness encoding condition. More precisely, we observed higher DLPFC activation in the survival encoding condition than in the pleasantness condition. Furthermore, and in line with previous results on the encoding of verbal material as well as with the HERA model (Tulving et al. 1994), we found that this activation occurs primarily in the left hemisphere. The novel finding that DLPFC is activated more during survival encoding is very important at the theoretical level since it provides considerable support for accounts of the survival processing advantage that assume that the mechanisms underpinning this effect are resource-dependent (Erdfelder and Kroneisen 2013; Nouchi 2012).

More precisely and importantly, our findings strongly support the hypothesis that the survival effect is underpinned by relational processing (Burns et al. 2011) among other proximate mechanims which have also been assumed to play a role (e.g., elaboration (Nouchi 2012, 2013), item-specific processing (Burns et al. 2011), self-reference (Cunningham et al. 2013)). In effect, the observation of a stronger activation of the DLPFC in survival encoding than in pleasantness encoding fits nicely with recent fMRI studies that have shown that the DLFPC is recruited, not for all types of effortful memory processes, but for encoding processes that promote the building of links among items, namely relational processing (Burns et al. 2011). As already set out in the Introduction, it has been shown that the DLPFC, and the left hemisphere in particular, plays a crucial role for organizational, associative (Ranganath 2010; Murray and Ranganath 2007) and semantic (Innocenti et al. 2010) memory encoding. Moreover, DLPFC activation seems to be more specifically sensitive to organizational processing demands and it may support long term memory by building associations among items that are active in memory (Blumenfeld and Ranganath 2007). The present findings strongly support this interpretation since the survival advantage, which has been assumed to be underpinned by relational processing (Burns et al. 2011) among other memory processes, was found to be associated with greater activation of the DLPFC.

In the literature on the survival processing advantage, certain researchers have assumed that, given that this effect can be accounted for by proximate mechanisms (e.g., self-encoding, richness of encoding, item-specific/relational process), any evolutionary account of this phenomenon has to be rejected. Such a claim is certainly due to a failure to distinguish between proximate and ultimate causes in the explanation of the survival-processing

[1] It could be argued that a schematic control condition (e.g., moving condition) could have been used instead of the pleasantness condition. However, as mentioned in the Introduction, pleasantness is thought to be a quintessential form of deep processing (Nairne et al. 2015). This condition is therefore an appropriate control condition for the evaluation of survival processing in memory performance and indeed is still used as a control condition for assessing survival processing (e.g., Nairne et al. 2015). Interestingly, it should be recalled that memory performance in the pleasantness condition in the original Nairne et al. (2007) study did not differ signicantly from performance in the "moving" schematic control condition.

advantage (Nairne 2013). It should be remembered that ultimate explanations are *"statements about the function of a trait and "why" it would have been selected by nature during an evolutionary process"* while proximate explanations *"focus on the mechanisms that produced the trait — that is, they are statements about "how" the trait works and the condition under which the trait is likely to be expressed"* (Nairne 2013). Indeed, proximate and ultimate causes should be conceived as complementary and not as competing levels of explanation. Indeed, both are necessary for a complete explanation of an effect (Buss 2010).

Conclusion

To conclude, the present study has turned the spolight on the survival processing advantage and has revealed the involvement of a neural substrate, the DLPFC, which underpins a proximate mechanism – relational processing - involved in this memory effect. From a methodological point of view, our study illustrates how fNIRS can be used to test hypotheses about the mechanisms that underlie the long-term encoding of information. Although there are clear limitations to the use of this technique, for instance the fact that deep brain structures cannot be tracked, we hope we have convinced readers that this technique can be used successfully by providing complementary evidence contributing to the understanding of complex human behavior such as remembering information. Our study offers further evidence that, whatever the precise nature of the proximate mechanisms involved in the survival processing advantage ultimately turn out to be, these mechanisms are truly strategic and resource-demanding since they are underpinned by a brain network known to be involved in strategic and resource-demanding processes, namely the DLPFC.

Acknowledgments

The first author wishes to thank the Institut Universitaire de France for funding this research. This work was supported by a grant from the Conseil Régional de Bourgogne and FEDER to the last author.

References

Blumenfeld, R. S., Parks, C. M., Yonelinas, A. P. and Ranganath, C. (2010). Putting the pieces together: The role of dorsolateral prefrontal cortex in relational memory encoding. *Journal of Cognitive Neuroscience*, 23, 257-65.

Blumenfeld, R. C. and Ranganath, C. (2007). Prefrontal cortex and long-term memory encoding: An integrative review of findings from neuropsychology and neuroimaging. *Neuroscientist*, 13, 280-291.

Bonin, P. and Bugaiska, A. (2014). "Survivre pour se souvenir." Une approche novatrice de la mémoire épisodique: la mémoire adaptative. *L'Année Psychologique*, 114, 571-610.

Bonin, P., Peereman, R., Malardier, N., Méot, A. and Chalard, M. (2003). A new set of 299 pictures for psycholinguistic studies: French norms for name agreement, image agreement, conceptual familiarity, visual complexity, image variability, age of acquisition, and naming latencies. *Behavior Research Methods, Instruments, and Computers*, 35, 158-167.

Bugaiska, A., Mermillod, M. and Bonin, P. (2015). Does the thought of death contribute to the memory benefit of encoding with a survival scenario? Memory, 23, 213-232.

Burns, D. J., Burns, S. A. and Hwang, A. J. (2011). Adaptive memory: Determining the proximate mechanisms responsible for the memorial advantages of survival processing. *Journal of Experimental Psychology: Learning, Memory, and Cognition*, 37, 206-218.

Buss, D. M. (2010). Why students love evolutionary psychology and how to teach it. *Psychology Teacher Network*, 20, 1-6.

Craik, F. I. M. and Tulving, E. (1975). Depth of processing and the retention of words in episodic memory. *Journal of Experimental Psychology: General*, 104, 268-294.

Cui, X., Bray, S., Bryant, D. M., Glover, G. H. and Reiss, A. L. (2011). A quantitative comparison of NIRS and fMRI across multiple cognitive tasks. *NeuroImage*, 54, 2808-2821.

Cunningham, S. J., Brady-Van den Bos, M., Gill, L. and Turk, D. J. (2013). Survival of the selfish: Contrasting self-referential encoding and survival processing. *Consciousness and Cognition*, 22, 237-244.

Cutini, S., Basso Moro, S. and Bisconti, S. (2012). Functional near infrared optical imaging in cognitive neuroscience: an introductory review. *J. NearInfrared Spec.*, 20, 75-92.

Duncan, A., Meek, J. H., Clemence, M., Elwell, C. E., Fallon, P., Tyszczuk, L. et al. (1996). Measurement of Cranial Optical Path Length as a Function of Age Using Phase Resolved Near Infrared Spectroscopy. *Pediatr. Res.*, 39, 889-894.

Erdfelder, E. and Kroneisen, M. (2013). Proximate cognitive mechanisms underlying the survival processing effect. In: B. L. Schwartz, M. L. Howe, M. P. Toglia and H. Otgaar (Eds.). *What is adaptive about adaptive memory?* (pp. 172-198). New York: Oxford University Press.

Fellner, M.-C., Bäuml, K.-H. T. and Hanslmayr, S. (2013). Brain oscillatory subsequent memory effects differ in power and long-range synchronization between semantic and survival processing. *NeuroImage*, 79, 361-370.

Ferrari, M., Quaresima, V. (2012). A brief review on the history of human functional near-infrared spectroscopy (fNIRS) development and fields of application. *NeuroImage*, 63, 921-935.

Ferreri, L., Aucouturier, J. J., Muthalib, M., Bigand, E. and Bugaiska, A. (2013). Music improves verbal memory encoding while decreasing prefrontal cortex activity: an fNIRS study. *Frontiers in Human Neuroscience*, 7:779.

Ferreri, L., Bigand, E., Muthalib, M., Perrey, S., Bard, P. and Bugaiska, A. (2014). Less effort, better results: How does music act on prefrontal cortex in older adults during verbal encoding? A fNIRS study. *Frontiers in Human Neuroscience*, 8:301.

Ferreri, L., Bigand, E., Perrey, S. and Bugaiska, A. (2014). The promise of Near-Infrared Spectroscopy (NIRS) for psychological research: a brief review. *Topics in Cognitive Psychology/L'Année Psychologique*, 114, 537-569.

Hunt, R. R. and Einstein, G. O. (1981). Relational and item-specific information in memory. *Journal of Verbal Learning and Verbal Behavior*, 20, 497-514.

Innocenti, I., Giovannelli, F., Cincotta, M., Feurra, M., Polizzotto, N. R., Bianco et al. (2010). Event-related rTMS at encoding affects differently deep and shallow memory traces. *NeuroImage*, 53, 325-330.

Jersild, A. T. (1927). Mental set and shift. *Archives of Pyschology*, 89, 5-82.

Jobsis, F. F. (1977). Noninvasive, infrared monitoring of cerebral and myocardial oxygen sufficiency and circulatory parameters. *Science*, 198 (4323), 1264-1267.

Jurcak, V., Tsuzuki, D., Dan, I. (2007). 10/20, 10/10, and 10/5 systems revisited: Their validity as relative head-surface-based positioning systems. *NeuroImage* 34, 1600-1611.

Kazanas, S. A. and Altarriba, J. (2015). The survival advantage: Underlying mechanisms and extant limitations. *Evolutionary Psychology*, 13, 360-396.

Kroneisen, M. and Erdfelder, E. (2011). On the plasticity of the survival processing effect. *Journal of Experimental Psychology: Learning, Memory, and Cognition*, 37, 1553-1562.

Kubota, Y., Toichi, M., Shimizu, M., Mason, R. A., Findling, R. L., Yamamoto et al. (2006). Prefrontal hemodynamic activity predicts false memory - A near-infrared spectroscopy study. *NeuroImage*, 31, 1783-1789.

Manenti, R., Cotelli, M., Robertson, I. H. and Miniussi, C. (2012). Transcranial brain stimulation studies of episodic memory in young adults, elderly adults and individuals with memory dysfunction: A review. *Brain Stimul.*, 5, 103-109.

Murray, L. J. and Ranganath, C. (2007). The dorsolateral prefrontal cortex contributes to successful relational memory encoding. *Journal Neurosci.*, 27, 5515-5522.

Nairne J. S. (2013). Adaptive memory: Controversies and future directions. In: B. L. Schwartz, M. L. Howe, M. P. Toglia and H. Otgaar (Eds.). *What is adaptive about adaptive memory?* (pp. 308-321). Oxford: Oxford University Press.

Nairne, J. S. (2010). Adaptive Memory: Evolutionary constraints on remembering. In: B. H. Ross (Ed.), *The psychology of learning and motivation* (Vol. 53), (pp. 1-32). Burlington: Academic Press.

Nairne, J. S. and Pandeirada, J. N. S. (2008a). Adaptive memory: Remembering with a stone - age brain. *Current Directions in Psychological Science*, 17, 239-243.

Nairne, J. S. and Pandeirada, J. N. S. (2008b). Adaptive memory: Is survival processing special? *Journal of Memory and Language*, 59, 377-385.

Nairne, J. S., Pandeirada, J. N. S. and Thompson, S. R. (2008). Adaptive memory: The comparative value of survival processing. *Psychological Science*, 19, 176-180.

Nairne, J. S., Thompson, S. R. and Pandeirada, J. N. S. (2007). Adaptive memory: Survival processing enhances retention. *Journal of Experimental Psychology: Learning, Memory, and Cognition*, 33, 263-273.

Nairne, J. S., Pandeirada, J. N. S., VanArsdall, J. E. and Blunt, J. (2015). Source-constrained retrieval and survival processing. *Memory and Cognition*, 43, 1-13.

New, B., Pallier, C., Brysbaert, M. and Ferrand, L. (2004). Lexique 2: A new French lexical database. *Behavior Research Methods Instruments and Computers*, 36, 516-524.

Nouchi, R. (2012). The effect of aging on the memory enhancement of the survival judgment task. *Japanese Psychological Research*, 54, 210-217.

Nouchi, R. (2013). Can the memory enhancement of the survival judgment task be explained by the elaboration hypothesis? Evidence from a memory load paradigm. *Japanese Psychological Research*, 55, 58-71.

Okamoto, M., Dan, H., Shimizu, K., Takeo, K., Amita, T., Oda, I. et al. (2004). Multimodal assessment of cortical activation during apple peeling by NIRS and fMRI. *Neuroimage*, 21, 1275-1288.

Okamoto, M., Wada, Y., Yamaguchi, Y., Kyutoku, Y., Clowney, L., Singh, A. K. et al. (2011). Process-specific prefrontal contributions to episodic encoding and retrieval of tastes: a functional NIRS study. *NeuroImage*, 54, 1578-1588.

Ranganath, C. (2010). Binding Items and Contexts: The Cognitive Neuroscience of Episodic Memory. *Current Directions in Psychological Science*, 19, 131-137.

Salthouse, T. A., Toth, J. P., Hancock, H. E. and Woodard, J. L. (1997). Controlled and automatic forms of memory *The Journal of Gerontology. Series B, Psychological sciences and social sciences*, 52, 216-28.

Snodgrass, J. G. and Vanderwart, M. (1980). A standardized set of 260 pictures: Norms for name agreement, image agreement, familiarity, and visual complexity. *Journal of Experimental Psychology: Human Learning and Memory*, 6, 174-215.

Spaniol, J., Davidson, P. S. R., Kim, A., Han, H., Moscovitch, M., Grady, C. L. (2009). Event-related fMRI studies of episodic encoding and retrieval: Meta-analyses using activation likelihood estimation. *Neuropsychologia*, 47, 1765-1779.

Spector, A. and Bierdeman, I. (1976). Mental set and mental shif revisited. *American Journal of Psychology*, 89, 669-679.

Tulving, E., Kapur, S., Craik, F. I. M., Moscovitch, M., Houle, S. (1994). Hemispheric encoding/retrieval asymmetry in episodic memory: Positron emission tomography findings. *P. Natl. Acad. Sci. US*, 91, 2016-2020.

Varela, F., Lachaux, J.-P., Rodriguez, E., Martinerie, J. (2001). The brain web: Phase synchronization and large-scale integration. *Nat. Rev. Neurosci.*, 2, 229-239.

Weinstein, Y., Bugg, J. M. and Roediger, H. L., III. (2008). Can the survival recall advantage be explained by basic memory processes? *Memory and Cognition*, 36, 913-919.

In: Spatial, Long-and Short-Term Memory
Editor: Edward A. Thayer

ISBN: 978-1-63484-148-1

Chapter 9

METHODS FOR IMPROVING NEUROPLASTICITY AND MEMORY FUNCTION IN THE AGING OR COMPROMISED BRAIN

John A. Bellone[1,2,*] ***and Karen J. Miller***[1]

[1]University of California, Los Angeles,
Semel Institute for Neuroscience & Human Behavior, Longevity Center, CA, US
[2]Loma Linda University, Department of Psychology, CA, US

ABSTRACT

The role of neuroplasticity, or the brain's ability to modify neural processes as a result of environmental changes, is crucial to normal memory functioning. Furthermore, this capacity of the central nervous system to adapt is essential for healthy aging and for recovery following trauma or disease states. In this chapter, we will identify the synaptic and structural mechanisms that drive plasticity, as well as describe the purported processes responsible for short- and long-term memory. We will then review the literature regarding the role of neuroplasticity in the aging brain and in recovery following various types of injury (e.g., traumatic brain injury and stroke). Particular focus will be placed on the implications of lifestyle factors, such as diet, exercise, and environmental enrichment, and formal cognitive training or rehabilitation strategies as potential methods for facilitating neuroplasticity and maintaining healthy memory functioning.

INTRODUCTION

The notion that the brain is set in stone following the initial developmental period has long since been replaced by the knowledge that the structure and function of each person's brain is highly malleable throughout all stages and conditions of life. This understanding is

* Manuscript correspondence: John A. Bellone, M.A., Loma Linda University, School of Behavioral Health, Department of Psychology, 11130 Anderson St., Suite 106, Loma Linda, CA 92350, email: jbellone@llu.edu.

central to the practice of healthy aging and recovery following injury. It is also essential for comprehending and maximizing one of the most fundamental and important cognitive abilities: memory. Over the course of this chapter we will distinguish between different types of memory, describe the synaptic and structural changes that comprise neuroplasticity, explain its purported role in memory, explain how memory and neuroplasticity are affected by aging and brain injury, and review a variety of methods that can be taken to sustain and enhance neuroplasticity and memory.

DEFINING MEMORY

Before delving into a description of neuroplasticity, we first need to unpack the term "memory." Memory is not a unitary concept, but an umbrella term that encompasses different systems and processes. These abilities can be broken down into two broad categories: short- and long-term memory. Short-term, or primary, memory refers to the ability to hold a limited amount of information for a temporary period of time. Together with attention and a concept called "the central executive," short-term memory allows for working memory, or the ability to manipulate information in one's mind (Mcallister, Flashman, Sparling & Saykin 2004). Subsumed under working memory is the capacity to hold and manipulate verbal information, named the "phonological loop," and visual and spatial information, named the "visuo-spatial sketchpad" (Baddeley & Hitch 1974). Another system has also been proposed for kinesthetic information (i.e., memory for body postural movements; Dolman, Roy, Dimeck & Hall 1999).

Long-term, or secondary, memory refers to the retention of potentially unlimited information for a long, even indefinite, period of time. This type of memory has two subdivisions: implicit and explicit memory. Implicit memory includes the concept of priming (i.e., being subconsciously prepared to behave a certain way), and procedural memory, or the ability to engage in a familiar task without conscious awareness (e.g., tying one's shoes, reading, or riding a bicycle after the initial acquisition phase). Explicit, or declarative, memory is the intentional recollection of facts (i.e., semantic memory) or experiences (i.e., episodic memory). Prospective memory, or the ability to plan and execute future actions (i.e., remembering that one needed to do something), and source memory, or the capacity to remember where or from whom one was exposed to a particular piece of information, are two other types of memory that do not fit neatly into any of the above categories. Although these are the main subclasses of memory, this list is not meant to be exhaustive (see Figure 1 for a schematic of the main types memory). Furthermore, although frequently used interchangeably, "learning" is the process of acquiring new skills or knowledge through experience and requires the ability to hold information in one's short-term memory store, while "memory" (synonymous with the phrase "long-term memory") is the retention of that information.

Although the mechanisms underlying memory are not fully understood, there have been significant gains in understanding one particularly important brain area: the hippocampus. The hippocampus is a structure in the medial temporal lobe that plays a crucial role in the consolidation of new information, particularly explicit/declarative information. This consolidation process entails the transferring of information from short-term memory into long-term memory (Dudai 2004). Other brain regions have also been implicated in different types of memory (M. Lynch 2004; Vakil 2005), but this chapter will mainly pertain to hippocampally-mediated memory since most of the literature has focused its efforts on this structure and the plasticity that takes place within it.

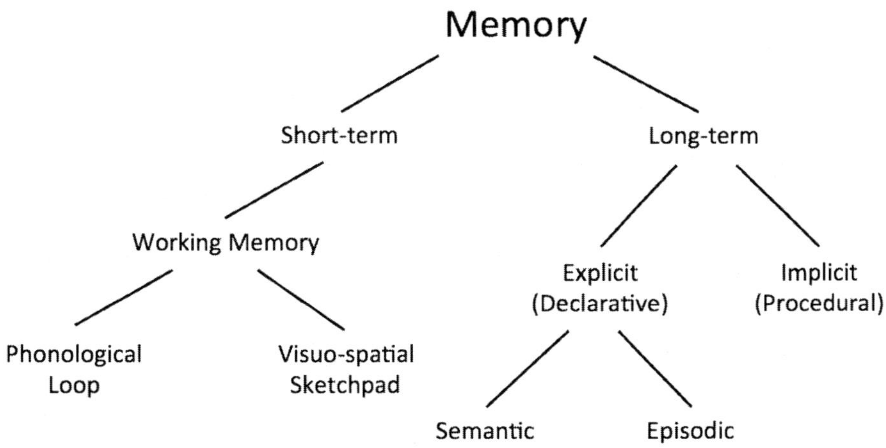

Figure 1. Schematic of the different types of memory.

Defining Neuroplasticity

"Neuroplasticity" is the overarching term for the many different processes that maintain functional adaptation and underlie learning and memory. Although there is no universally agreed-upon definition (Warraich & Kleim 2010), it can be viewed as the complex mix of structural and functional changes the brain undergoes in response to environmental, or even mental, stimuli.

This capacity for learning-dependent neural plasticity is universal in the animal kingdom, and is a fundamental property of the central nervous system (Kleim 2011; Warraich & Kleim 2010). We will briefly touch upon the most commonly studied mechanisms comprising the synaptic and structural levels of neuroplasticity (refer to Table 1 for relevant examples of these mechanisms), as well as discuss its role in memory. Note that the following is a simplified explanation of the general mechanisms comprising neuroplasticity, since numerous complex processes occur, the mechanisms are sometimes different in different brain regions, and many of the specifics are still unknown.

Table 1. Examples of neuroplasticity mechanisms initiated by neural activity

Synaptic	Structural
Long-term potentiation	Dendrite growth and density
Number of receptors	Axonal sprouting
CREB	Neurogenesis
Neurotrophins (e.g., BDNF)	Neural network formation
Trk receptors (e.g., TrkB)	

Synaptic Changes

Donald Hebb (1949), following the work of Santiago Ramón y Cajal (1889) and William James (1890), formulated the concept of synaptic plasticity by suggesting that neuronal synapses receiving frequent activity (i.e., action potentials) would become stronger (more "connected") than those receiving less activity. Over two decades later, Bliss and Lømo (1973) reported their findings on what would become known as long-term potentiation (LTP), a prime candidate for the biological substrate of learning and memory. LTP has been called a "neural analogue of long-term memory formation" (Hillman, Erickson & Kramer, 2008), and thousands of articles have been written on the topic. LTP is responsible for numerous molecular and structural changes that will briefly be discussed throughout this section (see M. Lynch, 2004, for an extensive review of LTP).

Normal synaptic communication occurs when one neuron (called the "pre-synaptic" neuron) sends chemicals (i.e., neurotransmitters) across the synapse (the "space" between neurons) to a second neuron (called the "post-synaptic" neuron). Excitatory neurotransmitters (i.e., glutamate) released by the pre-synaptic neuron bind to receptors (e.g., AMPA and NMDA) on the post-synaptic neuron, causing an influx of ions into the dendritic spine (branch-like projections) of the post-synaptic neuron (Malenka & Bear 2004). LTP gets triggered if the amount of activity (i.e., the frequency of action potentials) differs from the typical frequency of activity at that particular synapse (e.g., as a result of exposure to a novel experience or piece of information), leading to calcium influx (Bienenstock, Cooper & Munro, 1982). AMPA receptors can be added to the membrane of the post-synaptic neuron as a result of the increased calcium, thus modifying the number of ion channels and altering the probability of a neuron's subsequent firing (i.e., making it more likely to fire). These changes are usually referred to as "early-phase" LTP, and the specific manner in which this process works depends largely on the brain region, magnitude and timing of the calcium signal, history of activity at that particular synapse, and many other factors (Bear 1995; Jacob, Brasier, Erchova, Feldman & Shulz 2007; Montgomery & Madison 2004). As will be clarified shortly, these processes are vital for memory functioning.

"Late-phase" LTP occurs through gene expression and protein synthesis, which happens in a calcium-dependent manner (G. Lynch 1998) long after the receptor modifications have been made. One of the main gene transcription factors implicated in synaptic plasticity is the cAMP-response element-binding protein, or CREB (Marie, Morishita, Yu, Calakos & Malenka 2005), which is "turned on" (i.e., phosphorylated) by activity-dependent calcium influx (Tao, Finkbeiner, Arnold, Shaywitz & Greenberg 1998). CREB activates brain-derived neurotrophic factor (BDNF; Tao et al., 1998), which has been referred to as the "plasticity molecule" (Berchtold, Chinn, Chou, Kesslak & Cotman 2005) because of its role in initiating several neuroplastic processes. BDNF is part of the neurotrophin (i.e., growth factor) family and specifically activates TrkB receptors, which modulate plasticity in the hippocampus (Egan et al., 2003; Webster, Herman, Kleinman & Weickert 2006) among many other areas of the brain and body. BDNF-TrkB signaling also influences transmitter systems projecting to the hippocampus, one example being cholinergic innervation (Ward & Hagg 2000).

Structural Changes

In addition to the changes that occur at the level of the receptors, structural changes can occur on a larger scale, involving changes in neuronal morphology and cortical volume. One way this occurs is as a consequence of the aforementioned process of LTP (specifically the late phase), where extensions from the cell body, such as axonal sprouting, augmented dendritic branching (also referred to as arborization), and increased dendritic spine density can be generated (Tolwani et al., 2002; Tyler & Pozzo-Miller 2003; von Bohlen und Halbach 2010). Some of these hippocampal structural changes occur as quickly as 10-30 minutes following the application of an LTP-inducing stimulation protocol (Engert & Bonhoeffer 1999). As a result, new connections are formed with neighboring cells, and existing connections get stronger.

Adding new neurons also contributes to these structural changes. Although most neurons are formed during development, certain areas of the adult brain (i.e., the subventricular zone and the dentate gyrus of the hippocampus) maintain the ability to grow new neurons, a process termed "neurogenesis" (see Lillard & Erisir 2011, for a review of the mechanistic differences between juvenile and adult neuroplasticity). Many of these new neurons grow axons and dendrites (Markakis & Gage 1999) and are fully functional (Leuner & Gould 2010). LTP stimulates neurogenesis (Bruel-Jungerman, Davis, Rampon & Laroche 2006), as does BDNF (Bath, Akins & Lee 2012), and fosters the generation of new synapses in the hippocampus (Toni, Buchs, Nikonenko, Bron & Muller 1999).

Through the processes of increased synaptic efficacy (i.e., strength), neuronal extensions, and neurogenesis, networks of neurons form that are solidly "wired" to each other (Dupret et al., 2007). Thus, it is through the incremental, complex process of adding and subtracting axons, dendrites, synapses, receptors, and even whole neurons that neural networks are sculpted and certain parts of the nervous system get structurally reorganized.

Role in Memory

The synaptic and structural changes triggered by neuronal activity (i.e., altered action potential frequency due to exposure to new experiences or information) are especially important in how they relate to behavioral changes. Fortunately, there is substantial evidence that LTP, BDNF, and all the aforementioned downstream effects influence, if not define, learning and memory. However, although much is known about these processes, they are not yet fully understood (Costa-Mattioli et al., 2007; M. Lynch 2004), and any causal statements regarding the underpinnings of short- or long-term memory would be premature. Thus, this section will only offer a few of the potential mechanisms behind each type of memory.

The flux in neurotransmitters, modification of proteins, and addition of receptors as an outcome of early-phase LTP likely enables the short-term storing of information (i.e., short-term memory; Costa-Mattioli et al., 2007; Costa-Mattioli, Sossin, Klann & Sonenberg 2009). Since some of these changes in synaptic efficacy are temporary (on the order of milliseconds), the information would only be held in mind until one's attention is diverted. If not maintained through repetition, which leads to increased activity and strength of those circuits, these connections quickly degrade (Ohno et al., 2011). Although this type of synaptic plasticity is necessary for memory, it is still uncertain whether it is sufficient (S. Martin,

Grimwood & Morris 2000). Furthermore, other proposed synaptic correlates, such as a change in firing rate due to the accumulation of pre-synaptic calcium (Mongillo, Barak & Tsodyks 2008), are probably also involved in short-term memory function.

Long-term memory likely relies on processes different from those involved in short-term memory, and requires a greater amount of activity to initiate mechanisms that stabilize the synaptic changes (Costa-Mattioli et al., 2007). The most probable candidates are structural changes (e.g., dendritic growth as a result of late-phase LTP) brought about by gene transcription (e.g., by CREB; A. Chen et al., 2003) and protein synthesis (e.g., BDNF; Costa-Mattioli & Sonenberg 2008; McClung & Nestler 2008). The turnover dynamics of these processes (i.e., the balance of synaptic synthesis and degredation) is thought to be of extreme importance for memory consolidation (Attardo, Fitzgerald & Schnitzer 2015). A large body of evidence also suggests that continued hippocampal neurogenesis is required for both short- and long-term memory (Aimone, Wiles & Gage 2009; Deng, Aimone & Gage 2010; Imayoshi et al., 2008; Kernie & Parent 2010; Leuner, Gould & Shors, 2006; Saxe et al., 2006; Tashiro, Makino & Gage 2007), with hippocampus-dependent tasks shown to alter the rate of neurogenesis (Dupret et al., 2007; Dupret et al., 2008; Lillard & Erisir 2011; Olariu, Cleaver, Shore, Brewer & Cameron 2005). Refer to Barco and colleagues (2006) for a review of other potential neural and molecular candidates for the mechanisms underlying long-term memory formation.

Effects of Aging and Age-Related Conditions on Neuroplasticity and Memory

Many changes take place over the life course that alter the mechanisms underlying neuroplasticity and typically negatively affect memory functioning. Although we will review common changes that occur as we age, it is important to remember that heterogeneity is the norm. There are numerous factors that contribute to the level of functioning of an older adult, and it is therefore difficult to pinpoint how aging will affect specific individuals. Thus, we will report about what is generally regarded as "normal aging" and also touch upon the changes that occur in age-related pathologies such as mild cognitive impairment (MCI) and dementia. Understanding these processes is crucial to guiding older individuals toward positive adaptation, which we will discuss later.

Normal Aging

It is common knowledge that cognitive abilities typically decline with age, with particular functional loss in the domain of memory. These changes are associated with molecular and structural alterations in certain brain regions. Although cortical thickness decreases globally (Drachman 2006), the hippocampus is especially prone to shrinkage with age (Du et al., 2006). From age 55 on, it has been reported that the hippocampus atrophies at a rate of approximately 1.5% per year, on average, in individuals without dementia (Jack et al., 1998). It has been difficult to explain specifically why these structural changes occur, but it has been posited that cell death, decreased dendritic arborization, reduced neurogenesis, shrinkage of cells, and the loss of surrounding cortical areas that innervate the hippocampus are all contributing factors (von Bohlen und Halbach 2010).

All markers of neuroplasticity also show age-associated decline, with altered BDNF and neurogenesis being the most salient. For example, BDNF levels decrease with advancing age (Erickson, Miller & Roecklein 2012; Lommatzsch et al., 2005), as do the levels of TrkB (Webster et al., 2006). These decreases lead to significantly impaired LTP within the hippocampus (Gooney, Messaoudi, Maher, Bramham & Lynch 2004). Not surprisingly, BDNF-deficient aged mice show an inability to learn spatial tasks (Linnarsson, Björklund & Ernfors 1997). The age-related decreases in BDNF have also been associated with poor memory ability in humans (Erickson et al., 2010).

Decreased neurogenesis is another culprit in the aging process (Bernal & Peterson 2004), with substantial reductions occurring progressively from mid-life to old age (Bizon & Gallagher 2003). However, the mechanisms underlying this problem are still unknown (Hamilton, Joppé, M Cochard & Fernandes 2013). Furthermore, the neurons that do remain become more simplified, with decreased number and density of spines and less connections (Dickstein et al., 2007). Aging is also marked by a reduction in the number of synapses (Shimada, Keino, Satoh, Kishikawa & Hosokawa 2003) and alterations in synaptic transmission (Dickstein et al., 2007).

Immune mechanisms play a role in affecting neurogenesis, and thus contribute to the aging process (Yirmiya & Goshen 2011). In normal conditions, the immune system promotes healthy neuroplasticity and memory, with microglia producing inflammatory markers (e.g., cytokines) that regulate neurogenesis. However, high levels of these inflammatory mediators and changes in glial-neuron communication by a disruption in key regulators, such has been shown in aging (Krabbe, Pedersen & Bruunsgaard 2004), initiate a chronic inflammatory state that is deleterious to neurogenesis, hippocampal LTP, and memory consolidation (Gemma, Bachstetter & Bickford 2010; Yirmiya & Goshen 2011).

As is expected, the molecular and structural decrements seen in aging lead to functional declines in the area of memory. For example, the degree of neurogenesis is directly correlated with spatial memory ability, where animals that show larger increases in new neurons perform better on memory tests than those with less neurogenesis (Drapeau et al., 2003). Additionally, cholinergic fibers that project to the hippocampus are involved in moderating short-term spatial memory (Everitt & Robbins 1997), so the aforementioned loss in cortical areas such as these bodes poorly for memory ability. Although the most pronounced declines have been found in working memory (Salthouse & Babcock 1991; M. Wang et al., 2011), other types of memory, such as prospective memory (Zimmermann & Meier 2006) and episodic memory (Rioux et al., 1995), also show disturbances. Furthermore, it is important to realize that memory complaints could also be attributable to problems in other domains, such as attention/concentration, executive functions, or word-finding ability, which are commonly observed in older adults (Lindeboom & Weinstein 2004). See Rogers and colleagues (2007) for a review of cognitive profiles in aging.

Despite all the evidence suggesting molecular, structural, and functional decrements in older adults, a discussion of resilience in late adulthood is warranted. As aforementioned, the capacity for plasticity is retained throughout the lifespan (Jellinger & Attems 2013) and there is a subgroup of individuals who maintain relatively conserved cognitive abilities well into their 80's (Howieson et al., 1997). There is also evidence that the risk of developing dementia may stabilize or even decrease after the age of 90 in certain subgroups (Lautenschlager et al.,

1996). Furthermore, certain types of memory remain relatively preserved in old age, such as remote memory, semantic memory, and procedural memory (Rogers et al., 2007). It is important to remember these points, so as not to perpetuate stereotypes that lead to ageism and not to forget that there are neuroprotective measures that can be taken to maintain healthy functioning (see below).

Age-Related Conditions

Although most abilities decline with age, certain pathologies lead to a far larger degree of neuroplastic and functional decline that are not a part of normal aging. Older individuals who perform significantly worse than their same-age peers (typically in the domain of memory) but are still able to perform activities of daily living and do not meet criteria for dementia often receive a diagnosis of MCI (Petersen et al., 1999). MCI is generally referred to as the transitional stage between healthy cognition (i.e., normal aging) and dementia. Estimates of the percentage of individuals over age 65 with MCI range from 3-19% (Gauthier et al., 2006), with approximately 15% of those individuals projected to convert from MCI to dementia each year (Ritchie 2004).

In terms of the neuroplastic pathology, individuals with MCI tend to have greater deficits than the "normal aging" group. For example, they exhibit reduced BDNF levels (Mufson, Counts, Fahnestock & Ginsberg 2007) and disruption in hippocampal connectivity (Ikonomovic et al., 2003). The majority of individuals with MCI have also been found to have less synapses in the hippocampus compared to those with no cognitive impairment, with the number of synapses being correlated with performance on delayed recall tasks (Scheff, Price, Schmitt & Mufson 2006). However, despite these disturbances, many individuals with MCI retain the capacity to learn new information, which suggests some plasticity remains (Calero & Navarro 2004). It is also important to realize that this is a very heterogeneous group, with a large proportion of individuals remaining stable or reverting back to normal (Ganguli, Dodge, Shen & DeKosky 2004).

Much more attention has been given to the neuroplastic changes that occur in dementia, which is diagnosed when more severe cognitive deficits lead to an interference with one's daily functioning. Alzheimer's disease (AD), the most common type of dementia, has been thought of as a failure of neuroplasticity (Ma & Klann 2012; Mesulam 1999), implying that a major part of the functional impairments are due to underlying neuroplastic changes (or lack thereof). Several lines of evidence substantiate this claim. For example, amyloid beta oligomers (i.e., clumps of amyloid beta peptides implicated in AD) have been shown to impair synaptic plasticity by inhibiting LTP (Lambert et al., 1998), impeding axonal sprouting (Roher, Ball, Bhave & Wakade 1991), decreasing dendritic spine density (Shankar et al., 2008), and reducing dendritic arborization (H. Wu et al., 2010). Additionally, some of the major risk factors for AD, such as the APOE4 allele and presenilin-1 mutation, further inhibit dendritic plasticity and growth (Arendt et al., 1997; Furukawa, Guo, Schellenberg & Mattson 1998). As expected, these effects have been linked to the memory deficits characteristic of AD (Jellinger & Attems 2013).

Other common features of impaired neuroplasticity are also found in neurodegenerative disorders. For example, BDNF is reduced in AD (Narisawa-Saito, Wakabayashi, Tsuji, Takahashi & Nawa 1996; Zuccato & Cattaneo 2009), and certain polymorphisms of BDNF have been linked to increased risk of AD (Kunugi et al., 2001; Riemenschneider et al., 2001). There is also a reduction in a variety of other synaptic proteins (Counts, Nadeem, Lad, Wuu & Mufson 2006) and decreased neurogenesis in AD patients (Demars, Hu, Gadadhar & Lazarov 2010). Substantial hippocampal volume loss, possibly from the reductions in dendritic arborization and density, is a common finding (Price et al., 2001), with rates of atrophy estimated at 4% per year, over twice the rate of age-matched controls without AD (Jack et al., 1998). Chronic inflammation, as was discussed above, is also implicated in reducing markers of neuroplasticity and impairing memory in individuals with neurodegenerative diseases (Gemma et al., 2010; Yirmiya & Goshen 2011).

Effects of Injury on Neuroplasticity and Memory

The brain is organized in a manner that permits extensive recovery following injury. In this section, we will discuss two common types of acquired brain injury that have received the most attention in the neuroplasticity literature: traumatic brain injury (TBI) and stroke. These injuries typically have a negative impact on memory functioning but are highly amenable to rehabilitation, which largely aims to boost adaptive neuroplasticity. Like in aging, the changes that occur following injury depend on multiple factors and are highly heterogeneous. The time since injury, specifics of the lesion (e.g., volume, location, cause), demographics, and premorbid cognitive status are just a few of the many variables that can substantially alter the individual's presentation. Due to this uniqueness, rehabilitation following brain injury is optimized when techniques are tailored to the person's specific needs and goals. Although brain injuries can be devastating, with the proper help nearly everyone can maximize their neuroplastic potential and improve their functional status.

Traumatic Brain Injury

A TBI is an externally inflicted impact to the head that results in neuropathology. The main physical effects of such forces include immediate cell death and diffuse axonal injury (i.e., shearing of myelin, or white matter; Kraus et al., 2007). A direct disruption of brain tissue caused by the actual trauma is followed by secondary injury from a number of processes, such as inflammation, oxidative stress, blood-brain barrier disruption, intracranial pressure, and neurochemical changes (Ray, Dixon & Banik 2002). These biochemical cascades also harm cells in the area surrounding the impact site (Lu, Mahmood & Chopp 2003) and lead to neuronal degeneration and hemorrhage, among other deleterious changes (Kaplan, Vasterling & Vedak 2010). The effects of moderate to severe TBI can be devastating to physical and cognitive functioning, especially in the acute post-injury period.

The hippocampus is particularly vulnerable to TBI, with there being a high rate of mortality among its cells and a marked reduction in neurogenesis in the acute post-injury phase (Grady, Charleston, Maris, Witgen & Lifshitz 2003; Rola et al., 2006). One study found that half of boxers and mixed martial arts fighters show hippocampal atrophy as a result of repeated blows to the head (Orrison Jr et al., 2009). Other sports (most famously American football) have also come under scrutiny for the association between repeated mild injuries (i.e., concussions) and hippocampal damage (Guskiewicz et al., 2005; Slemmer, Matser, De Zeeuw & Weber 2002). Although beyond the scope of this chapter, the controversial field of chronic traumatic encephalopathy (CTE) links this repetitive brain trauma (including concussions) to long-term brain changes that may impact not only cognition but also emotional and behavioral functioning (Stern et al., 2011). Military-based trauma from blast waves caused by the detonation of explosive devices is another type of TBI and may result in a down-regulation of the genes involved in synaptic transmission and reduced neurogenesis immediately following the event, as well as contribute to cell death and neurotransmitter alterations within the hippocampus (Risling et al., 2011).

Memory problems are among the most common complaints from TBI patients and their families (Mcallister et al., 2004), and these difficulties can be particularly disabling (Brooks, McKinlay, Symington, Beattie & Campsie 1987). TBI has been shown to affect many different facets of memory, such as working memory (Christodoulou et al., 2001; McDowell, Whyte & D'Esposito 1997), verbal memory (Kersel, Marsh, Havill & Sleigh 2001), visual memory (Reid & Kelly 1993), prospective memory (Groot, Wilson, Evans & Watson 2002), spatial memory (Skelton, Bukach, Laurance, Thomas & Jacobs 2000), source memory (Vakil & Tweedy 1994), procedural memory (Vakil, Kraus, Bor & Groswasser 2002), and episodic memory (Zec et al., 2001). See Vakil (2005) for a comprehensive review of the topic. Furthermore, the degree of white matter damage correlates with learning and memory ability, where more damage leads to worse performance (Salmond et al., 2006).

Despite the large number of individuals who become disabled and/or have long-lasting cognitive decrements as a result of a severe TBI, many individuals recover, and a substantial amount of data have been accumulated on the various mechanisms of recovery. Plasticity is particularly amplified in the area surrounding the injury site, as new regions are recruited and existing circuitry is reorganized to compensate for the lost or damaged cells (H. Chen, Epstein & Stern 2010). Clinical findings suggest that spontaneous recovery (i.e., the natural neuroplastic response following injury) tends to plateau approximately 6 months after more severe injuries (Nakamura, Hillary & Biswal 2009), although it may continue for much longer periods (Stein & Hoffman 2003). Furthermore, studies have shown significant variability in cognitive and functional status when looking at TBI patients up to 5 years post-injury, with some patients showing no measureable impairment and some still experiencing severe deficits (Millis et al., 2001; Olver, Ponsford & Curran 1996).

Different markers of neuroplasticity have been assessed for their role in this recovery process. For example, neurotrophins have a big impact in improving conditions during the secondary injury period. BDNF is substantially increased (up to 75%) in the hippocampus and other brain regions following the acute post-injury phase (Griesbach, Hovda, Molteni & Gomez-Pinilla 2002) and likely plays a major role in repairing connectivity and restoring function (Gao, Smith & Chen 2009). This increase in growth-promoting factors also causes an axonal sprouting response in the peri-contused areas (i.e., area surrounding the impact site; Harris, Mironova, Hovda & Sutton 2010). Additionally, neurogenesis is stimulated in both the hippocampus and sub-ventricular zone after the acute phase, with some of the new neurons migrating to injured regions (Kernie & Parent 2010).

Although spontaneous reorganization plays a large role in functional recovery, training-induced changes accelerate and further the degree of restoration (H. Chen et al., 2010). This is the rationale behind any type of rehabilitation. These relearning techniques aimed at increasing adaptive plasticity have been shown to improve motor and cognitive functioning, including memory (Warraich & Kleim 2010). For example, one form of rehabilitation, teaching compensatory strategies, improved both immediate and delayed recall in severe TBI patients (Berg, Koning-Haanstra & Deelman 1991). Methods using different rehabilitation strategies, such as restoration (i.e., resuscitating damaged areas), recruitment (i.e., enlisting intact, related areas), and retraining (i.e., adapting typically non-related circuits or functions) have all been successfully applied to TBI patients (see Kleim 2011, for a review). Pharmacological treatment that helps bolster plasticity is another method being looked at as a potential intervention for this population (H. Wu et al., 2008).

Stroke

Stroke is a cerebrovascular accident that results in a disruption of blood flow to the brain. This disruption can occur in the form of a reduction or complete blockage of blood flow (i.e., ischemia), or an excess of blood flow (i.e., hemorrhage). Because neurons have a high metabolic rate compared to other types of cells, they are particularly susceptible to drastic changes in the level of oxygen and glucose (Attwell & Laughlin 2001; Laughlin, van Steveninck & Anderson 1998). The hypo-perfusion (i.e., decreased blood flow) and nutrient deficiencies often lead to a cascade of events that result in neuronal damage and death in the immediate area and in the penumbra (i.e., area around lesion that survives the infarct). Dysfunction can also occur in remote areas (termed "diaschisis") that relied on connection with the now-damaged portion (Y. Kim et al., 2005).

As a result of the oxidative stress, chronic inflammation, and toxicity caused by neuronal damage and alterations in ion concentrations, stroke patients often experience memory disturbances (Tatemichi et al., 1994). The type of memory impairment after stroke is typically specific to the infarct location, rather than a general memory issue (Stewart, Sunderland & Sluman 1996). Studies have found impairments in many different memory classes, including prospective memory (H. Kim, Craik, Luo & Ween 2009), working memory (Vallat et al., 2005), and episodic memory (H. Kim et al., 2009). Patients report that these problems are a major reason they experience a reduction in their quality of life (Doornhein & De Haan 1998).

Many of the neuroplastic changes that occur after a stroke are similar to that seen following TBI. For example, the non-affected neurons in the area around the infarct send new branches toward the lesion site in an effort to re-organize connections and rescue function (C. Brown, Aminoltejari, Erb, Winship & Murphy 2009). Increases in BDNF (J. Chen et al., 2005), neurogenesis (Zhang, Zhang & Chopp 2008), and the formation of new synapses (Warraich & Kleim 2010) have also been shown after stroke.

As with TBI, formal rehabilitation is key for recovery following stroke. Although a great deal of spontaneous recovery occurs, it has been shown that early initiation of medical and rehabilitation services, as well as rehabilitation in an interdisciplinary setting, drastically improves functional outcome (Katherine Salter, Mark Hartley & Norine Foley 2006; Paolucci et al., 2000). Traditionally, research relating to neuroplasticity following stroke has pertained mainly to motor learning (especially constraint-induced therapy) for those with hemiparesis (i.e., weakness of one side of their body). However, these services also show beneficial effects for memory functioning. For example, working memory is highly amenable to rehabilitation (Klingberg 2010; Westerberg et al., 2007), which is fortunate because improvements in working memory are important, if not required, for other forms of learning to take place (Malouin, Belleville, Richards, Desrosiers & Doyon 2004). Other types of memory have also been amenable to remediation and compensatory strategies (Cuesta 2002; Doornhein & De Haan 1998). However, despite these optimistic outcomes and the availability of intensive rehabilitation programs to help treat stroke patients, over two-thirds of survivors do not receive any therapy (CDC 2007). We hope the specific rehabilitation training strategies discussed below will prove beneficial to these individuals and their families.

METHODS FOR MAINTAINING HEALTHY NEUROPLASTICITY AND MEMORY FUNCTION

The human brain has the amazing capacity to change with experience. Although certain aspects of neuroplasticity slow down or get disrupted in the aged or compromised brain, the overwhelming message from research over the past several decades is that anyone can improve their neurobiology, at any age and in any condition. Maintaining a healthy diet and remaining physically, socially, and mentally active are just a few ways to drive neuroplasticity and improve both long- and short-term memory function. Here, we review the literature from animal and human studies related to these topics.

Lifestyle Factors

Diet

Dietary supplementation with foods and beverages rich in polyphenols (a subclass of phytochemicals that are abundant in a variety of plant sources) has received much attention from consumers and manufacturers over the past several years as a way to promote overall health, and has increasingly been investigated for its utility in preventing or improving numerous disease states. Although polyphenols have mainly been touted for their antioxidant and anti-inflammatory properties, mounting evidence suggests that they also play a role in driving neuroplasticity.

Different types of fruits and teas have been assessed for their utility in promoting plasticity. Short-term blueberry supplementation, for example, has been shown to increase different parameters of hippocampal neuronal plasticity (e.g., neurogenesis) in aged rats (Casadesus et al., 2004). A grape polyphenol preparation comprised of grape seed extract, Concord purple grape juice extract, and resveratrol also showed promise, rescuing the LTP deficits found in a diet-induced animal model of metabolic syndrome (J. Wang et al., 2013). Additionally, one polyphenol-rich component in green tea (i.e., EGCG) has led to enhanced levels of LTP, both in hippocampal slices from normal mice and in a Down's syndrome mouse model (Xie, Ramakrishna, Wieraszko & Hwang, 2008). LTP was similarly promoted following administration of an extract from a traditional Chinese herb (i.e., *Polygonum multiflorum*; T. Wang et al., 2011).

Curcumin, a polyphenol-laden spice found in turmeric, was shown to incorporate into neural stem cells and induce neurogenesis in the dentate gyrus of the hippocampus (S. Kim et al., 2008; Tiwari et al., 2013). Curcumin also has neuroprotective effects that are likely mediated by its ability to activate TrkB and increase BDNF (R. Wang et al., 2008; R. Wang et al., 2010). For example, it has protected against the deleterious effects of TBI on markers of neuroplasticity (A. Wu, Ying & Gomez-Pinilla 2006) and prevented a stress-induced decrease in BDNF and CREB (Xu et al., 2006), as well as increased hippocampal neurogenesis in this stress-induced model (Xu et al., 2007).

Nutrients outside of the polyphenol family have also garnered attention as potential promoters of neuroplasticity. Omega-(n)-3 fatty acids (n-3 FAs) are polyunsaturated fatty acids found in oily fish (e.g., salmon, trout, tuna, sardines, anchovies), plant sources (e.g., certain types of seeds and nuts), and some animal products in which the animals were grass-fed or fed grains rich in n-3 FAs. One study found that n-3 FAs boosted the levels of BDNF and CREB (A. Wu, Ying & Gomez-Pinilla 2008). Administration of n-3 FAs in that study was also shown to enhance the effects of exercise, so that each of those benefits was intensified by the combination. The same group further demonstrated that n-3 FAs normalize BDNF levels following TBI (A. Wu, Ying & Gomez-Pinilla 2004a).

Of course, the ability of dietary modification to improve neuroplasticity is only useful if it also leads to demonstrable benefits to cognition. Fortunately, there is a rich literature supporting this relationship, especially pertaining to polyphenols and aging. Since several reviews have been completed on this topic (Lau, Shukitt-Hale & Joseph 2005; Lau, Shukitt-Hale & Joseph 2006; L. Rossi, Mazzitelli, Arciello, Capo & Rotilio 2008; Spencer 2010), we will only briefly mention a few representative studies. For example, aged rats fed either spinach, strawberry, or blueberry extracts for 8 weeks had improved short-term memory compared to the control group (Joseph et al., 1999). An aforementioned study using blueberry supplementation also showed that increased plasticity correlated with improved spatial learning ability (Casadesus et al., 2004). Furthermore, curcumin reversed learning and memory deficits in an animal model of Alzheimer's disease (Tiwari et al., 2013) and following restraint-induced stress, preventing adverse changes in hippocampal neurons in a dose-dependent manner (Xu et al., 2009).

Our labs have had success in using pomegranate products to improve memory functioning in various populations, likely because pomegranates have been shown to have a particularly large amount and variety of phenol compounds (Gil, Tomás-Barberán, Hess-Pierce, Holcroft & Kader 2000; Seeram et al., 2008). For example, pomegranate juice ameliorated the neuropathological and learning and memory deficits in an animal model of Alzheimer's disease (Hartman et al., 2006). Two recent pilot studies have also shown promising findings in clinical populations, suggesting that pomegranate polyphenols can be used to improve memory functioning following cardiac surgery (Ropacki, Patel & Hartman 2013) and for individuals with mild memory complaints (Bookheimer et al., 2013).

Although the cognitive benefits of n-3 FAs (consumed as fish or fish oils rich in eicosapentaenoic acid and docosahexaenoic acid or derived from alpha-linolenic acid from vegetable sources) are less clear than for polyphenols, there are still a number of studies demonstrating their utility, and several reviews on the subject (Denis, Potier, Vancassel, Heberden & Lavialle 2013; Dyall & Michael-Titus 2008; Luchtman & Song 2013; Su 2010). A meta-analysis (i.e., study analyzing the pooled, weighted results from other studies) of the effects of n-3 FAs on neuropsychological functioning in individuals with cognitive decline showed a modest benefit to immediate recall (Mazereeuw, Lanctôt, Chau, Swardfager & Herrmann 2012). Studies using n-3 FAs have also found improved spatial learning ability (A. Wu et al., 2008) and cognitive functioning following TBI (A. Wu, Ying & Gomez-Pinilla

2004). However, this topic has garnered a fair amount of scientific skepticism over the past few years, and it is possible that some populations may serve to benefit while others may not (Grey & Bolland 2014).

So far we have explored the benefits of dietary supplementation with polyphenols and n-3 FAs in maintaining healthy neuroplasticity and cognitive functioning. However, the literature also suggests that reducing intake of certain products can be equally beneficial. For example, diets with high levels of sugars and saturated fats can have the effect of decreasing synaptic plasticity and impairing memory function (Raffaella Molteni, Barnard, Ying, Roberts & Gomez-Pinilla 2002; A. Wu, Ying & Gomez-Pinilla 2004b). This high-fat diet has also been shown to exacerbate the neuroplasticity dysfunction (i.e., decreases in BDNF and CREB) and learning and memory deficits after TBI (A. Wu, Molteni, Ying & Gomez-Pinilla 2003). Reductions in BDNF, dendritic spine density, and LTP, as well as impaired spatial learning ability, were also observed in an animal model of diabetes (Stranahan et al., 2008).

Exercise

Like diet, the effects of exercise on neuroplasticity and memory function have received extensive attention from researchers. It is now well established that, in addition to promoting overall health, exercise prompts numerous molecular processes that support neural growth and boost memory ability. Increased synthesis of neurotrophins, especially BDNF, caused by physical activity is one of the main processes that confers these beneficial effects in animals (Gomez-Pinilla, Vaynman & Ying 2008) and humans (reviewed in Knaepen, Goekint, Heyman & Meeusen 2010). It has also been suggested that, in addition to facilitating neurogenesis (Van Praag, Kempermann & Gage 1999), exercise primes the hippocampus for a future response to BDNF and other key molecules involved in the acquisition of new information (Berchtold et al., 2005).

Although the literature shows a strong association between exercise and learning and memory in rodents (Ang, Dawe, Wong, Moochhala & Ng 2006; Van Praag, Christie, Sejnowski & Gage 1999; Vaynman, Ying & Gomez-Pinilla 2004), the findings in humans have been somewhat mixed. For example, a meta-analysis on the relationship of physical activity on cognitive and academic performance in school-age children found small to moderate positive effects for all outcomes except for memory (with 7 studies included; Sibley & Etnier 2003). However, another meta-analysis looking at randomized clinical trials involving aerobic exercise and cognition over the past 40 years (with 29 studies meeting criteria for inclusion) showed "modest" improvements in memory (P. Smith et al., 2010). In this analysis, working memory was only significantly affected if aerobic exercise was combined with strength training. The authors concluded that more clinical trials were needed with longer follow-up periods, larger sample sizes, and more appropriate controls. Other authors have suggested that moderating variables, such as the length of time one spends exercising and degree of exertion, may alter the effects on cognition (Tomporowski 2003). Refer to Hötting and Röder (2013) for a contemporary review of this literature.

One potential explanation for the mixed results is that the aforementioned meta-analyses were mainly interested in studies assessing young, healthy populations, while the beneficial effects of exercise have been particularly strong for older adults and adults with age-related cognitive impairments (Hayes, Hayes, Cadden & Verfaellie 2013; Hillman et al., 2008; Kraft 2012). Higher levels of physical activity are associated with increased cerebral gray matter volume and improved memory encoding in this population (Flöel et al., 2010). Adults in their

60's also show increased hippocampal volume and perfusion and improved spatial memory following aerobic exercise (Erickson et al., 2011). An aforementioned meta-analysis concluded that, although exercise exerts moderate benefits to memory for healthy individuals, those with mild cognitive impairment are especially affected (P. Smith et al., 2010). Furthermore, individuals who engage in regular physical activity have been shown to be at a significantly reduced risk for cognitive impairment and dementia (Laurin, Verreault, Lindsay, MacPherson & Rockwood 2001). Among individuals with a diagnosis of dementia or related cognitive decrements, a meta-analysis showed that exercise improves cognitive functioning (Heyn, Abreu & Ottenbacher 2004). It has been suggested that exercise acts by "reinstating" hippocampal function in this population through the promotion of synaptic changes, neurogenesis, and even angiogenesis (i.e., the formation of new blood vessels; Intlekofer & Cotman 2013).

Exercise has also been used as a therapeutic intervention following injury. One study found that exercise up-regulated BDNF in the hippocampus and improved learning ability in rats subjected to TBI, but only when the exercise occurred after a short healing period (Griesbach, Hovda, Molteni, Wu & Gomez-Pinilla 2004). A follow-up study clarified that the therapeutic time window following TBI is severity-dependent, where rats given a moderate TBI showed increases in BDNF after a longer healing period than rats given a mild TBI (Griesbach, Gómez-Pinilla & Hovda 2007). The same group stressed that exercise performed too acutely following injury could have deleterious consequences to plasticity (Griesbach, Gomez-Pinilla & Hovda 2004). These findings are similar to those conducted with humans, where one study found that athletes who engaged in high levels of activity following a concussion performed worse on measures of visual and verbal memory than those with a moderate level of activity (Majerske et al., 2008). These data suggest that exercising following TBI leads to improved neuroplasticity and memory so long as it is done in moderation after a short time window (reviewed in Griesbach 2011).

The utility of exercise has also been implicated after stroke and other disease states. For example, improvements in working memory (Kluding, Tseng & Billinger 2011) and recall of information following a long delay (Rand, Eng, Liu-Ambrose & Tawashy 2010) were shown after exercise training in stroke patients (for a recent review of the effects of exercise on neuroplasticity after stroke, see Ploughman, Austin, Glynn & Corbett 2015). Furthermore, exercise has been demonstrated to reverse the negative effects of a high-fat diet on neuroplasticity and spatial learning in an animal model (R Molteni et al., 2004). It may also prove neuroprotective in Parkinson's disease, preventing or reducing the cognitive deficits typically seen later on in the course of the malady (Ahlskog 2011). Additionally, the pro-neuroplastic effects of exercise have been implicated in the treatment or prevention of psychiatric issues such as depression (Heyman et al., 2012; Laske et al., 2010) and anxiety (Marais, Stein & Daniels 2009).

Environmental Enrichment

Leading an active and engaged life is important for health at any age, but is especially imperative for older adults and individuals recovering from brain injury. Often the tendency following retirement or injury is to withdraw from complex forms of mental stimulation and social interaction. However, as the results from animal and human studies suggest, remaining in an environment of novelty, where one is constantly engaging in new, challenging tasks has repeatedly been shown to improve neuroplasticity and memory ability.

Most of the original literature on the effects of environmental enrichment came from animal studies, where rodents were placed in cages several times larger than the typical laboratory cage and given toys, running wheels, tubes, and other material that would enhance their living situation. Rodents placed in these settings had increased nerve growth factor (a type of neurotrophin) and BDNF levels in a variety of brain regions (including the hippocampus) as compared to animals in typical laboratory conditions, even when controlling for the effects of exercise (Ickes et al., 2000; C. Rossi et al., 2006). They also showed increased hippocampal neurogenesis (J. Brown et al., 2003; Van Praag, Kempermann, et al., 1999) and volume (Kempermann, Kuhn & Gage 1997), with denser dendritic arborization, which was linked to improved working memory, procedural competency, and speed of navigational strategy acquisition (Leggio et al., 2005). Several groups found improved spatial learning and memory ability as a result of enrichment (Kempermann et al., 1997; Schrijver, Bahr, Weiss & Würbel 2002; Wainwright, Levesque, Krempulec, Bulman-Fleming & McCutcheon 1993). For a review of this original literature, see Van Praag and colleagues (2000).

Older animals profit even more from these enriched environments. Aging mice living in enriched conditions show a substantial (up to fivefold) increase in hippocampal neurogenesis and improved learning ability compared to mice in an impoverished environment (Kempermann, Gast & Gage 2002; Kempermann, Kuhn & Gage 1998). Older enriched rats have increased levels of synaptophysin, a protein that typically decreases with age, and outperform their non-enriched peers on tests of spatial learning and memory, performing similar to younger rats (Frick & Fernandez 2003). Similarly, short-term memory is improved by enrichment (Soffié, Hahn, Terao & Eclancher 1999).

There is evidence that short periods of enrichment can make a difference, and that the effects are reversible. For example, aged rats housed for 3 months in an impoverished environment showed poorer learning and memory ability than those housed in an enriched environment (Winocur 1998). At 3 months, the conditions of the mice were reversed, so that those previously in the enriched group switched to impoverished and vice versa. The author found a decline in the performance of older rats moving from the enriched to impoverished environment and an improvement in those moving from impoverished to enriched.

A large body of research has also demonstrated the utility of environmental enrichment as an intervention following stroke and TBI in animal models. For example, being housed in an enriched environment can alter nerve growth factor-induced gene expression (Dahlqvist et al., 1999; Zhao, Mattsson & Johansson 2000) and increase spine density in post-ischemic brains (Johansson & Belichenko 2002). It has also been shown to decrease infarct size and reduce the long-term spatial memory impairments commonly seen after stroke (Buchhold et al., 2006; Dahlqvist, Rönnbäck, Bergström, Söderström & Olsson 2004). Similarly, many studies have demonstrated that enrichment enhances spatial learning and memory retention following TBI (Hicks et al., 2002; Kline et al., 2010; Kovesdi et al., 2011; Passineau, Green & Dietrich 2001).

Humans can enrich their environments too, by remaining mentally stimulated and engaging in novel, complex tasks (Carey, Bhatt & Nagpal 2005). For example, language acquisition enhances neuroplasticity. Bilingual speakers have been shown to have increased gray matter density in areas linked to phonological working memory compared to monolinguals (Mechelli et al., 2004). Authors have suggested that being bilingual may decrease the rate of gray matter volume loss in older adulthood and protect against age-related cognitive decline (Abutalebi et al., 2014; P. Li, Legault & Litcofsky 2014). Even short-term training with a second language can increase hippocampal volume (Mårtensson et al., 2012) and other markers of neuroplasticity (Hosoda, Tanaka, Nariai, Honda & Hanakawa 2013).

Other activities, such as learning a musical instrument, or increasing one's musical competence, can also improve neuroplasticity and memory. Music training leads to functional changes in the adult hippocampus (Herdener et al., 2010), and there have been numerous studies showing superior verbal and visual memory in individuals with musical experience (reviewed in Rodrigues, Loureiro & Caramelli 2010). Even novices engaging in short-term musical training, such as two weeks of learning to play a musical sequence on the piano, is sufficient to see changes in cortical plasticity (Lappe, Herholz, Trainor & Pantev 2008). Music therapy has also aided the recovery of function following neurological trauma (Baker & Roth 2004). Dancing is another activity that promotes plasticity and healthy cognition (Kattenstroth, Kalisch, Holt, Tegenthoff & Dinse 2013), and may act as a rehabilitation tool in certain populations (Horowitz 2013). These are just a few of the thousands of activities one can engage in to drive adaptive structural and functional changes in his or her brain.

A major part of an enriched environment is the availability of positive social stimulation. Social influences are among the most powerful drivers of neuroplastic change. In animals, being raised in isolation has been associated with fewer newborn neurons and decreased long-term potentiation in the hippocampus, as well as impaired performance on tasks of spatial learning and memory (L. Lu et al., 2003). Pro-social behavior and well-being may also promote neuroplasticity (Davidson & McEwen 2012). In a pilot study, older adults who volunteered in an elementary school to promote children's literacy and academic achievement showed signs of enhanced neuroplasticity (Carlson et al., 2009).

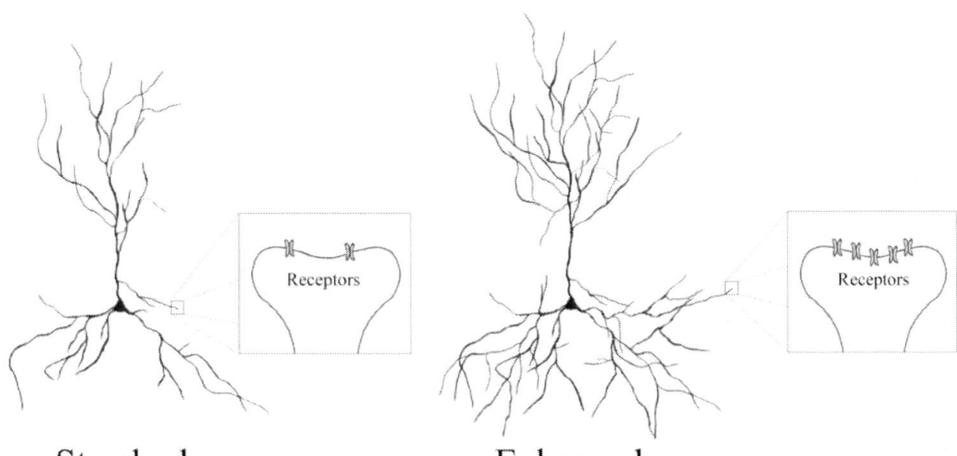

Figure 2. Hypothetical, simplified comparison of a standard neuron compared to a neuron that has benefited from neuroplastic changes (e.g., as a result of diet, exercise, or enrichment). Notice the increased dendritic arborization and number of receptors on the latter neuron.

In contrast, negative social interactions can have the opposite effect on certain markers of neuroplasticity. For example, subordinate tree shrews that experience a stressful social encounter with a dominant tree shrew show marked reductions in the number of newborn cells in the dentate gyrus compared to unstressed tree shrews (Gould, McEwen, Tanapat,

Galea & Fuchs 1997). These subordinate animals also show decreased dendritic length and branching in hippocampal cells (Magariños, McEwen, Flügge & Fuchs 1996). Similarly, humans exposed to traumatic experiences who go on to develop posttraumatic stress disorder (PTSD) have been found to have reduced hippocampal volume (O'Doherty, Chitty, Saddiqui, Bennett & Lagopoulos 2015) and other adverse neuroplastic consequences (Deppermann, Storchak, Fallgatter & Ehlis, 2014; Kolassa & Elbert 2007).

Maintaining emotional health (e.g., keeping a positive mood and reducing stress; Duman, 2004; Duman & Monteggia, 2006; Pittenger & Duman 2008), getting adequate sleep (Hobson & Pace-Schott, 2002; Maquet, 2001; Walker & Stickgold 2004), engaging in meditation practices (Chan et al., 2005; Davidson & Lutz, 2008; Newberg et al., 2014), and avoiding substance abuse (Kalivas & O'Brien 2008; Koob & Le Moal 2005), among other factors, also portend healthy neuroplasticity and memory functioning, but are outside the scope of this chapter. See Merrill and Small (2011) for a review of the effects of lifestyle factors on cognition.

Cognitive Training and Rehabilitation

In addition to the simple lifestyle changes that can boost neuroplasticity and maintain, or recover, memory function that we just reviewed, there are many formal programs designed especially for this purpose. Many of these are structured, standardized programs aimed at teaching strategies and skills in a classroom-type setting. They typically use compensatory techniques (e.g., memory notebooks, assistive technology, and visual imagery) to enhance strengths and recover areas of weakness (Mowszowski, Batchelor & Naismith 2010; Tsaousides & Gordon 2009). Other programs are computerized and mainly use games and exercises to target specific cognitive abilities depending on the individual's needs (for reviews, see Kueider, Parisi, Gross & Rebok 2012, and Miller, Geirland, Gomez, Dye & Ercoli 2015). While all under the umbrella of "cognitive remediation," and often used interchangeably, the term "cognitive training" is typically used for healthy or normal aging populations and "cognitive rehabilitation" used to refer to training following brain injury or in age-related conditions (Mowszowski et al., 2010).

Several programs have been assessed for their utility in improving learning and memory in healthy older adults, but the results have been somewhat mixed (Miller et al., 2015). Some meta-analyses and reviews have found beneficial effects on memory (Verhaeghen, Marcoen & Goossens 1992; Zehnder, Martin, Altgassen & Clare 2009) and some have not (Kelly et al., 2014; M. Martin, Clare, Altgassen, Cameron & Zehnder 2011), with the conclusions being largely contingent upon the types and quality of control groups of the studies included in the analysis. However, working memory has been shown to be particularly amenable to training (Klingberg 2010; Zinke et al., 2014), and more challenging computerized tasks may be especially beneficial among the normal aging population (Mahncke et al., 2006; G. Smith et al., 2009). Training designed to improve other cognitive domains, such as attention, could also indirectly benefit memory (Park & Ingles 2001; Sturm et al., 2003). Furthermore, signs of increased neuroplasticity, such as white matter changes, have been observed following training (Engvig et al., 2012).

Use of cognitive training strategies, both compensatory and computerized, have been expanded from individuals with normal aging to those with age-related conditions. Although more studies are needed, a recent meta-analysis using participants with mild cognitive impairment showed that these types of interventions mildly benefited working memory, episodic memory, and semantic memory, as well as self-rated memory and quality of life (H. Li et al., 2011). Evidence of neuroplasticity, such as increased brain activation in areas important to memory (e.g., hippocampus), has been observed in this population (Belleville et al., 2011; Rosen, Sugiura, Kramer, Whitfield-Gabrieli & Gabrieli 2011).

Existing literature is even more limited for those with dementia (Bahar-Fuchs, Clare & Woods 2013), as many individuals may find these techniques too challenging. Cognitive stimulation strategies (more related to environmental enrichment), such as playing Mahjong (a popular Chinese game) or practicing tai chi, have been found to be better tolerated and beneficial for this population (Cheng et al., 2014; Cheng, Chan & Yu, 2006; Mapelli, Di Rosa, Nocita & Sava 2013). However, preliminary findings suggest that computerized cognitive rehabilitation can at least benefit short-term memory in individuals with moderate to severe dementia (Mate-Kole et al., 2007).

The findings regarding the use of formal programs to improve memory following injury have also been encouraging. For example, a review of studies implementing memory retraining or restoration techniques following TBI or stroke has found these interventions, as a whole, to be effective (Cicerone et al., 2011). Regarding working memory, studies using computerized rehabilitation programs have shown improvements for both TBI (Lundqvist, Grundström, Samuelsson & Rönnberg 2010) and stroke patients (Westerberg et al., 2007). It has been suggested that the types of remediation techniques used may be more beneficial for those with more mild deficits (Ryan & Ruff 1988). Results also vary widely based on the type of program/strategy, intensity of training, severity of injury, time post injury, and a number of other factors (Miller et al., 2015). Overall, however, cognitive training shows promise as a way to enhance neuroplasticity and memory functioning for both healthy individuals and those compromised by aging or injury. Upcoming research will likely clarify which types of programs work best for which populations.

CONCLUSION

The brain is malleable throughout the life course. The synaptic and structural changes collectively referred to as "neuroplasticity" define this malleability, and are intimately involved in learning and memory. Different mechanisms are likely responsible for short- and long-term memory, and both abilities are compromised during aging, especially when there is a neurodegenerative process occurring, and following brain injury. There are, however, many empirically-supported methods for maintaining healthy neuroplasticity and memory throughout one's life or following injury. Lifestyle factors, such as maintaining a healthy diet (i.e., consuming foods rich in polyphenols and other nutrients and avoiding foods high in sugar and saturated fats), exercising, and enriching one's environment (i.e., engaging in novel, complex activities and maintaining positive social connections) can boost neuroplasticity and correspondingly improve memory function. Formal cognitive training or rehabilitation techniques also show promise toward this end. Although research continues to elucidate new methods for optimizing neuroplasticity and memory, the current message from the literature is overwhelmingly optimistic, suggesting that everyone can make a meaningful change in his or her current functioning.

ACKNOWLEDGMENTS

We would like to thank Raquel Bellone for creating Figure 2 and Dr. Roman Vlkolynský for his helpful comments regarding parts of the manuscript.

REFERENCES

Abutalebi, J., Canini, M., Della Rosa, P. A., Sheung, L. P., Green, D. W. & Weekes, B. S. (2014). Bilingualism protects anterior temporal lobe integrity in aging. *Neurobiology of aging, 35*(9), 2126-2133.

Ahlskog, J. E. (2011). Does vigorous exercise have a neuroprotective effect in Parkinson disease? *Neurology, 77*(3), 288-294.

Aimone, J. B., Wiles, J. & Gage, F. H. (2009). Computational influence of adult neurogenesis on memory encoding. *Neuron, 61*(2), 187-202.

Ang, E.-T., Dawe, G. S., Wong, P. T., Moochhala, S. & Ng, Y.-K. (2006). Alterations in spatial learning and memory after forced exercise. *Brain research, 1113*(1), 186-193.

Arendt, T., Schindler, C., Brückner, M. K., Eschrich, K., Bigl, V., Zedlick, D. & Marcova, L. (1997). Plastic neuronal remodeling is impaired in patients with Alzheimer's disease carrying apolipoprotein ε4 allele. *The Journal of Neuroscience, 17*(2), 516-529.

Attardo, A., Fitzgerald, J. E., & Schnitzer, M. J. (2015). Impermanence of dendritic spines in live adult CA1 hippocampus. *Nature.*

Attwell, D. & Laughlin, S. B. (2001). An energy budget for signaling in the grey matter of the brain. *Journal of Cerebral Blood Flow & Metabolism, 21*(10), 1133-1145.

Baddeley, A. D. & Hitch, G. J. (1974). Working memory. *The psychology of learning and motivation, 8*, 47-89.

Bahar-Fuchs, A., Clare, L. & Woods, B. (2013). Cognitive training and cognitive rehabilitation for persons with mild to moderate dementia of the Alzheimer's or vascular type: a review. *Alzheimers Res Ther, 5*(4), 35.

Baker, F. & Roth, E. A. (2004). Neuroplasticity and functional recovery: training models and compensatory strategies in music therapy. *Nordic Journal of Music Therapy, 13*(1), 20-32.

Barco, A., Bailey, C. H. & Kandel, E. R. (2006). Common molecular mechanisms in explicit and implicit memory. *Journal of neurochemistry, 97*(6), 1520-1533.

Bath, K. G., Akins, M. R. & Lee, F. S. (2012). BDNF control of adult SVZ neurogenesis. *Developmental psychobiology, 54*(6), 578-589.

Bear, M. F. (1995). Mechanism for a sliding synaptic modification threshold. *Neuron, 15*(1), 1-4.

Belleville, S., Clément, F., Mellah, S., Gilbert, B., Fontaine, F. & Gauthier, S. (2011). Training-related brain plasticity in subjects at risk of developing Alzheimer's disease. *Brain, 134*(6), 1623-1634.

Berchtold, N., Chinn, G., Chou, M., Kesslak, J. & Cotman, C. (2005). Exercise primes a molecular memory for brain-derived neurotrophic factor protein induction in the rat hippocampus. *Neuroscience, 133*(3), 853-861.

Berg, I. J., Koning-Haanstra, M. & Deelman, B. G. (1991). Long-term effects of memory rehabilitation: A controlled study. *Neuropsychological Rehabilitation, 1*(2), 97-111.

Bernal, G. M. & Peterson, D. A. (2004). Neural stem cells as therapeutic agents for age-related brain repair. *Aging cell, 3*(6), 345-351.

Bienenstock, E. L., Cooper, L. N. & Munro, P. W. (1982). Theory for the development of neuron selectivity: orientation specificity and binocular interaction in visual cortex. *The Journal of Neuroscience, 2*(1), 32-48.

Bizon, J. & Gallagher, M. (2003). Production of new cells in the rat dentate gyrus over the lifespan: relation to cognitive decline. *European Journal of Neuroscience, 18*(1), 215-219.

Bliss, T. V. & Lømo, T. (1973). Long-lasting potentiation of synaptic transmission in the dentate area of the anaesthetized rabbit following stimulation of the perforant path. *The Journal of physiology, 232*(2), 331-356.

Bookheimer, S. Y., Renner, B. A., Ekstrom, A., Li, Z., Henning, S. M., Brown, J. A., Small, G. W. (2013). Pomegranate juice augments memory and FMRI activity in middle-aged and older adults with mild memory complaints. *Evidence-Based Complementary and Alternative Medicine, 2013*.

Brooks, N., McKinlay, W., Symington, C., Beattie, A. & Campsie, L. (1987). Return to work within the first seven years of severe head injury. *Brain injury, 1*(1), 5-19.

Brown, C. E., Aminoltejari, K., Erb, H., Winship, I. R. & Murphy, T. H. (2009). In vivo voltage-sensitive dye imaging in adult mice reveals that somatosensory maps lost to stroke are replaced over weeks by new structural and functional circuits with prolonged modes of activation within both the peri-infarct zone and distant sites. *The Journal of Neuroscience, 29*(6), 1719-1734.

Brown, J., Cooper-Kuhn, C. M., Kempermann, G., Van Praag, H., Winkler, J., Gage, F. H. & Kuhn, H. G. (2003). Enriched environment and physical activity stimulate hippocampal but not olfactory bulb neurogenesis. *European Journal of Neuroscience, 17*(10), 2042-2046.

Bruel-Jungerman, E., Davis, S., Rampon, C. & Laroche, S. (2006). Long-term potentiation enhances neurogenesis in the adult dentate gyrus. *The Journal of Neuroscience, 26*(22), 5888-5893.

Buchhold, B., Mogoanta, L., Suofu, Y., Hamm, A., Walker, L., Kessler, C. & Popa-Wagner, A. (2006). Environmental enrichment improves functional and neuropathological indices following stroke in young and aged rats. *Restorative neurology and neuroscience, 25*(5-6), 467-484.

Calero, M. D. & Navarro, E. (2004). Relationship between plasticity, mild cognitive impairment and cognitive decline. *Archives of Clinical Neuropsychology, 19*(5), 653-660.

Carey, J. R., Bhatt, E. & Nagpal, A. (2005). Neuroplasticity promoted by task complexity. *Exercise and sport sciences reviews, 33*(1), 24-31.

Carlson, M. C., Erickson, K. I., Kramer, A. F., Voss, M. W., Bolea, N., Mielke, M., Fried, L. P. (2009). Evidence for neurocognitive plasticity in at-risk older adults: the experience corps program. *The Journals of Gerontology Series A: Biological Sciences and Medical Sciences*.

Casadesus, G., Shukitt-Hale, B., Stellwagen, H. M., Zhu, X., Lee, H.-G., Smith, M. A. & Joseph, J. A. (2004). Modulation of hippocampal plasticity and cognitive behavior by short-term blueberry supplementation in aged rats. *Nutritional neuroscience, 7*(5-6), 309-316.

Center for Disease Control (CDC) & Prevention. (2007). Outpatient rehabilitation among stroke survivors--21 States and the District of Columbia, 2005. *MMWR Morb Mortal Wkly Rep, 56*(20), 504.

Chan, A. S., Ho, Y., Cheung, M., Albert, M. S., Chiu, H. F., & Lam, L. C. (2005). Association Between Mind-Body and Cardiovascular Exercises and Memory in Older Adults. *Journal of the American Geriatrics Society, 53*(10), 1754-1760.

Chen, A., Muzzio, I. A., Malleret, G., Bartsch, D., Verbitsky, M., Pavlidis, P., Cepeda, I. (2003). Inducible enhancement of memory storage and synaptic plasticity in transgenic mice expressing an inhibitor of ATF4 (CREB-2) and C/EBP proteins. *Neuron, 39*(4), 655-669.

Chen, H., Epstein, J. & Stern, E. (2010). Neural plasticity after acquired brain injury: evidence from functional neuroimaging. *PM&R, 2*(12), S306-S312.

Chen, J., Zhang, C., Jiang, H., Li, Y., Zhang, L., Robin, A., Chopp, M. (2005). Atorvastatin induction of VEGF and BDNF promotes brain plasticity after stroke in mice. *Journal of Cerebral Blood Flow & Metabolism, 25*(2), 281-290.

Cheng, S. T., Chan, A. & Yu, E. (2006). An exploratory study of the effect of mahjong on the cognitive functioning of persons with dementia. *International journal of geriatric psychiatry, 21*(7), 611-617.

Cheng, S. T., Chow, P. K., Song, Y.-Q., Edwin, C., Chan, A. C., Lee, T. M., & Lam, J. H. (2014). Mental and physical activities delay cognitive decline in older persons with dementia. *The American Journal of Geriatric Psychiatry, 22*(1), 63-74.

Christodoulou, C., DeLuca, J., Ricker, J., Madigan, N., Bly, B., Lange, G., Diamond, B. (2001). Functional magnetic resonance imaging of working memory impairment after traumatic brain injury. *Journal of Neurology, Neurosurgery & Psychiatry, 71*(2), 161-168.

Cicerone, K. D., Langenbahn, D. M., Braden, C., Malec, J. F., Kalmar, K., Fraas, M., Bergquist, T. (2011). Evidence-based cognitive rehabilitation: updated review of the literature from 2003 through 2008. *Archives of physical medicine and rehabilitation, 92*(4), 519-530.

Costa-Mattioli, M., Gobert, D., Stern, E., Gamache, K., Colina, R., Cuello, C., Rosenblum, K. (2007). eIF2α phosphorylation bidirectionally regulates the switch from short-to long-term synaptic plasticity and memory. *Cell, 129*(1), 195-206.

Costa-Mattioli, M. & Sonenberg, N. (2008). Translational control of gene expression: a molecular switch for memory storage. *Progress in brain research, 169*, 81-95.

Costa-Mattioli, M., Sossin, W. S., Klann, E. & Sonenberg, N. (2009). Translational control of long-lasting synaptic plasticity and memory. *Neuron, 61*(1), 10-26.

Counts, S. E., Nadeem, M., Lad, S. P., Wuu, J. & Mufson, E. J. (2006). Differential expression of synaptic proteins in the frontal and temporal cortex of elderly subjects with mild cognitive impairment. *Journal of Neuropathology & Experimental Neurology, 65*(6), 592-601.

Cuesta, G. M. (2002). Cognitive rehabilitation of memory following stroke. Theory, practice, and outcome. *Advances in neurology, 92*, 415-421.

Dahlqvist, P., Rönnbäck, A., Bergström, S. A., Söderström, I. & Olsson, T. (2004). Environmental enrichment reverses learning impairment in the Morris water maze after focal cerebral ischemia in rats. *European Journal of Neuroscience, 19*(8), 2288-2298.

Dahlqvist, P., Zhao, L., Johansson, I.-M., Mattsson, B., Johansson, B., Seckl, J. & Olsson, T. (1999). Environmental enrichment alters nerve growth factor-induced gene A and glucocorticoid receptor messenger RNA expression after middle cerebral artery occlusion in rats. *Neuroscience, 93*(2), 527-535.

Davidson, R. J. & Lutz, A. (2008). Buddha's brain: Neuroplasticity and meditation. *IEEE signal processing magazine, 25*(1), 176.

Davidson, R. J. & McEwen, B. S. (2012). Social influences on neuroplasticity: stress and interventions to promote well-being. *Nature neuroscience, 15*(5), 689-695.

Demars, M., Hu, Y. S., Gadadhar, A. & Lazarov, O. (2010). Impaired neurogenesis is an early event in the etiology of familial Alzheimer's disease in transgenic mice. *Journal of neuroscience research, 88*(10), 2103-2117.

Deng, W., Aimone, J. B. & Gage, F. H. (2010). New neurons and new memories: how does adult hippocampal neurogenesis affect learning and memory? *Nature Reviews Neuroscience, 11*(5), 339-350.

Denis, I., Potier, B., Vancassel, S., Heberden, C. & Lavialle, M. (2013). Omega-3 fatty acids and brain resistance to ageing and stress: body of evidence and possible mechanisms. *Ageing research reviews, 12*(2), 579-594.

Deppermann, S., Storchak, H., Fallgatter, A. J. & Ehlis, A.-C. (2014). Stress-induced neuroplasticity:(Mal) adaptation to adverse life events in patients with PTSD–A critical overview. *Neuroscience, 283*, 166-177.

Dickstein, D. L., Kabaso, D., Rocher, A. B., Luebke, J. I., Wearne, S. L. & Hof, P. R. (2007). Changes in the structural complexity of the aged brain. *Aging cell, 6*(3), 275-284.

Dolman, R., Roy, E., Dimeck, P. & Hall, C. (1999). Age, gesture span, and dissociations among component subsystems of working memory. *Brain and cognition, 43*(1-3), 164-168.

Doornhein, K. & De Haan, E. H. (1998). Cognitive training for memory deficits in stroke patients. *Neuropsychological Rehabilitation, 8*(4), 393-400.

Drachman, D. A. (2006). Aging of the brain, entropy, and Alzheimer disease. *Neurology, 67*(8), 1340-1352.

Drapeau, E., Mayo, W., Aurousseau, C., Le Moal, M., Piazza, P.-V. & Abrous, D. N. (2003). Spatial memory performances of aged rats in the water maze predict levels of hippocampal neurogenesis. *Proceedings of the National Academy of Sciences, 100*(24), 14385-14390.

Du, A.-T., Schuff, N., Chao, L. L., Kornak, J., Jagust, W. J., Kramer, J. H., Chui, H. C. (2006). Age effects on atrophy rates of entorhinal cortex and hippocampus. *Neurobiology of aging, 27*(5), 733-740.

Dudai, Y. (2004). The neurobiology of consolidations, or, how stable is the engram? *Annu. Rev. Psychol., 55*, 51-86.

Duman, R. S. (2004). Role of neurotrophic factors in the etiology and treatment of mood disorders. *Neuromolecular medicine, 5*(1), 11-25.

Duman, R. S. & Monteggia, L. M. (2006). A neurotrophic model for stress-related mood disorders. *Biological psychiatry, 59*(12), 1116-1127.

Dupret, D., Fabre, A., Dobrossy, M., Panatier, A., Rodríguez, J. J., Lamarque, S., Abrous, D. N. (2007). Spatial learning depends on both the addition and removal of new hippocampal neurons. *PLoS Biol, 5*(8), e214.

Dupret, D., Revest, J.-M., Koehl, M., Ichas, F., De Giorgi, F., Costet, P., Piazza, P. V. (2008). Spatial relational memory requires hippocampal adult neurogenesis. *PloS one, 3*(4), e1959.

Dyall, S. & Michael-Titus, A. (2008). Neurological benefits of omega-3 fatty acids. *Neuromolecular medicine, 10*(4), 219-235.

Egan, M. F., Kojima, M., Callicott, J. H., Goldberg, T. E., Kolachana, B. S., Bertolino, A., Dean, M. (2003). The BDNF val66met polymorphism affects activity-dependent secretion of BDNF and human memory and hippocampal function. *Cell, 112*(2), 257-269.

Engert, F. & Bonhoeffer, T. (1999). Dendritic spine changes associated with hippocampal long-term synaptic plasticity. *Nature, 399*(6731), 66-70.

Engvig, A., Fjell, A. M., Westlye, L. T., Moberget, T., Sundseth, Ø., Larsen, V. A. & Walhovd, K. B. (2012). Memory training impacts short-term changes in aging white matter: A Longitudinal Diffusion Tensor Imaging Study. *Human brain mapping, 33*(10), 2390-2406.

Erickson, K. I., Miller, D. L. & Roecklein, K. A. (2012). The aging hippocampus interactions between exercise, depression, and BDNF. *The Neuroscientist, 18*(1), 82-97.

Erickson, K. I., Prakash, R. S., Voss, M. W., Chaddock, L., Heo, S., McLaren, M., Woods, J. A. (2010). Brain-derived neurotrophic factor is associated with age-related decline in hippocampal volume. *The Journal of Neuroscience, 30*(15), 5368-5375.

Erickson, K. I., Voss, M. W., Prakash, R. S., Basak, C., Szabo, A., Chaddock, L., White, S. M. (2011). Exercise training increases size of hippocampus and improves memory. *Proceedings of the National Academy of Sciences, 108*(7), 3017-3022.

Everitt, B. J. & Robbins, T. W. (1997). Central cholinergic systems and cognition. *Annual review of psychology, 48*(1), 649-684.

Flöel, A., Ruscheweyh, R., Krüger, K., Willemer, C., Winter, B., Völker, K., Breitenstein, C. (2010). Physical activity and memory functions: are neurotrophins and cerebral gray matter volume the missing link? *Neuroimage, 49*(3), 2756-2763.

Frick, K. M. & Fernandez, S. M. (2003). Enrichment enhances spatial memory and increases synaptophysin levels in aged female mice. *Neurobiology of aging, 24*(4), 615-626.

Furukawa, K., Guo, Q., Schellenberg, G. D. & Mattson, M. P. (1998). Presenilin-1 mutation alters NGF-induced neurite outgrowth, calcium homeostasis, and transcription factor (AP-1) activation in PC12 cells. *Journal of neuroscience research, 52*(5), 618-624.

Ganguli, M., Dodge, H. H., Shen, C. & DeKosky, S. T. (2004). Mild cognitive impairment, amnestic type An epidemiologic study. *Neurology, 63*(1), 115-121.

Gao, X., Smith, G. M. & Chen, J. (2009). Impaired dendritic development and synaptic formation of postnatal-born dentate gyrus granular neurons in the absence of brain-derived neurotrophic factor signaling. *Experimental neurology, 215*(1), 178-190.

Gauthier, S., Reisberg, B., Zaudig, M., Petersen, R. C., Ritchie, K., Broich, K., Chertkow, H. (2006). Mild cognitive impairment. *The Lancet, 367*(9518), 1262-1270.

Gemma, C., Bachstetter, A. D. & Bickford, P. C. (2010). Neuron-microglia dialogue and hippocampal neurogenesis in the aged brain. *Aging and disease, 1*(3), 232.

Gil, M. I., Tomás-Barberán, F. A., Hess-Pierce, B., Holcroft, D. M. & Kader, A. A. (2000). Antioxidant activity of pomegranate juice and its relationship with phenolic composition and processing. *Journal of agricultural and food chemistry, 48*(10), 4581-4589.

Gomez-Pinilla, F., Vaynman, S. & Ying, Z. (2008). Brain-derived neurotrophic factor functions as a metabotrophin to mediate the effects of exercise on cognition. *European Journal of Neuroscience, 28*(11), 2278-2287.

Gooney, M., Messaoudi, E., Maher, F. O., Bramham, C. R. & Lynch, M. A. (2004). BDNF-induced LTP in dentate gyrus is impaired with age: analysis of changes in cell signaling events. *Neurobiology of aging, 25*(10), 1323-1331.

Gould, E., McEwen, B. S., Tanapat, P., Galea, L. A. & Fuchs, E. (1997). Neurogenesis in the dentate gyrus of the adult tree shrew is regulated by psychosocial stress and NMDA receptor activation. *The Journal of Neuroscience, 17*(7), 2492-2498.

Grady, M. S., Charleston, J. S., Maris, D., Witgen, B. M. & Lifshitz, J. (2003). Neuronal and glial cell number in the hippocampus after experimental traumatic brain injury: analysis by stereological estimation. *Journal of neurotrauma, 20*(10), 929-941.

Grey, A. & Bolland, M. (2014). Clinical trial evidence and use of fish oil supplements. *JAMA internal medicine, 174*(3), 460-462.

Griesbach, G. S. (2011). Exercise after traumatic brain injury: is it a double-edged sword? *PM&R, 3*(6), S64-S72.

Griesbach, G. S., Gomez-Pinilla, F. & Hovda, D. A. (2004). The upregulation of plasticity-related proteins following TBI is disrupted with acute voluntary exercise. *Brain research, 1016*(2), 154-162.

Griesbach, G. S., Gómez-Pinilla, F. & Hovda, D. A. (2007). Time window for voluntary exercise-induced increases in hippocampal neuroplasticity molecules after traumatic brain injury is severity dependent. *Journal of neurotrauma, 24*(7), 1161-1171.

Griesbach, G. S., Hovda, D., Molteni, R., Wu, A. & Gomez-Pinilla, F. (2004). Voluntary exercise following traumatic brain injury: brain-derived neurotrophic factor upregulation and recovery of function. *Neuroscience, 125*(1), 129-139.

Griesbach, G. S., Hovda, D. A., Molteni, R. & Gomez-Pinilla, F. (2002). Alterations in BDNF and synapsin I within the occipital cortex and hippocampus after mild traumatic brain injury in the developing rat: reflections of injury-induced neuroplasticity. *Journal of neurotrauma, 19*(7), 803-814.

Groot, Y. C., Wilson, B. A., Evans, J. & Watson, P. (2002). Prospective memory functioning in people with and without brain injury. *Journal of the International Neuropsychological Society, 8*(05), 645-654.

Guskiewicz, K. M., Marshall, S. W., Bailes, J., McCrea, M., Cantu, R. C., Randolph, C. & Jordan, B. D. (2005). Association between recurrent concussion and late-life cognitive impairment in retired professional football players. *Neurosurgery, 57*(4), 719-726.

Hamilton, L. K., Joppé, S. E., M Cochard, L. & Fernandes, K. J. (2013). Aging and neurogenesis in the adult forebrain: what we have learned and where we should go from here. *European Journal of Neuroscience, 37*(12), 1978-1986.

Harris, N. G., Mironova, Y. A., Hovda, D. A. & Sutton, R. L. (2010). Pericontusion axon sprouting is spatially and temporally consistent with a growth-permissive environment after traumatic brain injury. *Journal of neuropathology and experimental neurology, 69*(2), 139.

Hartman, R. E., Shah, A., Fagan, A. M., Schwetye, K. E., Parsadanian, M., Schulman, R. N., Holtzman, D. M. (2006). Pomegranate juice decreases amyloid load and improves behavior in a mouse model of Alzheimer's disease. *Neurobiology of disease, 24*(3), 506-515.

Hayes, S. M., Hayes, J. P., Cadden, M. & Verfaellie, M. (2013). A review of cardiorespiratory fitness-related neuroplasticity in the aging brain. *Frontiers in aging neuroscience, 5.*

Hebb, D. (1949). *The organization of behavior.*

Herdener, M., Esposito, F., di Salle, F., Boller, C., Hilti, C. C., Habermeyer, B., Cattapan-Ludewig, K. (2010). Musical training induces functional plasticity in human hippocampus. *The Journal of Neuroscience, 30*(4), 1377-1384.

Heyman, E., Gamelin, F.-X., Goekint, M., Piscitelli, F., Roelands, B., Leclair, E., Meeusen, R. (2012). Intense exercise increases circulating endocannabinoid and BDNF levels in humans—possible implications for reward and depression. *Psychoneuroendocrinology, 37*(6), 844-851.

Heyn, P., Abreu, B. C. & Ottenbacher, K. J. (2004). The effects of exercise training on elderly persons with cognitive impairment and dementia: a meta-analysis. *Archives of physical medicine and rehabilitation, 85*(10), 1694-1704.

Hicks, R., Zhang, L., Atkinson, A., Stevenon, M., Veneracion, M. & Seroogy, K. (2002). Environmental enrichment attenuates cognitive deficits, but does not alter neurotrophin gene expression in the hippocampus following lateral fluid percussion brain injury. *Neuroscience, 112*(3), 631-637.

Hillman, C. H., Erickson, K. I. & Kramer, A. F. (2008). Be smart, exercise your heart: exercise effects on brain and cognition. *Nature Reviews Neuroscience, 9*(1), 58-65.

Hobson, J. A. & Pace-Schott, E. F. (2002). The cognitive neuroscience of sleep: neuronal systems, consciousness and learning. *Nature Reviews Neuroscience, 3*(9), 679-693.

Horowitz, S. (2013). The Healing Power of Music and Dance. *Alternative and Complementary Therapies, 19*(5), 265-269.

Hosoda, C., Tanaka, K., Nariai, T., Honda, M. & Hanakawa, T. (2013). Dynamic neural network reorganization associated with second language vocabulary acquisition: a multimodal imaging study. *The Journal of Neuroscience, 33*(34), 13663-13672.

Hötting, K. & Röder, B. (2013). Beneficial effects of physical exercise on neuroplasticity and cognition. *Neuroscience & Biobehavioral Reviews, 37*(9), 2243-2257.

Howieson, D. B., Dame, A., Camicioli, R., Sexton, G., Payami, H. & Kaye, J. A. (1997). Cognitive markers preceding Alzheimer's dementia in the healthy oldest old. *Journal of the American Geriatrics Society, 45*(5), 584-589.

Ickes, B. R., Pham, T. M., Sanders, L. A., Albeck, D. S., Mohammed, A. H. & Granholm, A.-C. (2000). Long-term environmental enrichment leads to regional increases in neurotrophin levels in rat brain. *Experimental neurology, 164*(1), 45-52.

Ikonomovic, M. D., Mufson, E. J., Wuu, J., Cochran, E. J., Bennett, D. A. & DeKosky, S. T. (2003). Cholinergic plasticity in hippocampus of individuals with mild cognitive impairment: correlation with Alzheimer's neuropathology. *Journal of Alzheimer's Disease, 5*(1), 39-48.

Imayoshi, I., Sakamoto, M., Ohtsuka, T., Takao, K., Miyakawa, T., Yamaguchi, M., Kageyama, R. (2008). Roles of continuous neurogenesis in the structural and functional integrity of the adult forebrain. *Nature neuroscience, 11*(10), 1153-1161.

Intlekofer, K. A. & Cotman, C. W. (2013). Exercise counteracts declining hippocampal function in aging and Alzheimer's disease. *Neurobiology of disease, 57*, 47-55.

Jack, C., Petersen, R. C., Xu, Y., O'Brien, P. C., Smith, G. E., Ivnik, R. J., Kokmen, E. (1998). Rate of medial temporal lobe atrophy in typical aging and Alzheimer's disease. *Neurology, 51*(4), 993-999.

Jacob, V., Brasier, D. J., Erchova, I., Feldman, D. & Shulz, D. E. (2007). Spike timing-dependent synaptic depression in the in vivo barrel cortex of the rat. *The Journal of Neuroscience, 27*(6), 1271-1284.

James, W. (1890). *The principles of psychology*: New York: Dover.

Jellinger, K. A. & Attems, J. (2013). Neuropathological approaches to cerebral aging and neuroplasticity. *Dialogues in clinical neuroscience, 15*(1), 29.

Johansson, B. B. & Belichenko, P. V. (2002). Neuronal Plasticity and Dendritic Spines: Effect of Environmental Enrichment on Intact and Postischemic Rat Brain. *Journal of Cerebral Blood Flow & Metabolism, 22*(1), 89-96.

Joseph, J. A., Shukitt-Hale, B., Denisova, N. A., Bielinski, D., Martin, A., McEwen, J. J. & Bickford, P. C. (1999). Reversals of age-related declines in neuronal signal transduction, cognitive, and motor behavioral deficits with blueberry, spinach, or strawberry dietary supplementation. *The Journal of Neuroscience, 19*(18), 8114-8121.

Kalivas, P. W. & O'Brien, C. (2008). Drug addiction as a pathology of staged neuroplasticity. *Neuropsychopharmacology, 33*(1), 166-180.

Kaplan, G. B., Vasterling, J. J. & Vedak, P. C. (2010). Brain-derived neurotrophic factor in traumatic brain injury, post-traumatic stress disorder, and their comorbid conditions: role in pathogenesis and treatment. *Behavioural pharmacology, 21*(5-6), 427-437.

Katherine Salter, B., Mark Hartley, B. & Norine Foley, B. (2006). Impact of early vs delayed admission to rehabilitation on functional outcomes in persons with stroke. *J Rehabil Med, 38*, 113-117.

Kattenstroth, J.-C., Kalisch, T., Holt, S., Tegenthoff, M. & Dinse, H. R. (2013). Six months of dance intervention enhances postural, sensorimotor, and cognitive performance in elderly without affecting cardio-respiratory functions. *Frontiers in aging neuroscience, 5*.

Kelly, M. E., Loughrey, D., Lawlor, B. A., Robertson, I. H., Walsh, C. & Brennan, S. (2014). The impact of cognitive training and mental stimulation on cognitive and everyday functioning of healthy older adults: a systematic review and meta-analysis. *Ageing research reviews, 15*, 28-43.

Kempermann, G., Gast, D. & Gage, F. H. (2002). Neuroplasticity in old age: Sustained fivefold induction of hippocampal neurogenesis by long-term environmental enrichment. *Annals of neurology, 52*(2), 135-143.

Kempermann, G., Kuhn, H. G. & Gage, F. H. (1997). More hippocampal neurons in adult mice living in an enriched environment. *Nature, 386*(6624), 493-495.

Kempermann, G., Kuhn, H. G. & Gage, F. H. (1998). Experience-induced neurogenesis in the senescent dentate gyrus. *The Journal of Neuroscience, 18*(9), 3206-3212.

Kernie, S. G. & Parent, J. M. (2010). Forebrain neurogenesis after focal Ischemic and traumatic brain injury. *Neurobiology of disease, 37*(2), 267-274.

Kersel, D. A., Marsh, N. V., Havill, J. H. & Sleigh, J. W. (2001). Neuropsychological functioning during the year following severe traumatic brain injury. *Brain injury, 15*(4), 283-296.

Kim, H. J., Craik, F. I., Luo, L. & Ween, J. E. (2009). Impairments in prospective and retrospective memory following stroke. *Neurocase, 15*(2), 145-156.

Kim, S. J., Son, T. G., Park, H. R., Park, M., Kim, M.-S., Kim, H. S., Lee, J. (2008). Curcumin stimulates proliferation of embryonic neural progenitor cells and neurogenesis in the adult hippocampus. *Journal of Biological Chemistry, 283*(21), 14497-14505.

Kim, Y. R., Huang, I. J., Lee, S.-R., Tejima, E., Mandeville, J. B., van Meer, M. P., Lo, E. H. (2005). Measurements of BOLD/CBV ratio show altered fMRI hemodynamics during stroke recovery in rats. *Journal of Cerebral Blood Flow & Metabolism, 25*(7), 820-829.

Kleim, J. A. (2011). Neural plasticity and neurorehabilitation: teaching the new brain old tricks. *Journal of communication disorders, 44*(5), 521-528.

Kline, A. E., McAloon, R. L., Henderson, K. A., Bansal, U. K., Ganti, B. M., Ahmed, R. H., Sozda, C. N. (2010). Evaluation of a combined therapeutic regimen of 8-OH-DPAT and environmental enrichment after experimental traumatic brain injury. *Journal of neurotrauma, 27*(11), 2021-2032.

Klingberg, T. (2010). Training and plasticity of working memory. *Trends in Cognitive Sciences, 14*(7), 317-324.

Kluding, P. M., Tseng, B. Y. & Billinger, S. A. (2011). Exercise and executive function in individuals with chronic stroke: a pilot study. *Journal of neurologic physical therapy: JNPT, 35*(1), 11.

Knaepen, K., Goekint, M., Heyman, E. M. & Meeusen, R. (2010). Neuroplasticity—exercise-induced response of peripheral brain-derived neurotrophic factor. *Sports Medicine, 40*(9), 765-801.

Kolassa, I.-T. & Elbert, T. (2007). Structural and functional neuroplasticity in relation to traumatic stress. *Current Directions in Psychological Science, 16*(6), 321-325.

Koob, G. F. & Le Moal, M. (2005). Plasticity of reward neurocircuitry and the 'dark side' of drug addiction. *Nature neuroscience, 8*(11), 1442-1444.

Kovesdi, E., Gyorgy, A. B., Kwon, S.-K. C., Wingo, D. L., Kamnaksh, A., Long, J. B., Agoston, D. V. (2011). The effect of enriched environment on the outcome of traumatic brain injury; a behavioral, proteomics, and histological study. *Frontiers in neuroscience, 5*, 42.

Krabbe, K. S., Pedersen, M. & Bruunsgaard, H. (2004). Inflammatory mediators in the elderly. *Experimental gerontology, 39*(5), 687-699.

Kraft, E. (2012). Cognitive function, physical activity, and aging: possible biological links and implications for multimodal interventions. *Aging, Neuropsychology, and Cognition, 19*(1-2), 248-263.

Kraus, M. F., Susmaras, T., Caughlin, B. P., Walker, C. J., Sweeney, J. A. & Little, D. M. (2007). White matter integrity and cognition in chronic traumatic brain injury: a diffusion tensor imaging study. *Brain, 130*(10), 2508-2519.

Kueider, A. M., Parisi, J. M., Gross, A. L. & Rebok, G. W. (2012). Computerized cognitive training with older adults: a systematic review. *PloS one, 7*(7), e40588.

Kunugi, H., Ueki, A., Otsuka, M., Isse, K., Hirasawa, H., Kato, N., Nanko, S. (2001). A novel polymorphism of the brain-derived neurotrophic factor (BDNF) gene associated with late-onset Alzheimer's disease. *Molecular psychiatry, 6*(1), 83-86.

Lambert, M. P., Barlow, A., Chromy, B. A., Edwards, C., Freed, R., Liosatos, M., Viola, K. L. (1998). Diffusible, nonfibrillar ligands derived from Aβ1–42 are potent central nervous system neurotoxins. *Proceedings of the National Academy of Sciences, 95*(11), 6448-6453.

Lappe, C., Herholz, S. C., Trainor, L. J. & Pantev, C. (2008). Cortical plasticity induced by short-term unimodal and multimodal musical training. *The Journal of Neuroscience, 28*(39), 9632-9639.

Laske, C., Banschbach, S., Stransky, E., Bosch, S., Straten, G., Machann, J., Eschweiler, G. W. (2010). Exercise-induced normalization of decreased BDNF serum concentration in elderly women with remitted major depression. *International Journal of Neuropsychopharmacology, 13*(5), 595-602.

Lau, F. C., Shukitt-Hale, B. & Joseph, J. A. (2005). The beneficial effects of fruit polyphenols on brain aging. *Neurobiology of aging, 26*(1), 128-132.

Lau, F. C., Shukitt-Hale, B. & Joseph, J. A. (2006). Beneficial effects of berry fruit polyphenols on neuronal and behavioral aging. *Journal of the Science of Food and Agriculture, 86*(14), 2251-2255.

Laughlin, S. B., van Steveninck, R. R. d. R. & Anderson, J. C. (1998). The metabolic cost of neural information. *Nature neuroscience, 1*(1), 36-41.

Laurin, D., Verreault, R., Lindsay, J., MacPherson, K. & Rockwood, K. (2001). Physical activity and risk of cognitive impairment and dementia in elderly persons. *Archives of neurology, 58*(3), 498-504.

Lautenschlager, N., Cupples, L., Rao, V., Auerbach, S., Becker, R., Burke, J., Glatt, S. (1996). Risk of dementia among relatives of Alzheimer's disease patients in the MIRAGE study: What is in store for the oldest old? *Neurology, 46*(3), 641-650.

Leggio, M. G., Mandolesi, L., Federico, F., Spirito, F., Ricci, B., Gelfo, F. & Petrosini, L. (2005). Environmental enrichment promotes improved spatial abilities and enhanced dendritic growth in the rat. *Behavioural brain research, 163*(1), 78-90.

Leuner, B. & Gould, E. (2010). Structural plasticity and hippocampal function. *Annual review of psychology, 61*, 111.

Leuner, B., Gould, E. & Shors, T. J. (2006). Is there a link between adult neurogenesis and learning? *Hippocampus, 16*(3), 216-224.

Li, H., Li, J., Li, N., Li, B., Wang, P. & Zhou, T. (2011). Cognitive intervention for persons with mild cognitive impairment: A meta-analysis. *Ageing research reviews, 10*(2), 285-296.

Li, P., Legault, J. & Litcofsky, K. A. (2014). Neuroplasticity as a function of second language learning: anatomical changes in the human brain. *Cortex, 58*, 301-324.

Lillard, A. S. & Erisir, A. (2011). Old dogs learning new tricks: neuroplasticity beyond the juvenile period. *Developmental review, 31*(4), 207-239.

Lindeboom, J. & Weinstein, H. (2004). Neuropsychology of cognitive ageing, minimal cognitive impairment, Alzheimer's disease, and vascular cognitive impairment. *European journal of pharmacology, 490*(1), 83-86.

Linnarsson, S., Björklund, A. & Ernfors, P. (1997). Learning deficit in BDNF mutant mice. *European Journal of Neuroscience, 9*(12), 2581-2587.

Lommatzsch, M., Zingler, D., Schuhbaeck, K., Schloetcke, K., Zingler, C., Schuff-Werner, P. & Virchow, J. C. (2005). The impact of age, weight and gender on BDNF levels in human platelets and plasma. *Neurobiology of aging, 26*(1), 115-123.

Lu, D., Mahmood, A. & Chopp, M. (2003). Biologic Transplantation and Neurotrophin-Induced Neuroplasticity After Traumatic Brain Injury. *The Journal of head trauma rehabilitation, 18*(4), 357-376.

Lu, L., Bao, G., Chen, H., Xia, P., Fan, X., Zhang, J., Ma, L. (2003). Modification of hippocampal neurogenesis and neuroplasticity by social environments. *Experimental neurology, 183*(2), 600-609.

Luchtman, D. W. & Song, C. (2013). Cognitive enhancement by omega-3 fatty acids from child-hood to old age: findings from animal and clinical studies. *Neuropharmacology, 64*, 550-565.

Lundqvist, A., Grundström, K., Samuelsson, K. & Rönnberg, J. (2010). Computerized training of working memory in a group of patients suffering from acquired brain injury. *Brain injury, 24*(10), 1173-1183.

Lynch, G. (1998). Memory and the brain: unexpected chemistries and a new pharmacology. *Neurobiology of learning and memory, 70*(1), 82-100.

Lynch, M. (2004). Long-term potentiation and memory. *Physiological reviews, 84*(1), 87-136.

Ma, T. & Klann, E. (2012). Amyloid β: linking synaptic plasticity failure to memory disruption in Alzheimer's disease. *Journal of neurochemistry, 120*(s1), 140-148.

Magariños, A. M. a., McEwen, B. S., Flügge, G. & Fuchs, E. (1996). Chronic psychosocial stress causes apical dendritic atrophy of hippocampal CA3 pyramidal neurons in subordinate tree shrews. *The Journal of Neuroscience, 16*(10), 3534-3540.

Mahncke, H. W., Connor, B. B., Appelman, J., Ahsanuddin, O. N., Hardy, J. L., Wood, R. A., Merzenich, M. M. (2006). Memory enhancement in healthy older adults using a brain plasticity-based training program: a randomized, controlled study. *Proceedings of the National Academy of Sciences, 103*(33), 12523-12528.

Majerske, C. W., Mihalik, J. P., Ren, D., Collins, M. W., Reddy, C. C., Lovell, M. R. & Wagner, A. K. (2008). Concussion in sports: postconcussive activity levels, symptoms, and neurocognitive performance. *Journal of Athletic Training, 43*(3), 265.

Malenka, R. C. & Bear, M. F. (2004). LTP and LTD: an embarrassment of riches. *Neuron, 44*(1), 5-21.

Malouin, F., Belleville, S., Richards, C. L., Desrosiers, J. & Doyon, J. (2004). Working memory and mental practice outcomes after stroke. *Archives of physical medicine and rehabilitation, 85*(2), 177-183.

Mapelli, D., Di Rosa, E., Nocita, R. & Sava, D. (2013). Cognitive stimulation in patients with dementia: randomized controlled trial. *Dementia and geriatric cognitive disorders extra, 3*(1), 263-271.

Maquet, P. (2001). The role of sleep in learning and memory. *Science, 294*(5544), 1048-1052.

Marais, L., Stein, D. J. & Daniels, W. M. (2009). Exercise increases BDNF levels in the striatum and decreases depressive-like behavior in chronically stressed rats. *Metabolic brain disease, 24*(4), 587-597.

Marie, H., Morishita, W., Yu, X., Calakos, N. & Malenka, R. C. (2005). Generation of silent synapses by acute in vivo expression of CaMKIV and CREB. *Neuron, 45*(5), 741-752.

Markakis, E. A. & Gage, F. H. (1999). Adult-generated neurons in the dentate gyrus send axonal projections to field CA3 and are surrounded by synaptic vesicles. *Journal of comparative neurology, 406*(4), 449-460.

Mårtensson, J., Eriksson, J., Bodammer, N. C., Lindgren, M., Johansson, M., Nyberg, L. & Lövdén, M. (2012). Growth of language-related brain areas after foreign language learning. *Neuroimage, 63*(1), 240-244.

Martin, M., Clare, L., Altgassen, A. M., Cameron, M. H. & Zehnder, F. (2011). Cognition-based interventions for healthy older people and people with mild cognitive impairment. *The Cochrane Library.*

Martin, S., Grimwood, P. & Morris, R. (2000). Synaptic plasticity and memory: an evaluation of the hypothesis. *Annual review of neuroscience, 23*(1), 649-711.

Mate-Kole, C., Fellows, R., Said, P., McDougal, J., Catayong, K., Dang, V. & Gianesini, J. (2007). Use of computer assisted and interactive cognitive training programmes with moderate to severely demented individuals: a preliminary study. *Aging & Mental Health, 11*(5), 485-495.

Mazereeuw, G., Lanctôt, K. L., Chau, S. A., Swardfager, W. & Herrmann, N. (2012). Effects of omega-3 fatty acids on cognitive performance: a meta-analysis. *Neurobiology of aging, 33*(7), 1482. e1417-1482. e1429.

Mcallister, T. W., Flashman, L. A., Sparling, M. B. & Saykin, A. J. (2004). Working memory deficits after traumatic brain injury: catecholaminergic mechanisms and prospects for treatment-a review. *Brain injury, 18*(4), 331-350.

McClung, C. A. & Nestler, E. J. (2008). Neuroplasticity mediated by altered gene expression. *Neuropsychopharmacology, 33*(1), 3-17.

McDowell, S., Whyte, J. & D'Esposito, M. (1997). Working memory impairments in traumatic brain injury: evidence from a dual-task paradigm. *Neuropsychologia, 35*(10), 1341-1353.

Mechelli, A., Crinion, J. T., Noppeney, U., O'Doherty, J., Ashburner, J., Frackowiak, R. S. & Price, C. J. (2004). Neurolinguistics: structural plasticity in the bilingual brain. *Nature, 431*(7010), 757-757.

Merrill, D. A. & Small, G. W. (2011). Prevention in psychiatry: effects of healthy lifestyle on cognition. *Psychiatric Clinics of North America, 34*(1), 249-261.

Mesulam, M.-M. (1999). Neuroplasticity failure in Alzheimer's disease: bridging the gap between plaques and tangles. *Neuron, 24*(3), 521-529.

Miller, K. J., Geirland, J., Gomez, M. E., Dye, R. V. & Ercoli, L. M. (2015). Memory training and aging. In *Complementary, Alternative, and Integrative Interventions for Mental Health and Aging.* Nova Science Publishers, Inc.

Millis, S. R., Rosenthal, M., Novack, T. A., Sherer, M., Nick, T. G., Kreutzer, J. S., Ricker, J. H. (2001). Long-term neuropsychological outcome after traumatic brain injury. *The Journal of head trauma rehabilitation, 16*(4), 343-355.

Molteni, R., Barnard, R., Ying, Z., Roberts, C. & Gomez-Pinilla, F. (2002). A high-fat, refined sugar diet reduces hippocampal brain-derived neurotrophic factor, neuronal plasticity, and learning. *Neuroscience, 112*(4), 803-814.

Molteni, R., Wu, A., Vaynman, S., Ying, Z., Barnard, R. & Gomez-Pinilla, F. (2004). Exercise reverses the harmful effects of consumption of a high-fat diet on synaptic and behavioral plasticity associated to the action of brain-derived neurotrophic factor. *Neuroscience, 123*(2), 429-440.

Mongillo, G., Barak, O. & Tsodyks, M. (2008). Synaptic theory of working memory. *Science, 319*(5869), 1543-1546.

Montgomery, J. M. & Madison, D. V. (2004). Discrete synaptic states define a major mechanism of synapse plasticity. *Trends in neurosciences, 27*(12), 744-750.

Mowszowski, L., Batchelor, J. & Naismith, S. L. (2010). Early intervention for cognitive decline: can cognitive training be used as a selective prevention technique? *International Psychogeriatrics, 22*(04), 537-548.

Mufson, E. J., Counts, S. E., Fahnestock, M. & Ginsberg, S. D. (2007). Cholinotrophic molecular substrates of mild cognitive impairment in the elderly. *Current Alzheimer Research, 4*(4), 340-350.

Nakamura, T., Hillary, F. G. & Biswal, B. B. (2009). Resting network plasticity following brain injury. *PloS one, 4*(12).

Narisawa-Saito, M., Wakabayashi, K., Tsuji, S., Takahashi, H. & Nawa, H. (1996). Regional specificity of alterations in NGF, BDNF and NT-3 levels in Alzheimer's disease. *Neuroreport, 7*(18), 2925-2928.

Newberg, A. B., Serruya, M., Wintering, N., Moss, A. S., Reibel, D. & Monti, D. A. (2014). Meditation and neurodegenerative diseases. *Annals of the New York Academy of Sciences, 1307*(1), 112-123.

O'Doherty, D. C., Chitty, K. M., Saddiqui, S., Bennett, M. R. & Lagopoulos, J. (2015). A systematic review and meta-analysis of magnetic resonance imaging measurement of structural volumes in posttraumatic stress disorder. *Psychiatry Research: Neuroimaging, 232*(1), 1-33.

Ohno, T., Hasegawa, T., Tsuruoka, T., Terabe, K., Gimzewski, J. K. & Aono, M. (2011). Short-term plasticity and long-term potentiation mimicked in single inorganic synapses. *Nature materials, 10*(8), 591-595.

Olariu, A., Cleaver, K. M., Shore, L. E., Brewer, M. D. & Cameron, H. A. (2005). A natural form of learning can increase and decrease the survival of new neurons in the dentate gyrus. *Hippocampus, 15*(6), 750-762.

Olver, J. H., Ponsford, J. & Curran, C. (1996). Outcome following traumatic brain injury: a comparison between 2 and 5 years after injury. *Brain injury, 10*(11), 841-848.

Orrison Jr, W. W., Hanson, E. H., Alamo, T., Watson, D., Sharma, M., Perkins, T. G. & Tandy, R. D. (2009). Traumatic brain injury: a review and high-field MRI findings in 100 unarmed combatants using a literature-based checklist approach. *Journal of neurotrauma, 26*(5), 689-701.

Paolucci, S., Antonucci, G., Grasso, M. G., Morelli, D., Troisi, E., Coiro, P. & Bragoni, M. (2000). Early versus delayed inpatient stroke rehabilitation: a matched comparison conducted in Italy. *Archives of physical medicine and rehabilitation, 81*(6), 695-700.

Park, N. W. & Ingles, J. L. (2001). Effectiveness of attention rehabilitation after an acquired brain injury: A meta-analysis. *Neuropsychology, 15*(2), 199.

Passineau, M. J., Green, E. J. & Dietrich, W. D. (2001). Therapeutic effects of environmental enrichment on cognitive function and tissue integrity following severe traumatic brain injury in rats. *Experimental neurology, 168*(2), 373-384.

Petersen, R. C., Smith, G. E., Waring, S. C., Ivnik, R. J., Tangalos, E. G. & Kokmen, E. (1999). Mild cognitive impairment: clinical characterization and outcome. *Archives of neurology, 56*(3), 303-308.

Pittenger, C. & Duman, R. S. (2008). Stress, depression, and neuroplasticity: a convergence of mechanisms. *Neuropsychopharmacology, 33*(1), 88-109.

Ploughman, M., Austin, M. W., Glynn, L. & Corbett, D. (2015). The Effects of Poststroke Aerobic Exercise on Neuroplasticity: A Systematic Review of Animal and Clinical Studies. *Translational stroke research, 6*(1), 13-28.

Price, J. L., Ko, A. I., Wade, M. J., Tsou, S. K., McKeel, D. W. & Morris, J. C. (2001). Neuron number in the entorhinal cortex and CA1 in preclinical Alzheimer disease. *Archives of neurology, 58*(9), 1395-1402.

Rand, D., Eng, J. J., Liu-Ambrose, T. & Tawashy, A. E. (2010). Feasibility of a 6-month exercise and recreation program to improve executive functioning and memory in individuals with chronic stroke. *Neurorehabilitation and neural repair, 24*(8), 722-729.

Ray, S., Dixon, C. & Banik, N. (2002). Molecular mechanisms in the pathogenesis of traumatic brain injury. *Histol Histopathol, 17*, 1137-1152.

Reid, D. B. & Kelly, M. P. (1993). Wechsler Memory Scale-Revised in closed head injury. *Journal of Clinical Psychology, 49*(2), 245-254.

Riemenschneider, M., Schwarz, S., Wagenpfeil, S., Diehl, J., Müller, U., Förstl, H. & Kurz, A. (2001). A polymorphism of the brain-derived neurotrophic factor (BDNF) is associated with Alzheimer's disease in patients lacking the Apolipoprotein E epsilon4 allele. *Molecular psychiatry, 7*(7), 782-785.

Rioux, P., Desgranges, B., Marchal, G., Petit-Taboué, M.-C., Dary, M., Lechevalier, B. & Baron, J.-C. (1995). Healthy aging, memory subsystems and regional cerebral oxygen consumption. *Neuropsychologia, 33*(7), 867-887.

Risling, M., Plantman, S., Angeria, M., Rostami, E., Bellander, B.-M., Kirkegaard, M., Davidsson, J. (2011). Mechanisms of blast induced brain injuries, experimental studies in rats. *Neuroimage, 54*, S89-S97.

Ritchie, K. (2004). Mild cognitive impairment: an epidemiological perspective. *Dialogues in clinical neuroscience, 6*(4), 401.

Rodrigues, A. C., Loureiro, M. A. & Caramelli, P. (2010). Musical training, neuroplasticity and cognition. *Dement. Neuropsychol, 4*, 277-286.

Rogers, S. A., Kang, C. H. & Miller, K. J. (2007). Cognitive profiles of aging and aging-related conditions. *Aging Health, 3*(4), 457-470.

Roher, A., Ball, M., Bhave, S. & Wakade, A. (1991). β-Amyloid from Alzheimer disease brains inhibits sprouting and survival of sympathetic neurons. *Biochemical and biophysical research communications, 174*(2), 572-579.

Rola, R., Mizumatsu, S., Otsuka, S., Morhardt, D. R., Noble-Haeusslein, L. J., Fishman, K., Fike, J. R. (2006). Alterations in hippocampal neurogenesis following traumatic brain injury in mice. *Experimental neurology, 202*(1), 189-199.

Ropacki, S. A., Patel, S. M. & Hartman, R. E. (2013). Pomegranate Supplementation Protects against Memory Dysfunction after Heart Surgery: A Pilot Study. *Evidence-Based Complementary and Alternative Medicine, 2013*.

Rosen, A. C., Sugiura, L., Kramer, J. H., Whitfield-Gabrieli, S. & Gabrieli, J. D. (2011). Cognitive training changes hippocampal function in mild cognitive impairment: a pilot study. *Journal of Alzheimer's Disease, 26*(Suppl 3), 349.

Rossi, C., Angelucci, A., Costantin, L., Braschi, C., Mazzantini, M., Babbini, F., Berardi, N. (2006). Brain-derived neurotrophic factor (BDNF) is required for the enhancement of hippocampal neurogenesis following environmental enrichment. *European Journal of Neuroscience, 24*(7), 1850-1856.

Rossi, L., Mazzitelli, S., Arciello, M., Capo, C. & Rotilio, G. (2008). Benefits from dietary polyphenols for brain aging and Alzheimer's disease. *Neurochemical research, 33*(12), 2390-2400.

Ryan, T. V. & Ruff, R. M. (1988). The efficacy of structured memory retraining in a group comparison of head trauma patients. *Archives of Clinical Neuropsychology, 3*(2), 165-179.

Salmond, C., Menon, D., Chatfield, D., Williams, G., Pena, A., Sahakian, B. & Pickard, J. (2006). Diffusion tensor imaging in chronic head injury survivors: correlations with learning and memory indices. *Neuroimage, 29*(1), 117-124.

Salthouse, T. A. & Babcock, R. L. (1991). Decomposing adult age differences in working memory. *Developmental psychology, 27*(5), 763.

Saxe, M. D., Battaglia, F., Wang, J.-W., Malleret, G., David, D. J., Monckton, J. E., Santarelli, L. (2006). Ablation of hippocampal neurogenesis impairs contextual fear conditioning and synaptic plasticity in the dentate gyrus. *Proceedings of the National Academy of Sciences, 103*(46), 17501-17506.

Scheff, S. W., Price, D. A., Schmitt, F. A. & Mufson, E. J. (2006). Hippocampal synaptic loss in early Alzheimer's disease and mild cognitive impairment. *Neurobiology of aging, 27*(10), 1372-1384.

Schrijver, N. C., Bahr, N. I., Weiss, I. C. & Würbel, H. (2002). Dissociable effects of isolation rearing and environmental enrichment on exploration, spatial learning and HPA activity in adult rats. *Pharmacology Biochemistry and Behavior, 73*(1), 209-224.

Seeram, N. P., Aviram, M., Zhang, Y., Henning, S. M., Feng, L., Dreher, M. & Heber, D. (2008). Comparison of antioxidant potency of commonly consumed polyphenol-rich beverages in the United States. *Journal of agricultural and food chemistry, 56*(4), 1415-1422.

Shankar, G. M., Li, S., Mehta, T. H., Garcia-Munoz, A., Shepardson, N. E., Smith, I., Lemere, C. A. (2008). Amyloid-β protein dimers isolated directly from Alzheimer's brains impair synaptic plasticity and memory. *Nature medicine, 14*(8), 837-842.

Shimada, A., Keino, H., Satoh, M., Kishikawa, M. & Hosokawa, M. (2003). Age-related loss of synapses in the frontal cortex of SAMP10 mouse: A model of cerebral degeneration. *Synapse, 48*(4), 198-204.

Sibley, B. A. & Etnier, J. L. (2003). The relationship between physical activity and cognition in children: a meta-analysis. *Pediatric Exercise Science, 15*(3), 243-256.

Skelton, R. W., Bukach, C. M., Laurance, H. E., Thomas, K. G. & Jacobs, J. W. (2000). Humans with traumatic brain injuries show place-learning deficits in computer-generated virtual space. *Journal of clinical and experimental neuropsychology, 22*(2), 157-175.

Slemmer, J. E., Matser, E. J., De Zeeuw, C. I. & Weber, J. T. (2002). Repeated mild injury causes cumulative damage to hippocampal cells. *Brain, 125*(12), 2699-2709.

Smith, G. E., Housen, P., Yaffe, K., Ruff, R., Kennison, R. F., Mahncke, H. W. & Zelinski, E. M. (2009). A cognitive training program based on principles of brain plasticity: Results from the Improvement in Memory with Plasticity-based Adaptive Cognitive Training (IMPACT) Study. *Journal of the American Geriatrics Society, 57*(4), 594-603.

Smith, P. J., Blumenthal, J. A., Hoffman, B. M., Cooper, H., Strauman, T. A., Welsh-Bohmer, K., Sherwood, A. (2010). Aerobic exercise and neurocognitive performance: a meta-analytic review of randomized controlled trials. *Psychosomatic medicine, 72*(3), 239.

Soffié, M., Hahn, K., Terao, E. & Eclancher, F. (1999). Behavioural and glial changes in old rats following environmental enrichment. *Behavioural brain research, 101*(1), 37-49.

Spencer, J. P. (2010). The impact of fruit flavonoids on memory and cognition. *British Journal of Nutrition, 104*(S3), S40-S47.

Stein, D. G. & Hoffman, S. W. (2003). Concepts of CNS plasticity in the context of brain damage and repair. *The Journal of head trauma rehabilitation, 18*(4), 317-341.

Stern, R. A., Riley, D. O., Daneshvar, D. H., Nowinski, C. J., Cantu, R. C. & McKee, A. C. (2011). Long-term consequences of repetitive brain trauma: chronic traumatic encephalopathy. *PM&R, 3*(10), S460-S467.

Stewart, F., Sunderland, A. & Sluman, S. (1996). The nature and prevalence of memory disorder late after stroke. *British Journal of Clinical Psychology, 35*(3), 369-379.

Stranahan, A. M., Norman, E. D., Lee, K., Cutler, R. G., Telljohann, R. S., Egan, J. M. & Mattson, M. P. (2008). Diet-induced insulin resistance impairs hippocampal synaptic plasticity and cognition in middle-aged rats. *Hippocampus, 18*(11), 1085-1088.

Sturm, W., Fimm, B., Cantagallo, A., Cremel, N., North, P., North, P., Rousseaux, M. (2003). Specific computerized attention training in stroke and traumatic brain-injured patients. *Zeitschrift für Neuropsychologie, 14*(4), 283-292.

Su, H.-M. (2010). Mechanisms of n-3 fatty acid-mediated development and maintenance of learning memory performance. *The Journal of nutritional biochemistry, 21*(5), 364-373.

Tao, X., Finkbeiner, S., Arnold, D. B., Shaywitz, A. J. & Greenberg, M. E. (1998). $Ca2^+$ influx regulates BDNF transcription by a CREB family transcription factor-dependent mechanism. *Neuron, 20*(4), 709-726.

Tashiro, A., Makino, H. & Gage, F. H. (2007). Experience-specific functional modification of the dentate gyrus through adult neurogenesis: a critical period during an immature stage. *The Journal of Neuroscience, 27*(12), 3252-3259.

Tatemichi, T., Desmond, D., Stern, Y., Paik, M., Sano, M. & Bagiella, E. (1994). Cognitive impairment after stroke: frequency, patterns, and relationship to functional abilities. *Journal of Neurology, Neurosurgery & Psychiatry, 57*(2), 202-207.

Tiwari, S. K., Agarwal, S., Seth, B., Yadav, A., Nair, S., Bhatnagar, P., Patel, D. K. (2013). Curcumin-loaded nanoparticles potently induce adult neurogenesis and reverse cognitive deficits in alzheimer's disease model via canonical Wnt/β-catenin pathway. *ACS nano, 8*(1), 76-103.

Tolwani, R., Buckmaster, P., Varma, S., Cosgaya, J., Wu, Y., Suri, C. & Shooter, E. (2002). BDNF overexpression increases dendrite complexity in hippocampal dentate gyrus. *Neuroscience, 114*(3), 795-805.

Tomporowski, P. D. (2003). Effects of acute bouts of exercise on cognition. *Acta psychologica, 112*(3), 297-324.

Toni, N., Buchs, P.-A., Nikonenko, I., Bron, C. & Muller, D. (1999). LTP promotes formation of multiple spine synapses between a single axon terminal and a dendrite. *Nature, 402*(6760), 421-425.

Tsaousides, T. & Gordon, W. A. (2009). Cognitive rehabilitation following traumatic brain injury: assessment to treatment. *Mount Sinai Journal of Medicine: A Journal of Translational and Personalized Medicine, 76*(2), 173-181.

Tyler, W. J. & Pozzo-Miller, L. (2003). Miniature synaptic transmission and BDNF modulate dendritic spine growth and form in rat CA1 neurones. *The Journal of physiology, 553*(2), 497-509.

Vakil, E. (2005). The effect of moderate to severe traumatic brain injury (TBI) on different aspects of memory: a selective review. *Journal of clinical and experimental neuropsychology, 27*(8), 977-1021.

Vakil, E., Kraus, A., Bor, B. & Groswasser, Z. (2002). Impaired skill learning in patients with severe closed-head injury as demonstrated by the serial reaction time (SRT) task. *Brain and cognition, 50*(2), 304-315.

Vakil, E. & Tweedy, J. R. (1994). Memory for Temporal Order and Spatial Position Information: Tests of the Automatic-Effortful Distinction. *Cognitive and Behavioral Neurology, 7*(4), 281-288.

Vallat, C., Azouvi, P., Hardisson, H., Meffert, R., Tessier, C. & Pradat-Diehl, P. (2005). Rehabilitation of verbal working memory after left hemisphere stroke. *Brain injury, 19*(13), 1157-1164.

Van Praag, H., Christie, B. R., Sejnowski, T. J. & Gage, F. H. (1999). Running enhances neurogenesis, learning, and long-term potentiation in mice. *Proceedings of the National Academy of Sciences, 96*(23), 13427-13431.

Van Praag, H., Kempermann, G. & Gage, F. H. (1999). Running increases cell proliferation and neurogenesis in the adult mouse dentate gyrus. *Nature neuroscience, 2*(3), 266-270.

Van Praag, H., Kempermann, G. & Gage, F. H. (2000). Neural consequences of enviromental enrichment. *Nature Reviews Neuroscience, 1*(3), 191-198.

Vaynman, S., Ying, Z. & Gomez-Pinilla, F. (2004). Hippocampal BDNF mediates the efficacy of exercise on synaptic plasticity and cognition. *European Journal of Neuroscience, 20*(10), 2580-2590.

Verhaeghen, P., Marcoen, A. & Goossens, L. (1992). Improving memory performance in the aged through mnemonic training: a meta-analytic study. *Psychology and aging, 7*(2), 242.

von Bohlen und Halbach, O. (2010). Involvement of BDNF in age-dependent alterations in the hippocampus. *Frontiers in aging neuroscience, 2.*

Wainwright, P., Levesque, S., Krempulec, L., Bulman-Fleming, B. & McCutcheon, D. (1993). Effects of environmental enrichment on cortical depth and Morris-maze performance in B6D2F 2 mice exposed prenatally to ethanol. *Neurotoxicology and teratology, 15*(1), 11-20.

Walker, M. P. & Stickgold, R. (2004). Sleep-dependent learning and memory consolidation. *Neuron, 44*(1), 121-133.

Wang, J., Tang, C., Ferruzzi, M. G., Gong, B., Song, B. J., Janle, E. M., Cheng, A. (2013). Role of standardized grape polyphenol preparation as a novel treatment to improve synaptic plasticity through attenuation of features of metabolic syndrome in a mouse model. *Molecular nutrition & food research, 57*(12), 2091-2102.

Wang, M., Gamo, N. J., Yang, Y., Jin, L. E., Wang, X.-J., Laubach, M., Arnsten, A. F. (2011). Neuronal basis of age-related working memory decline. *Nature, 476*(7359), 210-213.

Wang, R., Li, Y.-B., Li, Y.-H., Xu, Y., Wu, H.-l. & Li, X.-J. (2008). Curcumin protects against glutamate excitotoxicity in rat cerebral cortical neurons by increasing brain-derived neurotrophic factor level and activating TrkB. *Brain research, 1210*, 84-91.

Wang, R., Li, Y.-H., Xu, Y., Li, Y.-B., Wu, H.-L., Guo, H., Li, X.-J. (2010). Curcumin produces neuroprotective effects via activating brain-derived neurotrophic factor/TrkB-dependent MAPK and PI-3K cascades in rodent cortical neurons. *Progress in Neuro-Psychopharmacology and Biological Psychiatry, 34*(1), 147-153.

Wang, T., Yang, Y.-J., Wu, P.-F., Wang, W., Hu, Z.-L., Long, L.-H., Chen, J.-G. (2011). Tetrahydroxystilbene glucoside, a plant-derived cognitive enhancer, promotes hippocampal synaptic plasticity. *European journal of pharmacology, 650*(1), 206-214.

Ward, N. L. & Hagg, T. (2000). BDNF is needed for postnatal maturation of basal forebrain and neostriatum cholinergic neurons in vivo. *Experimental neurology, 162*(2), 297-310.

Warraich, Z. & Kleim, J. A. (2010). Neural plasticity: the biological substrate for neurorehabilitation. *PM&R, 2*(12), S208-S219.

Webster, M., Herman, M., Kleinman, J. & Weickert, C. S. (2006). BDNF and trkB mRNA expression in the hippocampus and temporal cortex during the human lifespan. *Gene Expression Patterns, 6*(8), 941-951.

Westerberg, H., Jacobaeus, H., Hirvikoski, T., Clevberger, P., Östensson, M.-L., Bartfai, A. & Klingberg, T. (2007). Computerized working memory training after stroke-A pilot study. *Brain injury, 21*(1), 21-29.

Winocur, G. (1998). Environmental influences on cognitive decline in aged rats. *Neurobiology of aging, 19*(6), 589-597.

Wu, A., Molteni, R., Ying, Z. & Gomez-Pinilla, F. (2003). A saturated-fat diet aggravates the outcome of traumatic brain injury on hippocampal plasticity and cognitive function by reducing brain-derived neurotrophic factor. *Neuroscience, 119*(2), 365-375.

Wu, A., Ying, Z. & Gomez-Pinilla, F. (2004a). Dietary omega-3 fatty acids normalize BDNF levels, reduce oxidative damage, and counteract learning disability after traumatic brain injury in rats. *Journal of neurotrauma, 21*(10), 1457-1467.

Wu, A., Ying, Z. & Gomez-Pinilla, F. (2006). Dietary curcumin counteracts the outcome of traumatic brain injury on oxidative stress, synaptic plasticity, and cognition. *Experimental neurology, 197*(2), 309-317.

Wu, A., Ying, Z. & Gomez-Pinilla, F. (2008). Docosahexaenoic acid dietary supplementation enhances the effects of exercise on synaptic plasticity and cognition. *Neuroscience, 155*(3), 751-759.

Wu, A., Ying, Z. & Gomez-Pinilla, F. (2004b). The interplay between oxidative stress and brain-derived neurotrophic factor modulates the outcome of a saturated fat diet on synaptic plasticity and cognition. *European Journal of Neuroscience, 19*(7), 1699-1707.

Wu, H., Lu, D., Jiang, H., Xiong, Y., Qu, C., Li, B., Chopp, M. (2008). Simvastatin-mediated upregulation of VEGF and BDNF, activation of the PI3K/Akt pathway, and increase of neurogenesis are associated with therapeutic improvement after traumatic brain injury. *Journal of neurotrauma, 25*(2), 130-139.

Wu, H.-Y., Hudry, E., Hashimoto, T., Kuchibhotla, K., Rozkalne, A., Fan, Z., Grosskreutz, C. L. (2010). Amyloid β induces the morphological neurodegenerative triad of spine loss, dendritic simplification, and neuritic dystrophies through calcineurin activation. *The Journal of Neuroscience, 30*(7), 2636-2649.

Xie, W., Ramakrishna, N., Wieraszko, A. & Hwang, Y.-W. (2008). Promotion of neuronal plasticity by (−)-epigallocatechin-3-gallate. *Neurochemical research, 33*(5), 776-783.

Xu, Y., Ku, B., Cui, L., Li, X., Barish, P. A., Foster, T. C. & Ogle, W. O. (2007). Curcumin reverses impaired hippocampal neurogenesis and increases serotonin receptor 1A mRNA and brain-derived neurotrophic factor expression in chronically stressed rats. *Brain research, 1162*, 9-18.

Xu, Y., Ku, B., Tie, L., Yao, H., Jiang, W., Ma, X. & Li, X. (2006). Curcumin reverses the effects of chronic stress on behavior, the HPA axis, BDNF expression and phosphorylation of CREB. *Brain research, 1122*(1), 56-64.

Xu, Y., Lin, D., Li, S., Li, G., Shyamala, S. G., Barish, P. A., Ogle, W. O. (2009). Curcumin reverses impaired cognition and neuronal plasticity induced by chronic stress. *Neuropharmacology, 57*(4), 463-471.

Ramón y Cajal, S. (1889). *Nuevas aplicaciones del método de coloración de Golgi.*

Yirmiya, R. & Goshen, I. (2011). Immune modulation of learning, memory, neural plasticity and neurogenesis. *Brain, behavior, and immunity, 25*(2), 181-213.

Zec, R. F., Zellers, D., Belman, J., Miller, J., Matthews, J., Ferneau-Belman, D. & Robbs, R. (2001). Long-term consequences of severe closed head injury on episodic memory. *Journal of clinical and experimental neuropsychology, 23*(5), 671-691.

Zehnder, F., Martin, M., Altgassen, M. & Clare, L. (2009). Memory training effects in old age as markers of plasticity: a meta-analysis. *Restorative neurology and neuroscience, 27*(5), 507.

Zhang, R. L., Zhang, Z. G. & Chopp, M. (2008). Ischemic stroke and neurogenesis in the subventricular zone. *Neuropharmacology, 55*(3), 345-352.

Zhao, L., Mattsson, B. & Johansson, B. (2000). Environmental influence on brain-derived neurotrophic factor messenger RNA expression after middle cerebral artery occlusion in spontaneously hypertensive rats. *Neuroscience, 97*(1), 177-184.

Zimmermann, T. D. & Meier, B. (2006). The rise and decline of prospective memory performance across the lifespan. *The Quarterly Journal of Experimental Psychology, 59*(12), 2040-2046.

Zinke, K., Zeintl, M., Rose, N. S., Putzmann, J., Pydde, A. & Kliegel, M. (2014). Working memory training and transfer in older adults: effects of age, baseline performance, and training gains. *Developmental psychology, 50*(1), 304.

Zuccato, C. & Cattaneo, E. (2009). Brain-derived neurotrophic factor in neurodegenerative diseases. *Nature Reviews Neurology, 5*(6), 311-322.

INDEX

A

B

C

D

E

F

G

H

I

J

L

M

N

O

P

S

T

U

V

W

Y

α